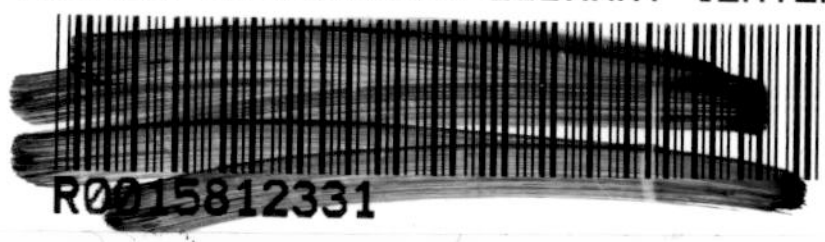

DATE			

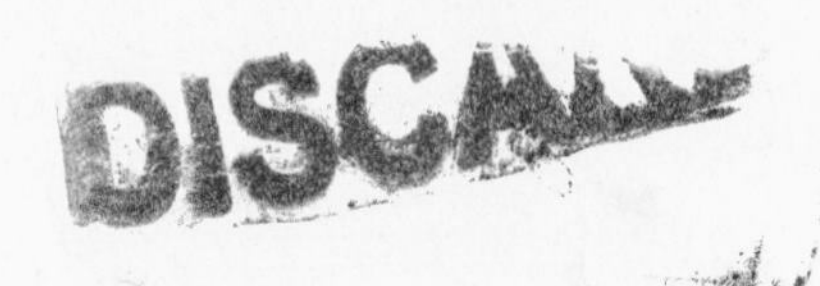

Health Care and Society

Health Care and Society

Arnold Birenbaum

LandMark Studies
ALLANHELD, OSMUN Montclair

ALLANHELD, OSMUN & CO. PUBLISHERS, INC.

Published in the United States of America in 1981
by Allanheld, Osmun & Co. Publishers, Inc.
6 South Fullerton Avenue, Montclair, New Jersey 07042

Library of Congress Cataloging in Publication Data

Birenbaum, Arnold.
Health care and society.

Bibliography: p.
Includes index.
1. Social medicine. 2. Social medicine—
United States. I. Title. [DNLM: 1. Sociology,
Medical—United States. 2. Delivery of health
care—United States WA30 B618h]
RA418.B57 362.1 80-67092
ISBN 0-916672-57-3

Printed in the United States of America

For
Jonathan and Steven
and their generation

Contents

Preface and Acknowledgments

Health Care and Society is a book that comes out of research and teaching. It is the work of a sociologist who would like to advance theoretical knowledge in order to understand and develop new ways of living. But new ways cannot be developed until the deep tensions and conflicts of our society are brought to the surface. Health care is one place where these problems are manifested.

Health care involves healing, an art and science with a long history. This practice seems like an unlikely subject for an excursion into modern living, but there are some features of health care in our time which justify the effort. Only in this century has medicine come to stand as the preferred system of healing, and there are some who say that its day is already past.

Despite the enormous growth of the health care field and the concomitant changes within it, [I sense that] it is losing its authority. In 1978, health care expenditures constituted 9.1 percent of the gross national product, surpassed only by defense spending. Although few would question the need for health care, are we any healthier as a result of this expense? Why should medical care price increases outdistance every item except food in the Consumer Price Index? There is a growing consumer skepticism about the established health care system. Do doctors, nurses, and hospitals do any good at all? Patients are turning to folk healing and self-care, and some physicians who recognize the growing distrust are willing to accept the alternative therapies; some physicians even practice holistic medicine, using a variety of healing techniques developed in many cultures.

Our society is changing very rapidly. The infusion of new people, new jobs, and new programs in the health care field is part of that social change. Despite the long history of healing, the professions and occupations that provide health services are new, being made up of individuals with little in the way of prior connections to health care. Few people can claim to come from a long line of X-ray technicians, health systems analysts, or oncologists.

Even occupations with lengthier histories in the health care field were given societal approval through licensing only some 65 years ago.

The rapid growth of the health care sector is unparalleled, particularly in the last decade. From 1970 to 1978, the number of jobs in the health care sector rose by 60 percent. "About one out of every seven jobs created in that time period was within the health industry. In 1978 there were 6.7 million health workers," says *The Nation's Health*, a monthly newsletter of the American Public Health Association. Who are these workers? Where do they come from? How do they fit into the system?

The health care consumer has reason to be confused. There is real difficulty in distinguishing between various medical specialties, nursing titles, and technicians. Patients are divided up by disease, task, and age but often do not have an identifiable physician who coordinates their care. Unnecessary services are provided when there is no one who can be identified as the major source of care.

To confuse matters even more, a new elite in the health care field has slipped quietly on the scene, challenging medical leadership and organizations. The new centers of power are found in insurance companies, health planning agencies, and government funding sources. Why are they so important, especially since they never see a patient? Who benefits from their services?

To make sense of the current system and the major roles performed within it requires a new perspective. In this book, health care is examined from the point of view of a sociologist looking at institutional development, the forces for change, and the unanswered challenges that remain.

The manuscript has benefited from the helpful criticism of Caroline Birenbaum, friend, wife, editor, and hospital administrator. My dear friend and co-worker in sociology, Edward Sagarin, provided me with stylistic assistance and, more important, sage advice at a time of great need. A number of anonymous reviewers along the way to publication were also very helpful in both strengthening crucial arguments and in forcing me to make my statements clearer. Phyllis Zammuto was an excellent and patient typist through various drafts.

Introduction

> . . . the individual can understand his own experience and gauge his fate only by locating himself within his period. . . . he can know his own chances in life only by becoming aware of those of all individuals in his circumstances.
>
> C. Wright Mills, *The Sociological Imagination*

This is a book about the human side of health care, how it is organized, why it is changing, and what the unresolved questions for the future are. For most of us contacts with health care providers are infrequent, and we receive direct services from a limited number of experts. But this is only the visible part of a complex set of arrangements, designed to meet certain human needs. The part that remains hidden is just as important. Decisions made in Congress, the national associations of hospitals, or at Blue Cross have great consequences for how much health care costs, who gets services, and whether physicians and others are trained to meet the current needs of the population.

A comprehensive view of health care requires investigation of its relationship to society. This book focuses on the social conditions that affect what happens when patients and practitioners interact within the ordinary settings of group practices, hospitals, and homes. The structure of past and current institutional arrangements shapes our lives and thoughts. Contemporary health care has certain built-in constraints and freedoms for patients and healers, so it is necessary to analyze the connections between institutions and individuals.

The common experience of going to the doctor and paying the bills has recently left many Americans wondering about whether services are for the benefit of the patients or for those who seek to heal them, operate hospitals, or manufacture and distribute pharmaceuticals. There are strong publicly expressed doubts that health services are equitably distributed, or even that people with moderate incomes can afford them. Yet most people still depend on medical care to meet their health needs, notwithstanding the criticisms and anger often voiced by our citizens.

And care is expected to improve as new diagnostic tests are introduced, techniques gain public attention, and as people become better educated. However, improving the overall health standards of the population depends less on sophisticated surgical procedures or diagnostic devices than upon adequate nutrition and the simple and effective technology of immunization. Despite this knowledge of what to do, still many children in impoverished urban areas have not been inoculated against measles, mumps and diphtheria.

WHAT IS HEALTH?

The concept of *health* is not easy to define because it includes both personal and group dimensions. Objectively, health is the absence of disease. For the purpose of understanding how human behavior affects a person's health, this definition is not clear and complete. People may either not recognize that they are affected by a disease and thereby *not* seek help, or they may believe strongly that they are subject to a disease and seek unnecessary or inappropriate treatment. A patient's beliefs may be supported or overturned by a health care provider. Healers sometimes identify disease when it is not present. Failure to identify disease or falsely identify it when absent make it evident that health is not simply a biological state, and its care is not based on ordinary routine technical processes. Health may be sociologically defined according to how the individual views himself in relation to others who have special social identities as healers. A person who is healthy would not see the need to acquire a special social identity. Reaching the point of seeing oneself as sick requires intervention by someone designated as having the duty to diagnose and treat disease.

Being considered by others and oneself as either subject or not subject to disease depends on many social factors that vary according to time and place, depending on the knowledge and beliefs held by a group or by society at large; it may even vary according to a person's rank and power. Regardless of this variability, the process of recognizing disease or its absence, whether based on biological realities or not, involves a social division of labor between at least two people—the patient and the healer—each with different rights and obligations.

Bundles of rights and obligations constitute *roles*, and the performances are guided by a generalized set of expectations, relative to the needs of patients and the expertise of healers. Therefore, providing care is a social process in which people mutually influence each other. The patient's capacity to cooperate with the healer and the healer's capacity to deal with the patient's needs are based upon mutually held assumptions which may not be fully warranted despite good will, trust, and expertise.

What kind of understanding and awareness is needed to cope with the complex institution of health care? New medical advances, the benefits of exercise, and the latest diets receive media coverage daily, as well as stories on the runaway costs of health care, the unwillingness or inability of professional associations to prevent incompetent physicians from practicing, and widespread fraud by owners of Medicaid-funded health facilities. Magazines devote space to articles on self-care, to personal testimony by cancer victims, and to the indignities and loneliness of living and dying in nursing homes.

The mass media are not alone in their criticism of health care; a national survey indicates that many Americans are ready for a change (Rensberger, 1978: A16). Yet this Harris poll, conducted early in 1978, reveals an enormous public ignorance of the basic facts concerning how much is spent on health care. Moreover, pollsters do not identify the basic factors or conditions built into the relationship between providers, patients, and insurance plans, which encourage high costs. The popular view may see greed as a root cause, but why is greed permitted and encouraged?

The Americans surveyed in the Harris poll were willing to pay more for improved care and saw consumers groups as a way to get more for their money. They were also opposed to further government regulation. But they seemed to identify government subsidization with regulation. The government contributes 40.6 percent of the total $192.4 billion spent in fiscal year 1978 on health care (Public Health Service, 1980: 237). Much of the federal dollar provides for services for the elderly and the poor, or for underwriting research. Little is spent on regulation, and further regulation might be in the taxpayer's interest, making it possible to avoid unnecessary spending.

Sociology can shed light on these issues by looking at how professions are created and organized and where they fit within the division of labor. The concepts of sociology provide a way of understanding how competition and even conflict occur between different professions that are supposedly dedicated to the same goals. The application of sociology also makes a greater command over one's working life possible, even deepening involvement with work, both important bases for life satisfaction.

This book is dedicated to improving health care in the United States, by providing information to the health care professional. Knowledge about the behavior of professionals can be very important. By taking into account the human side of work, improvements could be made at the points of contact between patients and healers.

Consider how day-to-day exchanges shape effective therapeutic intervention by a doctor. Physicians often demonstrate a lack of interest in patients and their troubles. Patients often cued by the doctor's demeanor will fail to ask important questions concerning their treatment and will stop taking a medication or maintaining dietary restrictions. These features of doctor-patient interaction have life and death consequences, and are not just examples of how human beings communicate.

A NEW WAY OF SEEING

Sociology is concerned with how the workings of society, on the interpersonal and the organizational level, influence health care and the health status of the consumer. In general, sociology creates scientific and valid explanations through theory, a body of abstract concepts, and propositions about how society works. Theory generates a pattern of inquiry leading to the collection of data that test these propositions. The study of sickness and disease and their professional or nonprofessional treatment is one important area of research in sociology.

Sociology not only tries to understand what exists in social arrangements but also seeks to suggest what *could* be. For example, if financial barriers were totally removed from receiving health care, would the general state of health of the American population improve, deteriorate, or remain the same?

The sociologist assumes that all social arrangements to meet certain human needs are alterable. Knowledge derived from the sociological study of health care may permit health care providers, and patients as well, to see things previously overlooked or unnoticed. Alvin Gouldner, a sociologist, describes this awareness as an emotional as well as an intellectual process, helping a person to get beyond his biases. Gouldner defines awareness as a state in which opposing ideas produce a new way of seeing. Dealing with opposing ideas teaches the learner how to learn.

> Awareness is access to hostile information born of a capacity to overcome one's own resistance to it and cannot, therefore be "retrieved" without a struggle—as can information. Since such resistance, is always based in some part upon the pain or fear of knowing, the struggle to overcome resistance and to attain awareness always requires a measure of valor. [1965: 271]

The struggle toward awareness requires recognition of how the American health care system is organized. In Part I, health care is approached as both an ordinary and extraordinary activity.

Health care may also be approached according to the ways in which the *terms* of relationships are set between providers and consumers. The major determinants of the doctor-patient relationship may be seen from several different theoretical perspectives. Four different social theories of this relationship are discussed in Chapter 3, each making different assertions about the origin and consequences of the role of the physician in modern society.

The earliest contribution of sociologists to the study of health care has been in the application of role concepts to the patient-practitioner relationship. The late Talcott Parsons developed concepts of the "sick role" and the professions, examining the nature of mutually held expectations that reduce the likelihood of deviant behavior. A person could malinger and thereby use the claim to being sick for illegitimate purposes. The clinical work of physicians also has high potential for deviant behavior, not being subject to direct monitoring and supervision, and thus providing opportunities for exploitation. In sum, Parson's work was concerned with the theoretical problem of how motivation for conformity is maintained when it may be equally as rewarding to deviate as to conform.

Parsons' theorizing focused on the unique moral authority of the physician. Eliot Freidson's study of the medical profession and its work is concerned with the application of knowledge to problematic situations. Professionalization means power as well as helping. Freidson specifically attends to the ways in which medicine has become the dominant profession in health care and how its group cohesion and political power are maintained. This analysis questions the importance of the internalization of altruism as a major source of social control in medicine and focuses more on the day-to-day social organization of doctoring. Given this uncertainty, Freidson makes a significant contribution in identifying the various role strains involved in managing what can be a set of conflicting demands on the physician.

While Freidson does make recommendations for bringing the profession more under the control of larger collectivities, it is David Mechanic who comes closest to the application of sociological knowledge and concepts in the service of planning a more adequate health care system. Mechanic has examined a variety of theoretical problems related to the impact of social organization on health and illness-related behavior; he has also studied the impact of diverse organization and delivery systems on the behavior and attitudes of physicians.

Other sociologists have attempted to look at who benefits from health care, dealing with the ways in which health and illness are used as the source of profits for corporations and individual entrepreneurs. Howard Waitzkin and Barbara Waterman follow this approach, taking off from current critical thinking about the articulation between monopoly capital, corporate development, and government guarantees for profits.

All of these theoretical points of view examine the nature of social relationships, and how certain patterns of behavior are permitted or constrained by them. When these theorists go beyond the patient-practitioner relationship, they are dealing with societal arrangements. These arrangements narrow the range of choices for members of society, encouraging the growth of some healing practices.

The delivery of health care services in any society is usually identified with specific healers. Part Two deals with the emergence of the profession of medicine as the legitimate healing source in American society. There are other healers of course, some practicing folk medicine within certain ethnic communities, and others, such as chiropractors, who model themselves after the physician but make different assumptions about the nature of disease and the human body. Despite the professional domination of medicine, change occurs in the American health care system. Paramedical and allied health personnel who use medical knowledge and implement the various technical decisions made by doctors are now part of the division of labor.

Any occupational group seeks both steady financial support and freedom from outside interference. Physicians in the United States are supported by fees paid directly by the patient for the service performed, through salaries received for caring for a fixed number of patients, or for providing consultations for a specified number of hours per week. Medicine is also self-regulating, based on the generalized belief that only *technical* considerations should determine what is done for a patient and only those with this expertise can exercise professional judgment. But what are the consequences of allowing self-regulation under new economic arrangements where insurance companies and government programs pay the bill rather than the patient? When the immediate cost to the patient is of no concern, do doctors perform unnecessary procedures?

The organization of medicine depends on the availability of various support services and technology. The hospital as the work place for modern medicine is examined as a special environment in which practitioners and patients are brought together, and where patients seek to maintain some control over their lives even when sick and in need.

The administration of the modern hospital is further complicated by its many purposes and tasks. Medical technology has also made it possible to create a highly differentiated division of labor, involving 200 health-related occupations, as listed in the Labor Department's *Dictionary of Occupational Titles*. How are these various roles coordinated in a hospital? Does hospital size account for this extreme specialization?

Since many health care workers, including doctors, are now subject to receiving compensation from a variety of remote sources and are subject to various administrative structures, they often join unions to protect their positions and livelihoods. Unions have become a major factor in determining costs, impeding or encouraging greater concern for patients, and setting the terms of employment. Even those reluctant to join unions are affected. Nurses have turned their state associations into collective bargaining agents in order to gain higher salaries and better working conditions. These organizations are part of the social structure of health care, affecting the behavior of management and planners as well as employees. What implications do these developments have for efforts to improve services?

The costs of being sick are determined, in part, by the fees charged by physicians and the hospitals' *per diem* rates for inpatient care. There have been many proposals to deliver health care by limiting these two expenditures, and they have evolved into new patterns of service. Part Three discusses the new practitioners and new practices created by the introduction of physician assistants and nurse practitioners. New programs of home care have also been constructed around their services, and community care networks have been designed and implemented to reduce the cost and adverse affects of long-term hospitalization for the chronically ill. How do patients respond to the new practitioners? What are the reactions of older professions to them? How well are the chronically ill cared for in the community, and what has been the reaction of those formerly hospitalized?

The development of allied health-worker roles and the extension of the roles of nurses and pharmacists also raises the possibility of the autonomy of these professionals to make medical decisions. The question of whether health care workers can be considered independent professionals will be discussed, and particular attention will be paid to the interesting phenomena of occupations acquiring the attitudes associated with professional identity without gaining control over their own work and the rules concerning admission to the craft. Central to this discussion is the importance of acquiring control over a specific sphere of responsibility and demonstrating competency. The particular case of pharmacy and its loss of control over the preparation of compounded prescriptions and the possibility of automated dispensing has had a deep impact both on current and future pharmacists. Leaders in the field have advocated the creation of new educational and clinical roles for pharmacists that would stabilize their position in a field where they may become obsolete.

Part Four deals with some emerging issues in the field of health care. These are matters of public policy and debate, i.e., whether to implement a national health insurance program or create a national health service. New debates on consumer participation such as the women's health movement are also discussed. This movement has been active and vocal regarding the lack of concern for the female patient's rights. The lessons learned here can be applied to any patients without resources to command respectful and concerned care.

Many questions can be raised about the implications of various proposals. If efforts are made to provide more equal access to health care and to control costs, can these goals be accomplished without setting up general rules for determining when a patient can be hospitalized and tests performed? Would such bureaucratic control interfere with the physician's autonomy in technical procedures? Would this form of control make doctors more accountable to the consumer and taxpayer? Chapter 14 discusses these questions.

Chapter 15 returns to the theme of awareness, or what the patient can learn from sickness. As in the case of many stressful events, this one both tests the individual and provides opportunities for growth. It is important to recognize this attribute of the patient's situation because it makes it possible for providers to pay attention to the strengths of the person in a social context. In becoming aware of these possibilities, it is hoped that the reader will become better able to see the role that providers of care play in a sociological perspective. Awareness makes health care more complicated because new questions about patients are raised, but it also makes it more humane as previously unseen features emerge.

REFERENCES

Gouldner, Alvin W. 1965. *Enter Plato: Classical Greece and the Origins of Social Theory.* New York: Basic Books.

Public Health Service. 1980. *Health United States: 1979.* Washington, D.C.: Department of Health, Education, and Welfare.

Rensberger, B. 1978. "Polls show concern about health costs." *New York Times,* June 6: A16.

Part One
A SOCIOLOGICAL APPROACH

1

A Sociology of Health and Illness

Sociological ideas or concepts, like concepts in the natural sciences, look for relationships between phenomena. The products of human activity—the groups formed, the ideas held about nature, and the efforts to make things—constitute the subject matter of sociology. The sociology of health and illness focuses on the impact of disease on human arrangements and the efforts and consequences of human beings to deal with illness, accident, and injury. The approach taken by sociologists is based on the scientific method. Underlying this approach is the belief that the physical world and human behavior and attitudes can be explained naturalistically. This means that ideas such as fate, luck, or the whims of the gods are not regarded as necessary to an understanding of how certain things come to pass.

A simple example of how this kind of thinking works is found in the commonplace observation that human beings have an impact on their environment. Human life depends on support from the natural systems that make up the physical environment of the earth. Human activity, mainly through efforts to wrest needed and desired objects from that environment, can alter it, producing conditions adverse for life. Yet the knowledge that dangerous environmental hazards exist would remain undiscovered without the concept of variability. Comparisons between before and after, here and there, even "them" and "us," make it possible to expand our knowledge of environmental pollution through human intervention. Air pollution, to name a common hazard, results in increased death rates during periods when inversions occur in the atmosphere. Comparisons among members of different groups also give us information about who is "at risk" with regard to a particular disease and make it possible to understand differences in the behavior of people in different sectors of society who are seeking health care. Finally, we can compare how different societies organize their health care resources.

Human life not only depends on support from natural systems but requires connection with our fellow human beings. Group membership fosters the survival of individuals and the species. In a group, a person can feel important—can be somebody. Recognition of the need to be accorded status or prestige by others is a condition that promotes cooperation and conflict as people trade and exchange money, work, or approval (Goode, 1979). Indirectly, the desire for status is sometimes a way of risking one's health. Advertising helps to depict certain activities, such as smoking cigarettes or consuming alcoholic beverages, as desirable and glamorous, (although there is advertising to the opposite effect).

While the mass media—television, radio, and newspapers—reach almost everyone in the United States and most other countries, individuals who belong to groups that share a common set of values and point of view filter and respond to these messages in different ways. Consumer research shows that people learn about products and acquire particular tastes as a result of membership in family, ethnic, neighborhood, and work groups (Katz and Lazarsfeld, 1964). Members of a group share not only a similar position in society but a common culture, which is defined as a way of life for a particular group with a common set of values, beliefs, knowledge, and rules (Kluckhohn and Kelly, 1945). Cultures provide different recipes for living, encouraging some behaviors and discouraging others. The Mormons, for example, prohibit their members from smoking and drinking, interdictions that have been shown to decrease their chances of contracting diseases to which their neighbors are subject (Fuchs, 1974). Living side by side in the same geographic areas, Mormons have lower rates of morbidity (presence of disease) and mortality than their non-Mormon counterparts of the same ages and sexes.

Cultures create rules of behavior for their members, but there are differences in what is expected, encouraged, and allowed for men and for women, for the young and for the old. In the United States as a whole it seems that younger people and males are more experimental and willing to take risks than older people and females. If this is true, it may account for the fact that automobile accidents are the leading cause of death in the United States among young adults (Sidel and Sidel, 1978) and that the death rate of males in the 25–34 age bracket is twice that of same aged females (World Health Organization, 1976).

Even though age and gender characteristics may be responded to differently, depending on the society, they are used in all cultures to provide guidelines for interaction and social selection, affecting whether people will receive one kind of upbringing or another, what jobs they will be regarded as capable of performing, what other roles they will be expected to perform, and what honor, respect, or deference they will be entitled to or required to give others (Harrison, 1974). In some portions of American society, for example, children are expected to show respect by saying hello first when meeting an adult whom they know. Even older children, through their gestures, seem to demand deference from younger children, and confusion reigns when two peers pass in the street. Even today, in an age of emancipation from outmoded gender stereotypes, among couples women enter an aisle of a theater ahead of men, walk on the inside, and exit from an elevator before men (Goffman, 1976). These unstated rules of social interaction continuously reinforce more basic divisions in society.

SOCIAL DIFFERENTIATION

Control over the sources of wealth (e.g., production, commerce, finance) is a primary basis for creating social relationships such as those between owners of factories and those who work for wages and salaries. Despite widespread acceptance of the doctrine that "all men are created equal," negotiations, struggles, and sometimes outright conflicts among people are basic efforts to gain or maintain greater control over the factors that produce wealth. Social relationships have an influence on human life and health that go far beyond the dictates of culture, extending the inquiry of sociology into circumstances that exist independent of values, beliefs, knowledge, and rules. The forms of group affiliation may be of greater importance in determining rates of death than the common culture of a society. First, the objective conditions of living encourage or prevent members of groups from reinforcing the rules or norms of the group, as when poverty discourages the maintenance of conventional family living (Lebow, 1967; Stack, 1974). Moreover, cultural preferences are also weakened by the infrequency of contact between members of a particular group, as when migration and assimilation of newcomers take place. Opportunities for members to feel connected to the groups to which they belong and thus to feel a sense of social solidarity may vary, depending on where people live and work. Second, a sense of belonging may be affected by the presence or absence of such noncultural factors as multiple group memberships, conflict with other groups, and the size of the group to which one belongs.

Americans believe in equality of opportunity, yet little is done to ensure it. The importance of family advantage, relative to opportunities for the children to acquire college educations and have access to income and prestige-generating jobs, has been demonstrated by sociologists for the past two decades (Bowles, 1972; Blau and Duncan, 1967). The work a person performs within the division of labor in society also creates a likelihood of exposure to environmental hazards and social stress. The environment in which miners work, for example, is known to be associated with high levels of disease and accident (Kitagawa and Hauser, 1973). Recently there has been much interest in the relationship between coronary heart disease and occupational stress (House, 1974).

The work environment is a social as well as a physical milieu. The response to pressures on the job, such as the need to work overtime or to organize and take action against unfair employers, has an impact on death rates. Cyclical trends in the economy, such as periods of business expansion or depression, can lead to opportunities for overwork, or alternatively, for social cohesion through strike action (Eyer, 1977).

The concept of culture must be complemented by an additional factor—*social structure*. Social structure refers to the conditions that make for repetitive and uniform patterns of conduct among people who are similarly situated. These conditions are built into the group life of a society, mainly in the institutions that accomplish tasks. Institutions affect the differential distribution of scarce resources in society, such as wealth, income, influence, the opportunities of members of society to conform or deviate from rules, and even opportunities to feel self-worth.

By examining social structure, sources of conflict, strain, and deviance can be determined, as well as conditions that promote the stability of social relationships and social control. Behavior is strongly associated with one's position or location in society, and patterned social activities have been used by observers to locate the origins and spread of disease (Susser and Watson, 1962).

The special field of epidemiology grew out of comparative observations on how some groups in society were more susceptible than others to certain diseases. In the eighteenth century, medical researchers noted that chimney sweeps were more prone than other men to cancer of the scrotum. In the nineteenth century, public health officials in London linked cholera in one district with use of a public water pump that had become contaminated with sewage. The isolation of this source of infection came about over a quarter of a century before Robert Koch found the bacillus that is the precise cause of the disease (MacMahon and Pugh, 1970 : 10).

Sometimes changes in behavior related to the adoption of new values or a new position in society influence health conditions. The emancipation of women in the twentieth century has been accompanied by increased use of tobacco and a concomitant increase in the incidence of lung cancer. Similarly, fuller sexual expression and the use of oral contraceptives have been accompanied by increased rates of venereal disease. (This increased incidence of disease is inferred to result also from more frequent sexual activity among multiple partners.) While antibiotics can control the severity of venereal disease, reported cases are difficult to trace back to the source when sex partners cannot be located. Therefore, in the absence of early treatment, the disease spreads (Public Health Service, 1978 : 243–47).

In sum, sociologists study the basic aspects of how people live in groups, how they deal with and relate to one another. As a special field of study, the sociology of health and illness can be particularly useful in understanding the dynamics of disease. Findings on the relationship among culture, social structure, and disease can be used to develop plans for intervention to eliminate a disease or reduce the severity of its consequences. In addition, knowledge of how health care services are created and delivered makes it possible to evaluate alternative forms of organizing these services. To better understand how contemporary health care services developed, certain important features of health care as an institution must be noted.

THE SOCIAL SIGNIFICANCE OF HEALTH AND ILLNESS

Health care practices in societies vary as to the extent of their organization and importance. Evidence found in the ruins of many early societies shows that sophisticated techniques were used in efforts to help people, relieve suffering, and learn more about injury and illness. Physicians in the southern highlands of Mexico, in the Valley of Oaxaca, practiced skull surgery 1,300 years ago. Similar archeological evidence of skull surgery has been found in the ancient civilizations of the Andes Mountains in South America and in Europe as well (Wilkinson, 1975).

Human intervention in matters of illness does not always await the development of a scientific body of verified knowledge. The personal ties among people and the social division of labor promote generalized concern with matters of illness and health. Group life is based on cooperation and interdependence among members in order to get things done. Thus the problems presented by illness, disease, and accidents have organizational consequences. Group life is also accompanied by bonds of affection and concern for others, including a sense of being abandoned or let down or feelings of anger when someone cannot live up to prior expectations. In turn, the person who is ill or injured may feel guilty about not being able to perform assigned tasks or angry that others do not show proper concern for his absence, suffering, or disability. Disease may also be contagious, and leaders in society encourage a variety of measures to counteract it, such as isolation, exile, or magical intervention.

In a sociological sense, illness, disease, and accident create social uncertainty that goes beyond individual interests or the interests of a small group such as a family or a work team. Consider what happens when a national leader dies unexpectedly in office. The death of such a figure produces general concern from all, not only because such figures are regarded as unique and strong, but because organized social life is considered a form of protection against unexpected disasters. If a powerful and important figure, particularly in the prime of life, cannot be protected by society, our security as members of society is called into question. We do not have to have any commitment to the values of the society to experience the diminution of security produced by an assassination or similar event. As for death from natural causes, national leaders are frequently replaced when they are old or in poor health.

The uncertainty created by illness, disease, and accident can take two forms: the structural uncertainty produced by the absence or incapacitation of someone with whom one is interdependent, and the *interpersonal* uncertainty that ensues because of the actual or anticipated loss. The second form of uncertainty deals with feelings among people. New questions are raised for two or more people who see themselves as yoked together by some common bond of affection, blood, or vow. These questions have to do with the intensity of feelings or the nature of obligations between people when one person is sick or disabled. It is hard to imagine a society that does not take some precaution against the possibility of such unforeseen events.

Intervention by an outside expert can help reduce uncertainty. The creation of "third-party roles," whether or not their intervention can influence the course of disease, can ease the transition back to the affected relationships. Those who are assigned to make the consequences of illness, disease, and accident more predictable and therefore more socially manageable, deal with this uncertainty as well as with the physical aspects of the sick person.

Whether physicians and nurses (or witch doctors and herbalists) actually help people to get well or simply see them through the various social and psychological disruptions, they deal with illness, disease, and accident in an organized way. In other words, the program of health care in any society is *institutionalized,* and rules dictate who is to perform what activities. In addition, justifications are established to prove that this is the *best way* to provide health care and transmit this system to the uninitiated.

Health care, an organized, concrete, practical activity found in all societies, is usually performed by those who can provide at *least* two services: diagnosis and treatment. In performing these essential activities, health care practitioners help relieve uncertainty, both on a structural and interpersonal level, in addition to relieving pain and effecting cures where possible. Healing may be regarded as much as an art as a science. Such a view does not aim to belittle medical knowledge but to emphasize the importance of looking at health care as a result of a relationship entered into by patient and practitioner. Implicit, if not explicit, in that relationship is the expectation that *something* be done about current complaints, even when no widely approved treatment exists.

While each society develops an approved way of handling matters related to health and illness and assigns roles to specialists equipped to deliver such services, there usually exist a number of alternative systems of health care, particularly in a pluralistic society with many different cultures. Alternative healers base their practices on knowledge and skills that are theoretically at odds with established health care providers. Urban folk medicine, for example, receives steady support from users in many industrialized and industrializing societies (Press, 1978). In nineteenth-century American medicine, there was a great deal of competition among physicians following diverse theories, and even competition among medical societies and medical schools over the question of which corporate body should issue licenses.

Eventually licensing became a power of the various states, and licensing agencies sought to prevent alternative providers from practicing medicine without a license. Regulating agencies regard these alternative specialists as less skilled than the socially approved providers, or as possessing less appropriate knowledge or treatment procedures. These judgments were often based on social exclusiveness rather than on technical effectiveness. While health care in the United States is based on the use of *medical* knowledge—and that knowledge is regarded as scientifically valid—there is still a great reliance in the United States on nonmedically trained doctors of chiropractic.

Chiropractic is based on a unique but scientifically unvalidated theory of how the body works ("Chiropractors," 1975). Nonetheless, many find relief from pain through spinal manipulation. There are also healers who rely on faith alone to help people. Spiritualists are believed by themselves and others to have special gifts of healing. These gifts are considered to be an expression of extraordinary power which flows from within the person. A person who uses a spiritualist for cure generally believes in the presence of psychic and divine powers that operate in this world to control or alter it.

Today, people in some parts of the United States (e.g. Appalachia) use healers because their parents and grandparents used them and they are considered part of the community. Yet in many cases, people who visit these nonmedical healers, whether spiritualists or chiropractors, do so because conventional medicine has failed to reverse a deteriorating physical condition. Others may use alternative health care systems simultaneously with conventional medical facilities. Because modern medicine is often distant and impersonal to patients and their families, a few modern physicians have learned to recognize that patient compliance can be gained if they do not reject the use of alternative healers, so long as the patient is not exposed to any new risks. When patients and their families believe strongly in an alternative system of healing, often physicians will use a tactful procedure of "working with" the spiritualist, thereby maintaining contact with the patient and the family by showing respect for their customs.

Yet even when physicians demonstrate a sophisticated point of view with respect to the beliefs of patients and their families, they do so within the limits of their own knowledge of the natural world. They continue to regard their own understanding of the natural world as the ascendant and superior knowledge. Physicians may regard alternative systems of health care as more of a threat to the health and safety of patients when exaggerated claims are made as to success or when these practitioners seek to compete directly. Chiropractic has the social appearance of conventional medicine, despite its different theory. Chiropractors see themselves as specialists concerned only with health care, conducting themselves in ways similar to medical doctors. In contrast, spiritualism tends to be relatively unspecialized, with healing being only one gift (Borrello and Mathias, 1977).

CARE AND SOCIAL CONTROL

Health care is not only a way of dealing with the private troubles that people have and the consequent uncertainties those troubles create, but it is also a mechanism for preserving existing social relationships and cultural patterns of belief. Because health care involves both practitioner and patient it reinforces the existing social order. As such, it functions as a form of regulation or *social control* (Birenbaum and Sagarin, 1976). The form of social control taken today by medicine is one of "professional management" of large numbers of people who are socially deviant such as drug addicts, alcoholics, child abusers and unwed teenage parents (Ehrenreich and Ehrenreich, 1974:29).

Within the established field of health care, the medical profession controls the organization and delivery of services (Freidson, 1970a). Physicians are without serious rival or challenge in most industrialized societies. Their authority is dominant, even when they are subject to state controls or work under a collective ideology, as in the People's Republic of China (Sidel, 1973). The specialized tasks of societally assigned health care agents in industrialized societies are similar insofar as they (1) help to determine when the sick person can return to full-time social roles; (2) define those who cannot be regarded as fully competent either because of permanent or temporary incapacities (e.g., the developmentally disabled and people recovering from open heart surgery); (3) coordinate activities for those who are incapacitated, either through some kind of management program and/or rehabilitation; and (4) coordinate the commencement of life through birth, or termination through death.

While enormous similarities in the regulatory tasks are assigned to health care providers in all societies with complex divisions of labor, there are also substantial differences. Every industrialized society organizes these services in accordance with its basic concepts of ownership, the fostering or prevention of accumulated advantages, the appropriateness of realizing profits from illness and accident, and a sense of what society owes to each member. Consequently, the organized field of health care in any society is integrated with other institutions, including the economic, legal, and education.

The United States is one of the few advanced industrialized countries without either a publicly financed, if not wholly subsidized, national health insurance program or a national health service (Terris, 1977). Health facilities and related services are generally in the control of the private and voluntary sector of the economy in the United States. However, there is a great deal of public financing of services and even direct subsidization, mainly by the federal government's involvement in care for the elderly and the poor and support for research and facilities development. Most insurance programs, as well as pharmaceutical manufacturing and dispensing, are in the private sector.

An established health care system is vital in every society. A fundamental concern in any society is getting work done both to guarantee survival and economic surplus. Every society has various ways of getting people to conform to the labor system. And the delivery of health care, both in the form of direct services and measures that support a healthy population, is necessary to maintain production. Since any production system requires a reliable work force, i.e., predictable, health care measures become all-important in ensuring the regular return of workers to their jobs. Hence health care will receive support from those who require an adequate work force. In modern or modernizing societies, disease is viewed as something that can be diminished through public health measures and education.

The history of industrialization in Europe and North America provides evidence of how this process works. First, public health measures that eliminate the threat of such deadly epidemics as cholera, smallpox, and typhus were extremely important to the advancement of industrialization. Second, badly nourished populations are more susceptible to infections and their consequences. Public health officials advocated programs to ensure that enough food was available to feed factory workers. This was not urged strictly for humanitarian reasons but because of the medical findings on the state of the laboring poor in nineteenth-century England. Their physical condition was so dreadful that England had difficulty in raising an army for the Crimean War in the 1850s. The push for restrictions on the exploitation of women and children among English liberals was a direct result of this experience (Mayhew, 1971).

Available food supplies also meant that the work force would not be distracted or demoralized by a day-to-day struggle to acquire sustenance. Yet the prevailing opinion was that people returned to work from day to day because of the fear of starvation. Nineteenth-century factory owners and political economists believed that the cost of food should be kept high so factory workers would be willing to work long hours, stay at their jobs, and return willingly the next day (Bendix, 1963).

It took the English elites some time to recognize that cheap food was a way of keeping the work force healthy and relatively happy. When the price of food became too high, riots ensued in England and France. Bakeries were broken into and bread and flour were distributed (Rudé, 1959). These hostile outbursts were reminders to the elites of England that sensitivity to the needs and rights of workers was required to maintain order. Factory owners often feared that their establishments would be the next to be "liberated" and that schedules of production would be disrupted.

In modern industrial society, where food shortages have been avoided, new problems arise in maintaining a disciplined and available work force. Here, physicians perform different social control functions, having to do with maintaining motivation. Depending on the sector of the work force, physicians deal with problems of underachievement and overachievement or become involved in many regulating tasks, such as determining the fitness of those who claim to be sick and request disability insurance payments, or caring for children in large families who are not always subject to adequate monitoring of their health. This work is important, but it covers up the need to educate people better to prevent illness. Although the commitment to treatment is strong in contemporary medical practice, instructions in self-care skills are rarely given by physicians, even when they are clearly called for.

Among the skilled manual and professional sectors of the work force, health deterioration results not from wanting to drop out, but from wanting to achieve and be productive. Some employment situations are demanding; "there is rather consistent evidence that job pressures (measured both objectively and subjectively), such as work overload, responsibility, and role conflict, significantly increase heart disease risk and actually coronary heart disease" (House, 1974 : 21). Middle-class Americans are conscious of their health because being healthy means being attractive and eligible for promotion. Competitive individualism sees health as a personal asset rather than a collective responsibility. The same drives that motivate people to come to work when ill may also help to infect everyone at the workplace. Appearing sick to others by staying out, however, means appearing to be vulnerable and unable to keep up with the work pace. Illness is often kept secret from others, lest one be regarded as weak and failing, or socially avoided, or discharged from work because of supposed incapacities.

People often fail to go to a physician when they have symptoms of illness because they do not want to be told the bad news. Illness can be an unsharable problem, and even some physicians succumb to this mentality when they are ill and treat themselves with painkilling narcotics, to which they become addicted. They do this not because they believe they are invulnerable to illness, but because they do not want to appear vulnerable to their colleagues and because they want to keep up their demanding and often overextended professional lives (Winick, 1963). Physicians may be among the most competitive professionals, and they provide good evidence of the meaning of the relationship between health care and social regulation.

Studies of the kinds of pressures on physicians and their responses to them reveal a good deal about the nature of medical practice and its reliance on medication as a solution to problems presented by patients. The response of physicians to others with similar problems is not significantly different from their response to their own problems. The way physicians deal with anxiety, a common patient complaint, provides a case in which the treatment selected is sometimes based on the physician's belief that recurrences cannot be prevented.

Many physicians are reluctant to refer patients for psychiatric assessments, both because mental illness is stigmatizing and because they feel that they should be able to heal, and not have to call another healer. Consequently, mood-changing drugs are prescribed. The single most prescribed drug in the United States, and one that is used extensively through Western Europe, is the mild tranquilizer Valium (diazepam), which has become a household word. The compound is a muscle relaxant and has other uses as well, but it is mainly prescribed for anxiety, and it is most often prescribed by general practitioners and internists rather than psychiatrists (Cant, 1976).

When psychiatrists prescribe Valium, it is to assist agitated patients in conjunction with psychotherapy, not in place of it. Other physicians readily admit that they prescribe Valium for patients whom they know will not use psychotherapeutic services or those whom they feel cannot benefit from them. In addition, patients have their own prejudices about seeking help for mental or emotional problems, and some feel they lack the time for psychotherapy. In general practice, tranquilizers are used simply to keep people functioning rather than to help them avoid future suffering (Cant, 1976).

Both major and minor tranquilizers are widely used, in institutional settings. Valium is given extensively in old-age homes and extended-care nursing homes as a way to make angry patients (who often have genuine complaints) more manageable. Instead of working with the administration to correct the environment, physicians prescribe drugs, and this is accepted by administrators (Mendelson, 1975).

The use of physicians as agents of social control indicates that the responsibilities (and sometimes the unnecessary consequences) of medicine often go far beyond combating illness. The successes of medicine in some aspects of health care (e.g., immunizations) have encouraged the profession to become involved in all sorts of activities, such as treating drug addiction, alcoholism, and child abuse. Medical intervention in the treatment of behavior problems is based on the *mystique* of the profession—the belief that medicine can do the job better than law enforcement officials or clergy.

The extraordinary contemporary influence of medicine and its model for tackling problems has also resulted from new forms of structural differentiation and specialization (e.g., the medical college, the hospital, the medical center), as well as the introduction of technologies that advanced training and some forms of treatment, e.g., anaesthesia, X-rays, and antibiotics (Freidson, 1970b). The process was as much social as technical. The upgrading of hospitals to respected places of care began in the late nineteenth century; but the middle-class public had to be convinced. The hospital as the work place for physicians and nurses was partly based on greater success in keeping people alive after surgical and medical treatment; it was also based on the idea that the treatment of disease could not be made predictable in domestic households. While nurses were hardly educated, they were trained to follow the doctor's orders. By the beginning of the twentieth century, the hospital was viewed by the doctor as a place where control over conditions could be maintained (Hartwell, 1973). Soon the growing ranks of the middle classes began to accept hospitals as respectable places. In families where there were few domestic servants, it was difficult to provide care for a bedridden person. Today, planners are developing out-patient or ambulatory care facilities, such as neighborhood health centers and health maintenance organizations. These services depend on the family for support to keep the patient out of the hospital.

SOCIAL ORGANIZATION

Hospitals are the most concrete symbols of the way the work and training of doctors, nurses, pharmacists, technicians, and other health care providers are organized. Obviously medical care exists outside of hospitals, such as group practices, solo practices, and health centers, but the hospital is the central foundation for the network of health services. Few physicians can practice effectively without the availability of bed space for patients. The right to admit patients to a hospital is earned by physicians, being based on their affiliation with these organizations whose standards they meet. Qualifications are based on having earned degrees in medicine and demonstrated competency. Only physicians have the right to admit patients to a hospital. Even when it appears that a nurse is admitting a patient, it is done under standing orders issued by a doctor.

The organization of medical work is based upon the physician's knowledge and the generalized belief by society that the task of health care should be under the direction of the medical profession (Larson, 1977). Current organization is strongly influenced by the ways physicians are trained and by the new knowledge that is acquired. Physicians are also expected to keep up with advances in medical practice. The acquisition and advancement of knowledge results from research concerning new therapies, the discovery of etiologies of various diseases, and the measurement of general effectiveness of health and medical practice, as reflected in reduced rates of morbidity and mortality. But some observers of medical colleges and their curricula have questioned whether this highly complex technical training is conducted at the expense of helping medical students to learn interpersonal skills necessary in communicating with patients and gaining their compliance. Students model themselves after physicians who stress technical intervention through drugs, surgery, or radiation treatment; and with good reason, these physicians often have a difficult time gaining the patient's trust (Shuval, 1979). The selection, recruitment, and education of students may therefore serve to reproduce the existing features of the medical profession.

The expertise that physicians as a group possess is backed by legal recognition. Professionals who provide services, such as doctors, lawyers, and engineers, are licensed by the state in order to protect unsuspecting and unknowledgeable clients. Essentially, the relationship between physician and patient is based on trust, since the latter seeks expert advice and services, the quality of which he cannot judge. In order to protect the public, licenses are granted only to professionals who have demonstrated competency in their field. Competency is established in each state by boards of professionals judged to be qualified to set standards of practice. Boards that license also have the power to revoke the licenses of those who engage in deceitful practices or are judged to be incompetent. Patients also may sue doctors, nurses, and hospitals for malpractice, a common occurrence today, and a basis for the high cost of insurance for the providers.

Despite the formal criteria for admission and maintenance of medical practice, group loyalty, or solidarity among peers, makes formal regulation less important in the organization of health care work than informal controls (Freidson, 1972). It is rare that one physician will bring charges against another physician, because there is both sympathy with the plight of a fellow doctor who makes a mistake and fear of ostracism by his colleagues (State of New York, 1976).

Thus medicine is organized on both a formal and an informal basis. The concept of social organization is useful for analyzing the foundations of relationships among doctors, between doctors and patients, and between doctors and paramedical personnel. The dominant position held by physicians is a result of the institutionalizing of the tasks of health care under the direction of the profession. This situation results as much from medicine's unified efforts to prevent the unregulated delivery of health care by those who had alternative training and knowledge, as from their claim apparently recognized by the public, that they have a monopoly on knowledge and skill in treatment. The licensing of physicians was the major form by which competition from chiropractors, osteopaths, herbalists, and spiritualists—some of the less exotic healers known in nineteenth-century America—was restricted (Larson, 1977). Recent developments in health care of both a technical and financial nature have influenced the creation of new social relationships between physicians and other professionals in the field and have altered relationships between doctors and patients.

The *social organization* of health care is defined as the general standards and specific rules that govern physicians and other health care deliverers (Blauner, 1964:9). These rules define the network of positions that exist and the rights and duties of occupants of those positions. Positions are identified by titles such as doctor, nurse, blood technician, and medical secretary.

Some positions are identified internally in an organization, so there may be chief residents, residents, and nursing supervisors as well as nurses in a hospital. There are also distinctive uniforms or other ways of indicating the title of the occupant, so that it is clear that the person has the right to issue an order. While uniforms serve to eliminate confusion, they also make it possible for intruders to impersonate a health care provider. Therefore, in most health care settings, written orders or standing orders also assist in ensuring that appropriate procedures are undertaken.

The titles, rules, and standing orders of a medical organization do not reveal the full range of activities that are undertaken by a particular nurse, technician, or pharmacist. A pharmacist in the community may perform first aid or give advice, tasks the doctor or nurse would perform in a clinic or hospital. The rights and obligations of patients may also vary from hospital to hospital, depending on policies and staffing patterns. Some maternity wards permit mothers and newborns to share the same room, allowing parenting to begin early in the life of the child. Other maternity services place newborns directly under the care of a nurse in the nursery.

THE DIVISION OF LABOR

The assignment of tasks in health care can vary from organization to organization. The division of labor in health care is influenced by the size of the organization, the size of the patient population, and the kinds of health care needs within the scope of the organization. The job description of a nurse in the solo practice office of a country doctor can be quite different from a nurse who works in a large voluntary hospital. The systematic assembling of tasks in different health care organizations is defined as the *division of labor* (Blauner, 1964:9) The more formal the rules and procedures, the more specific and narrow are the particular tasks performed by individuals who hold certain job titles. Generally, the larger an organization, the more bureaucratic the form by which work is distributed.

Job specialization is also influenced by the complexity of the organization. Hospitals that receive reimbursement for services rendered have to account for bills to insurers such as Blue Cross and Blue Shield. Therefore, hospital financing becomes a specialized set of tasks within the overall organization. Further, general hospitals also perform teaching and research functions, and planning and coordination is required in these areas as well. Staff allocation is planned and coordinated, new therapies and procedures are developed and tested, and even new ways of evaluating performance are built into the daily activities of the hospital.

Another division of labor in health care locates both pure and applied research in medical colleges, much of it supported by grants from the National Institutes of Health. Research and development have become so important and influential that modern medical practice has become totally dependent on the flow of information from these sources. Moreover, because researchers are able to bring in financial support for medical schools and other organizations, their influence in policy making has also increased.

Interestingly, in the 1920s, the solo practitioners in the American Medical Association were able to drive out research-oriented physicians, mainly over the issue of supporting health insurance legislation. Ironically, those research-oriented physicians who found refuge in medical schools now have been able to eclipse the AMA in influencing Congress and the Department of Health, Education, and Welfare (Alford, 1972).

Leadership from medical schools has opened up a redistribution of tasks in the division of labor in health care. Nurses, for example, have taken on many technical tasks that were delegated by physicians. Further, new roles such as physician assistants and nurse practitioners have been created to free the physician from doing certain routine procedures, with prescription writing under standing orders now delegated to such subordinates. The standardization of the treatment of certain acute illnesses, such as ear infections, is creating a new division of labor.

TECHNOLOGY OF HEALTH CARE

The technology of health care includes efforts to prevent disease as well as diagnostic and treatment procedures. The development of diagnostic machines, such as body scanners, and machines for keeping people alive, such as the kidney dialysis, has received the greatest public attention. These devices have had a large impact on the social organization, the division of labor, and the costs of health care. However, immunization and the use of antibiotics for treating infections have had a more decisive impact on eliminating acute illness as major cause of death.

Technology refers to the state of the art, the practices, procedures, tools, machines, and drugs used to produce a desired outcome (Blauner, 1964:6). Because of the human factor, the extent to which the work can be mechanized is limited. Moreover, clinical judgment and the involvement of patients will always be necessary to perform diagnoses and treatment. In the field of prevention, the active cooperation of the public will also be necessary, no matter what the state of the technology.

The advances in medical technology make rapid diagnosis of many illnesses possible and bring into existence a host of positions based on different specializations, such as blood technicians, X-ray technicians, and others. Similar technical specialties are found in surgery and in medical treatments that are dependent on machines to trace internal procedures. Most of these occupational specialists are found in the large and more complex health care organizations, such as hospitals and medical centers, with some being employed in independent service businesses. These laboratories work on a contract basis with physicians in private practice. By virtue of these new techniques, health care appears to be shifting from being a *labor intensive* industry to a *capital intensive* one. Yet often staff must be hired or retrained to use this machinery. These expenses, for equipment and labor, have pushed health care costs ever upward. To practice modern medicine, a doctor requires access to sophisticated machinery. Yet some expensive devices are infrequently or inappropriately used, even at general hospitals that see a wide variety of cases. The need to attract highly trained physicians to hospitals, a feature of social organization, leads to needless duplication of equipment and facilities in the same region.

Two aspects of technology significantly shape the nature of relationships between health care providers and patients, a subject most intensively examined in the structure of the doctor-patient relationship (Merton and Barber, 1976): (1) the type of medical problem, whether it is subject to routine procedures with few exceptions, and (2) the capacity of the physician and paramedical personnel to find the causes of the patient's dysfunction and suggest a remedy (Perrow, 1967).

Preventive technologies, such as the elimination of environmental hazards or immunization, constitute ways of protecting the public at large from risk. Preventive intervention is generally performed on a societal basis, precluding the relationship between physician and patient. Some forms of prevention, such as immunization of children, may be the basis for sporadic contact. And some preventive measures are specific to a high-risk group, as when amniocentesis is performed on older pregnant women to forecast a Down's Syndrome child.

Technology may also be considered as preparatory, involving efforts by the physician to avoid complicated medical problems, as illustrated by surgery for hernia repair as a way of avoiding possible blood poisoning when a piece of intestine becomes trapped in the muscle. Regular examinations of women during the last trimester of pregnancy are also performed to avoid unexpected circumstances at birth. Again, outcomes are improved by such intervention, and patients usually are coöperative and trusting of medical practitioners under these conditions.

Finally, there are remedial technologies—the most dramatic types of intervention practiced by doctors. Remedial interventions themselves may range from routine treatments of infections with antibiotics, the removal of an inflamed appendix, or the effort to treat malignant tumors through radiation or chemotherapy. Remedial technology does not always end in cure; intervention may or may not be successful, depending on the overall health of the patient, the time at which disease is diagnosed, and the state of knowledge in the field. Not only are interventions problematic, but a long, drawn-out relationship between doctor and patient often ensues, making patients sometimes feel that they are not always being helped. Patients often undergo treatment that is painful, experimental, ineffective, and costly. Under these conditions, partly induced by the availability of sophisticated although not always decisive technologies, medicine fails. The physician's failure in itself does not produce patient retaliation, but evasions, lies, and callousness do. Physicians lack knowledge and training in interpersonal skills, and this ineptitude is partially responsible for the increasing rate of malpractice suits (Bernstein, Bernstein, and Dana, 1974).

ECONOMIC STRUCTURE

Technology influences the economic as well as the social relationship between providers and consumers. The cost of current standards of treatment reflect the types of diseases brought to the attention of physicians, the labor necessary for treatment and the length of time patients receive services from medical and paramedical personnel. These costs are supposed to be basic to determining fees charged by doctors and rates for hospitalization.

Health care in the United States is financed through an amalgam of individual expenditures, private insurance plans offered as fringe benefits to employees, policies purchased on the open market, and federally funded Medicare and Medicaid programs for the elderly and the medically indigent. Both patients and their doctors have been known to "work the reimbursement system," sometimes cooperatively and sometimes in antagonistic relationships, to limit out-of-pocket costs of the former and maximize income for the latter. The use of "third-party payers" for 90 percent of hospital bills, for example, encourages unnecessary hospitalization, since patients are only reimbursed for care or services rendered on an inpatient basis (Public Health Service, 1978: 364). Similarly, unnecessary tests are often ordered and treatment performed when the costs are not directly borne by patients. Some states monitor doctors' bills sent to third-party payers to discourage unnecessary procedures and will not reimburse physicians who perform unwarranted tests.

The *economic structure* of health care is defined as the system of payment utilized, the extent to which control is concentrated or dispersed, the profit margins in the field, current and expected costs, rates of growth, and trends in demand. As of 1978, $863 per person was spent annually in the United States for health care (Public Health Service, 1980: 235). The demands on the system have increased as more Americans develop higher expectations of service. Figure 1 breaks down personal health care expenditures by type of service and source of funds.

Much of the health care system is paid for by third-party payers either through public agencies or insurance groups. Blue Cross, Medicare and Medicaid, other direct public funds, and other private insurance companies have a great influence on the delivery of health care, since their rules of reimbursement encourage remedial intervention and discourage preventive and preparatory work. Payments are made to providers for the procedure performed, not the amount of time spent in delivering the service. Thus it is not as profitable for an internist to perform a complete physical examination as it is to treat an illness.

In the 1970s, price rises in health care outstripped inflation in other spheres of the economy. The cost of supplies and machinery influences the rates charged in hospitals and medical centers. Drug companies, which seek to realize high profit, operate as any other large corporation. Labor costs also drive up hospital charges. In addition, physicians in group and solo practice have adopted modern corporate financial practices and management techniques to make sure they are paid for *all* services rendered.

Medical economics has become a growing field as hospitals and third-party payers become increasingly concerned about zooming costs, unnecessary services, and overutilization of hospitals for treatment. Efforts to reduce the cost of health care delivery have stimulated the development of new health care practitioners (physician assistants and nurse practitioners) and new practices (home care and the geriatric day hospital).

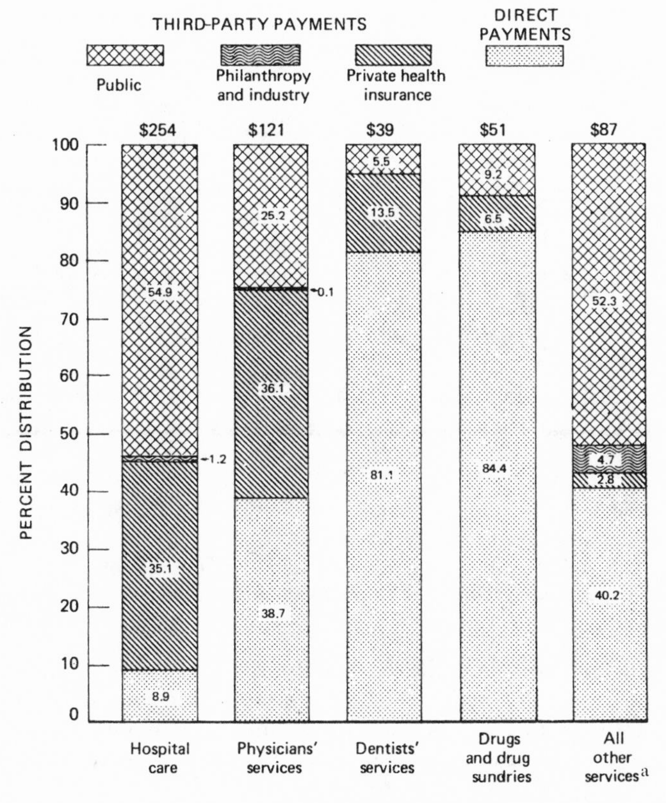

[a]Includes other professional services, eyeglasses and appliances, nursing home care, and other services not elsewhere classified.

Source: Gibson, R. M., and M. S. Mueller. National Health Expenditures. Fiscal Year 1976. *Social Security Bulletin* 40 (4):3–22, April 1977.

Figure 1 Percentage Distribution of Per Capita Personal Health Care Expenditures by Type of Expenditure and Source of Funds, Fiscal Year 1976

The availability of third-party payments varies by the type of expenditure, with hospitals being most likely to be supported by public funds and private health insurance and drugs most likely to be paid for directly by the consumer, as seen in Figure 1. Since hospitals are the most expensive part of the cost of health care, it follows that both public support and private insurance programs would be most heavily concentrated in this part of the almost 9 percent of the gross national product that goes for health care (see Figure 2).

The proportion of the health care dollar spent on hospitals has increased over the last forty years as a result of new techniques of treatment, the

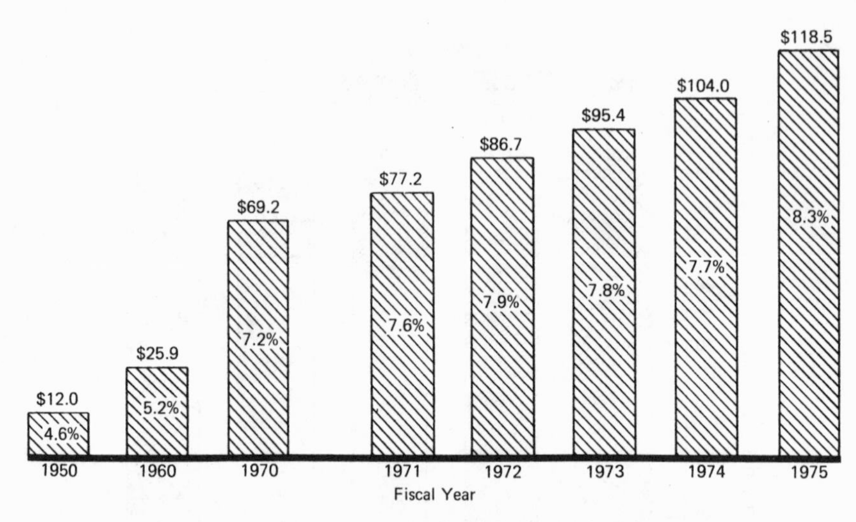

Source: Social Security Administration, Office of Research and Statistics.

Figure 2 National Health Expenditures and Percentage of Gross National Product, Selected Fiscal Years 1950–1975 (in billion dollars).

increasing division of labor, the availability of public funds for construction, and private and public insurance. As can be seen in Figure 3, more than 53 percent of the national expenditures in the area of health now go for hospitals, nursing homes, and the construction of research and medical facilities.

These financial arrangements have a major impact on consumer behavior and ultimately on the health status of individuals. People without private hospital insurance coverage are not randomly distributed throughout the population. Even though 78 percent of Americans are covered, there are sharp differences in the extent of coverage by income level, age, and color. It can be argued that those with lower incomes do not need private hospital insurance, since they are eligible for federally and state funded programs. Yet many people near or below the poverty level are excluded, given the great diversity of rules and levels of support for these programs from state to state. For example, California excludes only 6 percent of this group, whereas Mississippi defines 66 percent of its poor and near poor as ineligible (Public Health Service, 1978: 113).

When the costs of health care are prohibitive for those of limited means, their use of available services is affected, and consequently, their health status. Two findings highlight the fact that poorer people avoid visits to the doctor for preventive or preparatory procedures and wait longer before presenting symptoms, thus lowering the probability that remedial intervention will be effective.

> Visits to emergency rooms accounted for 4.5 percent of all physician contacts in 1975 in contrast with 2.5 percent in 1971. In 1975, 11 percent of all physician

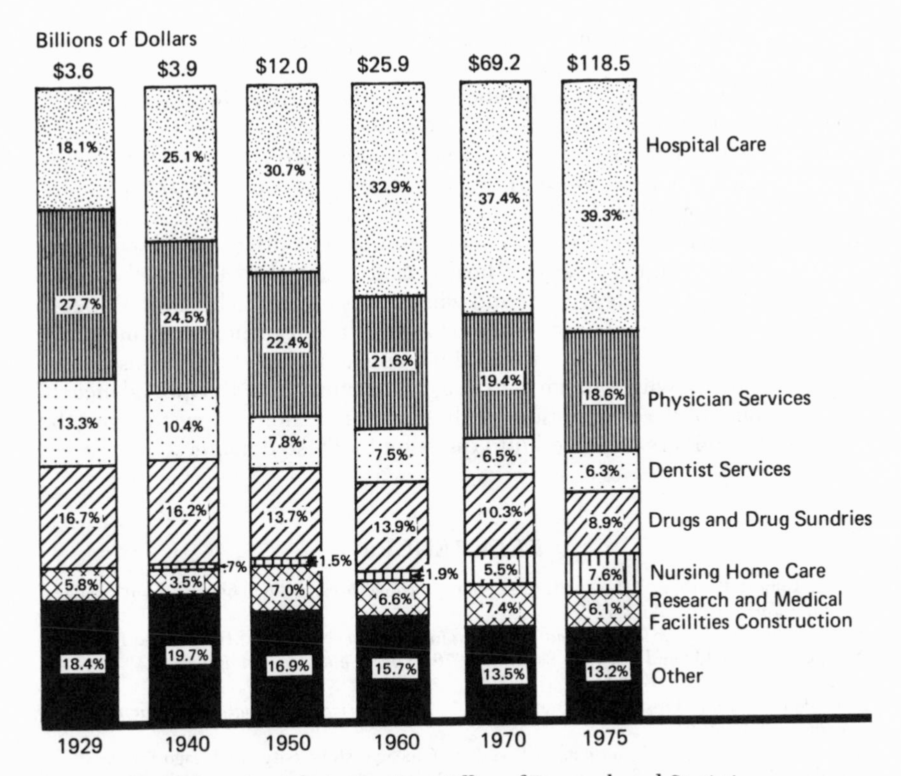

Source: Social Security Administration, Office of Research and Statistics.

Figure 3 Percentage Distribution of Aggregate National Health Expenditures by Type of Expenditure, Selected Fiscal Years 1929–1975

contacts of children under age 15 in low-income (less than $5,000) families were emergency room visits in contrast with 5.7 percent in 1971.

People in families with low incomes are hospitalized more often, and once hospitalized they remain in the hospital longer than people in families with higher incomes. [Public Health Service, 1978: vi]

Finally, focusing on the economic structure of health care makes it possible to examine the extent to which the concentration of resources is in the hands of a few producers of goods or services—as in the case of the drug industry's control over the production and distribution of pharmaceuticals on a retail and wholesale level—affect their price and, in turn, the willingness of consumers to pay for them, even when prescribed. Similarly, the near monopoly over health services held by physicians has also helped to account for increased costs. While more doctors are available for the population than twenty years ago, since the growth rate of the population has slowed considerably, the fees and incomes of physicians have climbed at a faster rate than any other occupation in the United States (Shabecoff, 1978). Economic concentration makes it more difficult to reorganize services so that they become available to all, regardless of ability to pay. Not only economic control but geographic concentration are factors in the health care field. Doctors abound in urban areas and in states where the mean income is higher than the national average (O'Donoghue, 1976). And paradoxically, fees are highest in areas where there are more doctors per 100,000 persons.

A sociology of health and illness is designed to introduce some basic concepts and to raise some critical questions about health care and society. Is the organization and delivery of health care adapted to the needs of our population? What needs are met and what needs remain to be met? To begin to understand contemporary issues in health care, the ways in which demographic changes affect the patient population have to be considered. Chapter 2 deals with our changing age structure and the prevalence of disease. Many of the assumptions of the health care delivery system and the training of providers are called into question by these dynamics.

REFERENCES

Alford, Robert R. 1972. "The political economy of health care: Dynamics without change." *Politics and Society* (Winter): 1–38.

Bendix, Rhinehardt. 1963. *Work and Authority in Industry.* New York: Harper and Row.

Birenbaum, Arnold, and Edward Sagarin. 1976. *Norms and Human Behavior.* New York: Praeger.

Blau, Peter M., and Otis Dudly Duncan. 1967. *The American Occupational Structure.* New York: John Wiley.

Blauner, Robert. 1964. *Alienation and Freedom.* Chicago: University of Chicago Press.

Borrello, Mary Ann and Elizabeth Mathias. 1977. "Botanicas: Puerto Rican Folk Pharmacies." *Natural History* 86 (August-September): 64–73.

Bowles, Samuel. 1972. "Unequal education and the reproduction of the social division of labor." Pp. 36–64 in M. Carnoy, ed. *Schooling in Corporate Society: The Political Economy of Education in America.* New York: McKay.

Cant, G. 1976. "Valiumania." *New York Times Magazine,* February 1. Pp. 34–44.

"Chiropractors: Healers or quacks?" Part I. 1975. *Consumer Reports* (September), Pp. 542–610.

Ehrenreich, Barbara, and John Ehrenreich. 1974. "Health care and social control." *Social Policy* (May/June): 26–40.

Eyer, J. 1977. "Does unemployment cause the death rate peak in each business cycle?" *International Journal of Health Services* 7: 625–62.

Freidson, Eliot. 1970a. *Professional Dominance: The Social Structure of Medical Care.* New York: Atherton Press.

———. 1970b. *The Profession of Medicine: A Study of the Sociology of Applied Knowledge.* New York: Dodd, Mead.

Freidson, Eliot, and Buford Rhea. 1972. "Processes of control in a company of equals." Pp. 185–201 in Eliot Freidson and Judith Lorber, eds., *Medical Men and Their Work: A Sociological Reader.* Chicago: Aldine.

Fuchs, Victor. 1974. *Who Shall Live? Health, Economics and Social Choice.* New York: Basic Books.

Gibson, R. M., and M. S. Mueller. 1977. "National health expenditures, fiscal year 1976." *Social Security Bulletin* 40 (April): 3–22.

Goffman, Erving. 1976. "Gender advertisements." *Studies in the Anthropology of Visual Communication* 3 (Fall).

Goode, William J. 1979. *The Celebration of Heroes: Prestige as a Social Control System.* Berkeley: University of California Press.

Harrison, Barbara Grizzuti. 1974. *Unlearning the Lie: Sexism in School.* New York: Morrow.

Hartwell, R. M. 1973. "The economic history of medical care." pp. 3–20 in Mark Perlman, ed., *The Economics of Health and Medical Care*. New York: Halsted Press.
House, James A. 1974. "Occupational stress and coronary heart disease: A review and theoretical integration." *Journal of Health and Social Behavior* 15 (March): 12–27.
Katz, Elihu, and Paul F. Lazarsfeld. 1964. *Personal Influence*. New York: Free Press.
Kett, Joseph F. 1968. *The Formation of the American Medical Profession, The Role of Institutions 1780–1860*. New Haven: Yale University Press.
Kitagawa, Evelyn M., and Philip M. Hauser. 1973. *Differential Mortality in the United States: A Study of Socioeconomic Epidemiology*. Cambridge: Harvard University Press.
Kluckhohn, Clyde, and William H. Kelly. 1945. "The concept of culture." in Ralph Linton, ed., *The Science of Man in World Crisis*. New York: Columbia University Press.
Larson, Magali Sarfatti. 1977. *The Rise of Professionalism: A Sociological Analysis*. Berkeley: University of California Press.
Lebow, Eliot. 1967. *Tally's Corner: A Study of Negro Street Corner Men*. Boston: Little, Brown.
MacMahon, Brian, and Thomas F. Pugh. 1970. *Epidemiology: Principles and Methods*. Boston: Little, Brown.
Mayhew, Henry. 1971. *Voices of the Poor*. Anne Humpherys, ed. London: Frank Cass.
Mendelson, Mary Adelaide. 1975 *Tender Loving Greed*. New York: Vintage.
Merton, R. K., and E. Barber. 1976. "Sociological ambivalence," Pp. 3–31 in Robert K. Merton, *Sociological Ambivalence and Other Essays*. New York: Free Press.
O'Donoghue, Patrick. 1976. "The influence of financial, educational and regional factors on the distribution of physicians." Pp. 285–316 in Elinor Ostrom, ed., *The Delivery of Urban Services: Outcomes of Change*, Vol. 10, Urban Affairs Annual Reviews. Beverly Hills, Sage Publications.
Perrow, C. 1967. "A framework for the comparative analysis of organizations." *American Sociological Review* 32: 194–208.
Press, Irwin. 1978. "Urban folk medicine: A functional overview." *American Anthropologist* 80: 71–84.
Public Health Service. 1978. *Health United States 1976–1977*. Washington, D.C.: Department of Health, Education, and Welfare.
———. 1980. *Health United States 1979*. Washington, D.C.: Department of Health, Education, and Welfare.
Rudé, George. 1959. *The Crowd in the French Revolution*. London: Oxford.
Shabecoff, Philip. 1978. "Doctors' fees rising at fastest U.S. rate." *New York Times*, March 23: pp. A1, B13.
Shuval, Judith T., and Israel Adler. 1979. "Health occupations in Israel: Comparative patterns of change during socialization." *Journal of Health and Social Behavior* 20 (March): 77–88.
Sidel, Victor. 1973. "Medical Personnel and their training." In Joseph R. Quinn, ed., *Medicine and Public Health in the People's Republic of China*. Washington, D.C.: Department of Health, Education, and Welfare.
Sidel, Victor W., and Ruth Sidel. 1978. *A Healthy State: An International Perspective on the Crisis in United States Medical Care*. New York: Pantheon.
Stack, Carole. 1974. *All Our Kin: Strategies for Survival in a Black Community*. New York: Harper and Row.
State of New York. 1976. Report of the Special Advisory Panel on Medical Malpractice. New York State.
Susser, Mervyn W., and W. Watson. 1962. *Sociology in Medicine*. London: Oxford University Press.
Terris, Milton. 1977. "The three world systems of medical care: Trend and prospects." Presented at the 105th annual meeting of the American Public Health Association. Washington, D.C.
Wilkinson, R. G. 1975. "Techniques of ancient skull surgery." *Natural History* (October), pp. 94–101.
Winick, C. 1963. "Physician drug addicts." Pp. 261–80 in Howard S. Becker, ed., *The Other Side: Perspectives on Deviance*. New York: Free Press.
World Health Organization. 1976. World Health Statistics Annual, 1973–1976, Vol. I, Vital Statistics and the Causes of Death. Geneva: World Health Organization.

2

Disease and the Changing Population

Sociological concepts describe and analyze institutional arrangements or the nature of interaction among people performing diverse tasks. These relationships may directly or indirectly involve health. As a characteristic of a population, health goes far beyond the direct activities of curing and caring found within hospitals and other service organizations. Concepts such as social organization, division of labor, technology, and financial structure are aids in explaining the sources of stability and change in health care institutions. Yet they must be supplemented by facts in examining the health status of the American people. The social conditions associated with certain types of disease require careful description and analysis.

Society, substantially a human construction, has objective consequences for human life. The conditions introduced by arrangements for survival between human beings influence the life chances of those subject to those conditions, and of future generations also. Life expectancy, for example, has increased enormously in advanced industrial societies, resulting far more from adequate nutrition than from advances in medical technology (McKeown, 1976). Health needs can change as a result of changing characteristics of the population, such as the new profile of the age distribution.

Viewing society as a human construction rather than as an eternal or natural force implies that different arrangements are possible through new forms of intervention. The dynamics of a changing population may sometimes obscure the inequities in the distribution of vital forms of support for families. Whether by circumstance or design, such maldistributions have significant consequences for the health status of the nation.

Defining the health needs of the population helps us learn how to make services more useful. The criticisms of health care services that laymen express are, in part, based on recognition that new forms of distribution and financing are required. The health needs of any population at any time, therefore, may be viewed as the combination of what laymen believe should be treated and what the medical profession believes can be treated with success. All of these expectations are subject to change. For instance, the dramatic success in treating infectious diseases has increased the demand on the medical profession to be equally productive in other areas of health and illness.

Medicine has an extraordinary capacity to treat injuries and illnesses effectively. But the expectation of effective treatment as routine medical behavior has not been constant throughout history. As recently as 1915, Lawrence J. Henderson, a faculty member at Harvard Medical School, commented critically about medicine, saying that the average patient "had no better than a 50-50 chance of benefitting from an encounter with the average physician" (Glazier, 1973: 19). But the success of contemporary medical practice is recognized by the population at large: National opinion surveys show that Americans have more confidence in health than in other social services. However, this faith has declined from 73 percent in 1966 to 43 percent in 1977 (Lyons, 1977).

Even within the same area, individuals in different sectors of society have divergent definitions of the kinds of symptoms that deserve medical attention. Koos (1954: 33) asked respondents from different social class backgrounds to determine whether 17 different physical symptoms required a visit to the doctor. He found wide differences in responses. Furthermore, women were less likely to seek medical attention than men of the same social class. Apparently, women reasoned that the incapacitation of a man would result in a loss of income, causing more disruption of family life than if they themselves became seriously ill. Today, with so many women in the work force and with greater equality between the sexes, one wonders whether the same findings would result.

With greater access to education and health benefits and with public adulation of the physician, the demand for care is intense. Today, there may be an excessive reliance on medical intervention, even when treatment does not work. Faith in the effectiveness of drugs to cure illness has resulted in patients demanding antibiotics for the common cold or flu, even when there are no actual cures for these illnesses.

The increased reliance on medical intervention may also result in higher fees, increased rates for medical insurance, and excessive patient loads for doctors. Mistakes and failures to communicate directly with the patient and the family increase under these conditions, resulting in dissatisfied patients, and, in some instances, malpractice suits. Sadusk found that in nine out of ten malpractice cases, the defendant was found to be not guilty of a technical error (1959: 137). Results of studies conducted for the California Medical Association came up with similar findings (Blum, 1960: 105). More recently, the Special Advisory Panel on Medical Malpractice, State of New York, reported that along with higher risks associated with more sophisticated technology and medications, the most important sources of increased malpractice litigation were

> . . . changes in the traditional doctor-patient relationship reflecting the impersonalized character of a more organized and speciality-oriented health care delivery system; new patient attitudes toward the provision of health services, stimulated in part by the general attitudes of consumerism, and a sharpened sensitivity to long ignored rights of individuals, and perhaps less than realistic expectations about the capacities of modern medicine to bring about "miracle cures." [1976: 10]

Despite the importance of subjective judgments that influence whether or not people seek treatment, and the greater accessibility of services resulting from private insurance plans and government programs, some ways of evaluating the overall health status of Americans should be found. It is also important to determine how the vast resources of the current system can be more effectively distributed.

Any assessment of needs requires that an examination of how this system compares with health care in other countries with similar social and economic characteristics. It makes little sense to compare the United States to newly emerging nations, such as Uganda, or to nations undergoing industrialization, such as Brazil, because birthrates and mortality rates will be vastly different. But the United States could be compared with countries like Sweden or England to see whether such fundamental measures of overall health status are similar or different. Given the enormous amount of money and proportion of our gross national product devoted to health care, the overall health of the American people could be improved. As of 1976, the United States had only the 15th lowest infant mortality rate of all nations, with varying rates for different sectors of the population. The death rate for white infants was 14.4 per 1,000 live births, while for nonwhite infants the rate was 22.9 (Public Health Service, 1976: 13). (See Figure 4.) The male mortality rate in the 45–54 age range in England was 78 percent of that found in the same population in the United States, and it was even lower in Sweden (Sidel and Sidel, 1978: 10).

While comparisons of this kind are important in understanding whether the resources of the United States are adequately distributed, more information is needed about the age structure in the United States and how health care personnel are organized to meet the changing rates of disease resulting from changes in the birth and death rate.

THE GRAYING OF AMERICA

The bicentennial year 1976 witnessed not only a celebration of the birth of the United States but the end of a time when more than half of the population was under the age of thirty. While the median age in 1977 was 28.9, it is anticipated that by the year 2030 more than half the population will be over 36 (Reinhold, 1977: 1).

The U.S. population could be characterized, as of the late 1970s, by its low birthrate and a lowering mortality rate. This means that, proportionately, more people are living into their seventies and eighties, and the health needs of the country must address the chronic diseases of old age, as can be

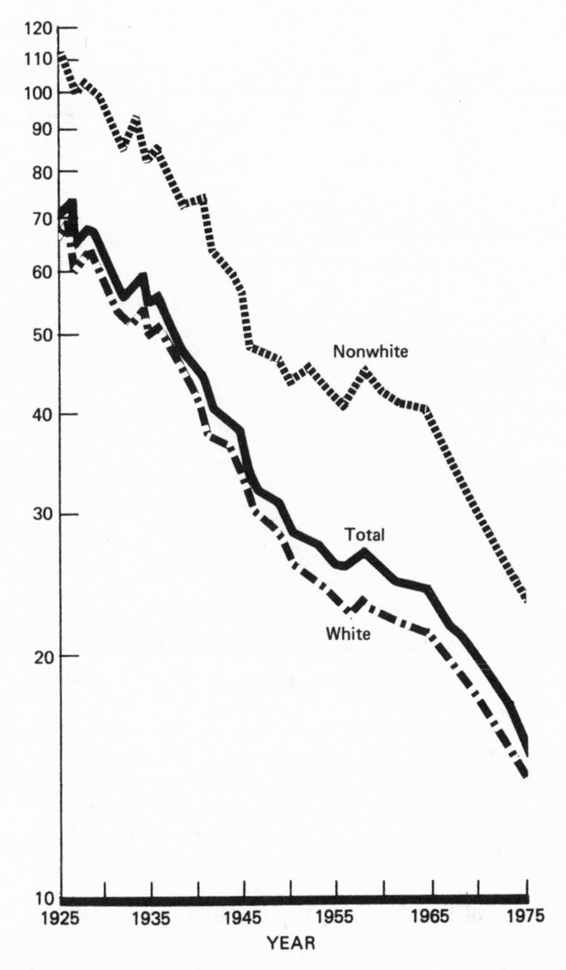

Note: Rates are the number of deaths under one year of age per 1,000 live births.
Source: National Center for Health Statistics.

Figure 4 Infant Mortality Rates by Color, United States 1925–1975

seen in Figures 5 and 6. Some of these changes are the result of the use of antibiotics, which reduce the consequences of infection, enabling more people to live longer when they become subject to long-term or chronic illnesses. Other changes are the result of new patterns of living, including fewer marriages, family planning, and more planned childless marriages.

Undoubtedly these changes in the age structure will promote a variety of social consequences. New lifestyles may develop, using the model of the commune or the group home, a concept being promoted by agencies that

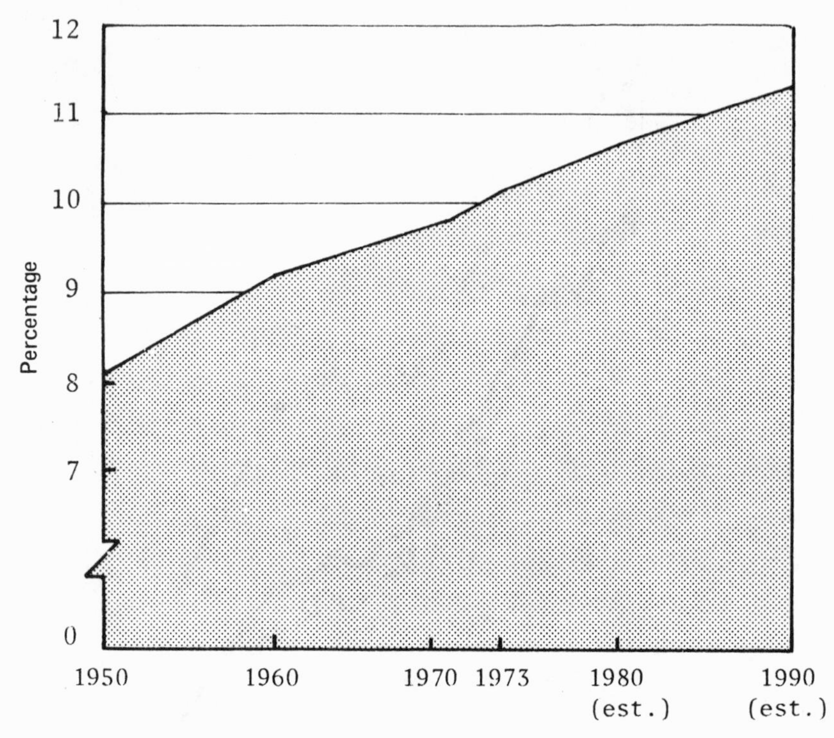

Source: U.S. Department of Commerce, Bureau of the Census, *Statistical Abstract of the United States: 1974* (Washington, D.C.: U.S. Government Printing Office, 1974), Tables 3 and 35. The 1980 and 1990 population projection is the Census Bureau's Projection under Series I–E, which assumes 2,100 births per 1,000 women upon completion of childbearing and continuation of 1960–1970 migration patterns.

Figure 5 Percentage of United States Population Aged 65 and Older, 1950–1990

care for semidependent people. These population changes will also make new demands on the health delivery system. Medical specialties will certainly be deeply affected by the reduction of the birth rate; for example less pediatricians will be needed. Many specialists are already starting to diversify, branching out into related areas such as child psychiatry. As many of the diseases of childhood are eliminated through immunization, pediatricians more frequently see children who manifest behavior problems at home or school, making training in psychiatry a useful way to retool.

Health care for the adult population can also shift, but with far more radical changes in the education, training, and deployment of health personnel. A major consequence of an aging population is the increased frequency of cardiovascular disease and hypertension, with physicians seeing fewer cases of injury and acute illness in their overall patient load. With the

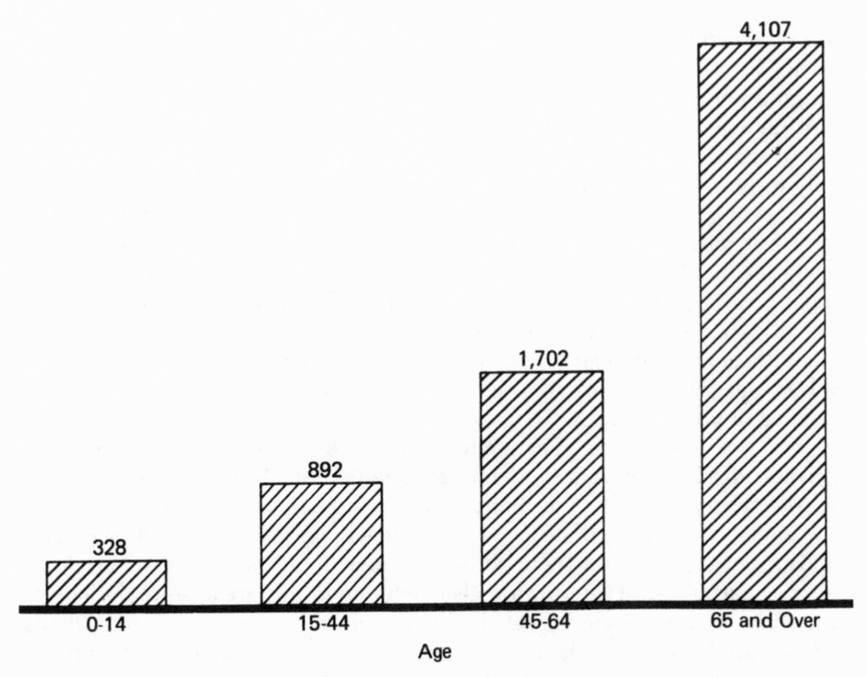

Source: National Center for Health Statistics, Hospital Discharge Survey.

Figure 6 Number of Short-Stay Hospital Days per 1,000 Population by Age, 1974

changing needs of the population comes a fundamental redefinition of the basic tasks of medicine. Medicine today emphasizes the treatment of trauma or acute illness, immediate life and death situations.

The education and training of physicians concentrate on immediate problem-solving situations, where physicians learn to recognize these life and death situations. But often the detection, followup, and monitoring of chronic illness is largely ignored (Ebert, 1977). Physicians in practice, particularly in internal medicine and among heart and cancer specialists, spend most of their time caring for patients who have a chronic illness such as hypertension (McDermott, 1977: 138). Other chronic illnesses result from serious bouts with acute illnesses, as in patients recovering from heart attacks or cancer surgery. Here the emphasis is on long-term recovery and management of the illness without giving up activities such as work or recreation. Finally, many physicians also care for the terminally ill patient whose recovery is unlikely but who may live for several years. The subject of death and dying is only beginning to become part of the medical school curriculum, and few practicing physicians or other health care practitioners are trained to handle the interpersonal dynamics or the psychological strain created by these situations (Kubler-Ross, 1969).

Several implications about health care and the aging population can be drawn. First, various kinds of redesign are necessary if the needs of a changing population are to be met. Enriching medical education to include more knowledge on the natural history and treatment of chronic illnesses may be easy to undertake. The social consequences of disability are less likely to be incorporated in the curriculum, however. Medicine is resistant to increasing the behavioral science content of medical school curricula because it raises questions about the current effectiveness of delivering and paying for health care. Further questions may be raised about the domination of health care by physicians. Redesign of the organization and delivery of health care to deal with chronic illness requires increased utilization of paramedical personnel and greater delegation of decision making to them, as well as the giving up of routine responsibilities that once were the sole province of physicians.

Second, new concepts of care and recovery are needed. Careful monitoring is required in the treatment and management of chronic illness to return the patient to a "normal" life. Rehabilitation medicine (or physical medicine) is a specialized area that focuses on teaching patients to use various appliances that will help them return to their homes and former activities. Exercise and physical therapy are also included in this area. More difficult to deal with are the psychological doubts during recovery on the part of the patient, family, and friends. Friends and family make up an informal support network, and they may or may not be capable of helping the patient to return to normal life. All of these considerations enter into the successful or unsuccessful management of a chronic illness or physical disability in the community rather than in a hospital. It requires a rethinking of the health care delivery system, and especially the role of the physician in it, in order to meet the needs of a population with high rates of chronic illness and the substantial numbers of people who are partially disabled. The late William Glazier, an astute observer of the American health care delivery system, summarized the problem very well:

> The medical system encounters several types of problems in dealing with the chronically ill. In the first place, it is essentially a passive system, that is, it does not go into operation until a patient takes the initiative by visiting a physician or a clinic. Often by the time a patient with a chronic illness takes this step it is late in the progress of the disease. For many of the chronic diseases much of the treatment is directed to symptoms rather than being curative. The regime of treatment is also likely to be protracted and costly. Another type of problem is that the system is geared to the one-to-one, episodic relationship in which the patient sees a physician, receives treatment and pays a fee. The system is unwieldy and inefficient when, as is often the case with chronic disease, the patient requires care by several physicians with different specialties, by other professional people such as nurses, therapists and social workers and by different institutions. Finally, the system is in a better position to take care of the patient who is so incapacitated that he has to be in a hospital bed than the patient who is ill but more or less able to go about his normal business—and such patients constitute about 85 percent of the total. [1973: 14–15]

To care effectively for the chronically ill in a team setting, with nurses, physician assistants, pharmacists, physical therapists, and social workers, might best be accomplished in mixed educational settings in which health care professionals and medical students learn together. Certain problems related to chronic illness are best studied in an interdisciplinary setting so that all health care professionals can learn to deal with their impact on members of the team as well as on the patient and family.

Wasting diseases such as cancer has increased 268 percent since 1900 (Glazier, 1973: 14). Furthermore, life is often prolonged by medical intervention in a hospital or nursing home, where the patient is surrounded by members of the staff rather than friends and family. Under such conditions, medical and nursing staff at times fail to support each other, let alone the patient. Quint reported that nurses and physicians used many ways of avoiding the questions of the terminally ill patient or lost interest in patients who had poor prognoses (1965: 119–32). Emerson's study of interaction on a hospital ward showed how patients were rebuffed in attempts to break through good-natured banter by nurses in order to find out about their condition (1973: 269–80). Nurses and doctors sometimes used their daily hospital routines as justifications for failing to continue conversations with concerned patients. (A more extended discussion of this subject is found in Chapter 6.)

Under certain conditions, death and dying can be made manageable for health care personnel. A study of a Dutch hospital found that nurses were able to deal directly with patient fears and anxieties when they had opportunities to express their own feelings in a supportive peer group (Casee, 1975: 224–34).

Health care personnel are better able to answer patients' questions when they are aware of patients' rights. Statements requiring informed consent on the part of patients for performance of medical and surgical procedures are manifestations of these rights. More significantly now, self-help groups formed among the terminally ill help to promote an open and dignified living space for those who are regarded as beyond medical help. For example, the organization "Make Today Count" helps cancer patients get together and talk about things that they cannot share with others (Pellman, 1976).

THE OTHER AMERICA

America is a land of social contradictions. A decade after the civil rights movement and the civil disorders of the late 1960s, the gap between a largely white middle class and a largely poor black, Puerto Rican, Mexican-American, and Native American population remain evident. Despite the rhetoric and activity of the 1960s, the median income of black families was 58 percent that of white families in 1974, an increase from the 1964 figure of only 4 percent (Burkey, 1978: 395). Even after the War on Poverty, 23 percent of all black families had incomes below the poverty line, compared with 7 percent of white families in 1974 (Burkey, 1978: 394).

Federal intervention has attempted to make food and medical services available to the poor through two major programs—the food stamp program and Medicaid. Eligible families receive a moderate amount of script in the form of stamps to purchase foods previously inaccessible because of their cost. However, many families who need it most do not take advantage of it. In some parts of the country, families do not have the cash to buy the stamps or cannot get to the offices that administer the program. Nutrition makes a difference in recovering quickly from bouts of acute infectious disease (Keusch, 1975). Physical growth disparities between poor and nonpoor children, as reflected in differences in height, have not been eliminated (Sidel and Sidel, 1978: 26).

Traditionally, utilization of physicians' services has directly correlated with income. While the Medicaid program has made physicians' services available to the poor without cost (and the number of office visits for poor persons is slightly larger on the average than for those better off), "high income persons are more likely to obtain preventive care than low income persons, particularly such patient-initiated care as routine physicals, eye examinations, Pap smear, breast examination and glaucoma tests" (Public Health Service, 1976: 19).

The effect of poverty clearly emerges in a widely used comparison of health status, the rate of infant mortality per 1,000 live births. The impact of poverty interacting with race and residence is associated with high rates of infant mortality.

> One such study, performed by the U.S. National Center for Health Statistics of infant mortality in poverty and nonpoverty areas of 19 large cities of the United States from 1969 to 1971, showed that "whites" living in poverty areas had an infant mortality rate almost 50 percent higher than that of "whites" living in nonpoverty areas, and that "blacks," while having a higher rate than the "whites" in either type of area, also have a far higher infant mortality rate in poor areas than in nonpoor areas. [Sidel and Sidel, 1978: 17]

The Sidels suggest that many of these deaths among infants are preventable, since Sweden, the country with the lowest infant mortality rate, provides a benchmark for comparison.

Poverty involves other risks for children, and in some instances it leads to a life of disability. Many preventable illnesses, such as measles, strike poor children in large numbers because the rates of immunization are low in poverty areas. Consequently, poor children are more likely to be absent from school or have other disruptions in living.

Chronic illness and disability are more frequently found among the poor than those who are better off. It is possible that two causes may be at work here: First, those who are subject to impaired health may not be as able to compete in the labor market and therefore earn less; second, life chances may produce more biological insult, resulting in more serious bouts of illness or long-term impairment. In a U.S. Public Health Service survey

> . . . people aged 17–44 with family incomes under $5000 in the early 1970s had a 30 percent higher prevalence rate of chronic conditions such as arthritis, and heart conditions, and a 50 percent higher rate of diabetes, hypertension, hearing

impairments and vision impairments than do those with incomes higher than $15,000. [Sidel and Sidel, 1978: 25]

Disability is strongly associated with absence from work, limited activity, and substantial numbers of days bedridden. In addition, mobility in this age group is more restricted among the poor (Sidel and Sidel, 1978: 25).

HEALTH NEEDS AND THE DISTRIBUTION OF SERVICES

Better nutrition and anti-biotics have been responsible for controlling acute infectious disease, thereby dramatically reducing the death rate in American society. The birthrate has also declined, mainly as the result of changing patterns of production and living. Children are simply not regarded as a form of "insurance" against the troubles of old age, an opinion often associated with traditional agricultural societies with limited economic surpluses.

Health care is also needed in modern societies to keep people at work. Services such as policing and fire fighting are provided by the state to ensure the even distribution of resources, since crime and fire can spread easily from unprotected to protected areas. Health services in many countries are operated by the government, determining their availability, the number of personnel to be trained, fees to be charged, and salaries paid. In the United States and some other countries, health services are only partially supported by government funding, with the more affluent purchasing health insurance from private companies. Disastrous and prolonged illnesses and injuries can wipe out the savings of affluent families even when they carry private health insurance.

Despite government reimbursement for services to the elderly and poor under Medicare and Medicaid and government support for research and training in medicine, the organization and delivery of health services in the United States is still subject to market conditions. Income criteria are important in determining where physicians set up practices, and an unequal distribution of physicians exists. Despite the dramatic narrowing of the gap between the poor and others, the frequency of physician visits not withstanding, inequities remain, as illustrated by the following findings:

> Residents of metropolitan areas report more physician visits per year than do nonmetropolitan residents. A greater proportion of the ambulatory physician visits among metropolitan residents are made to specialists as opposed to general practitioners.
>
> In 1974, there were 199 physicians providing patient care per 100,000 persons living in the largest metropolitan areas. The comparable ratio for small nonmetropolitan counties was 40 physicians for every 100,000. There is a direct association between the number of hospital beds available in an area, the number of physicians performing surgery, and the number of operations performed per 1000 population. [Public Health Service, 1976: 18–23]. (See Figure 7.)

One reason the health care system of the United States has been criticized is the uneven development of services, despite the great deal of money spent. The most advanced medical research in the world is done in this

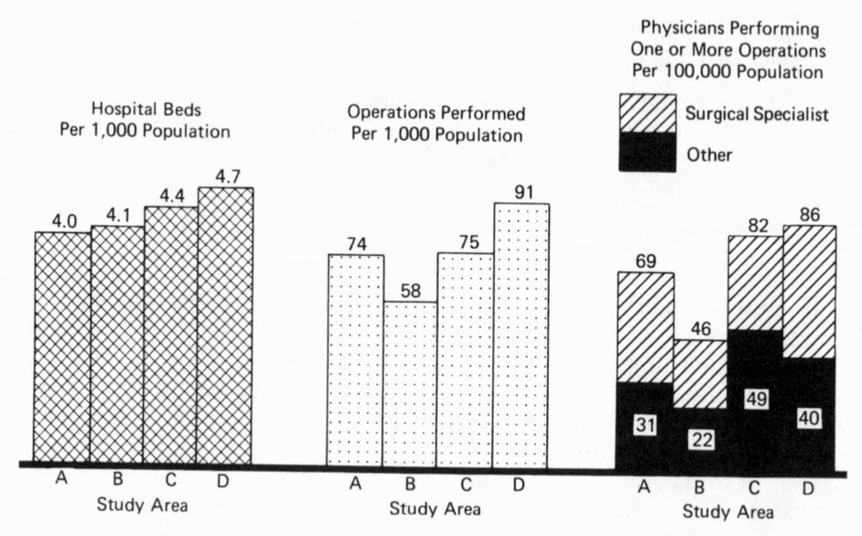

Figure 7 Hospital Beds, Operations Performed and Physicians Performing One or More Operations in Four Study Areas

country, as indicated by the number of Nobel prizes awarded to Americans. But many people have diseases that go untreated, and others are given unnecessary surgery or medication (Brody, 1976). The question remains, can Americans have both sophisticated research and minimal standards of care without the reorganization of all health services and related activities? Reorganization would still leave the technical criteria and their application to physicians and other experts. The distribution of physicians and other health care personnel would be encouraged on the basis of other than market criteria, with population concentration and regional planning used to ensure the equal access to services. A model for such a national program has been developed by Milton I. Roemer (1973), a public health planner. This program is organized by the number of people who could be served most effectively by a special health care unit and by the types of services required to meet all needs, ranging from the treatment of simple illnesses to complex procedures and serious illnesses.

A program of this kind would be most successful if it were organized for the entire nation and if resources were distributed according to population needs rather than ability to pay. Regional deployment of resources would also reduce unnecessary duplication of equipment and staff in the same region, as when hospitals and medical centers compete in order to attract "star" researchers and practitioners. Sometimes units are built and staffs assembled, and then later these resources go unused or are used rarely. Given their infrequent use, expensive diagnostic devices such as brain

Table 1 Roemer's Regionalized Network of Health Services

Type of unit	Personnel	Numbers served in region	Illnesses treated, procedures
Primary health center	Teams: internist, physician, assistants, nurse-practitioners	10,000	1. Common cold 2. Minor injury 3. Followup visits after serious illness or injury 4. Preventive services
District hospital (120–50 beds)	Teams: specialists, maternity teams using nurse–mid-wife	40,000–50,000	1. Maternity cases 2. Trauma 3. Abdominal surgery of lesser complexity 4. Cardiovascular diseases
Regional hospital (550 beds)	Full medical departments	500,000	1. Complex medical and surgical problems: e.g., chest surgery, complicated abdominal surgery, kidney dialysis, complex diagnostic workups 2. Medical research 3. Nursing and allied health training
University medical center	Academic departments	1.5 to 2.5 million	Complex and simple cases for teaching and research, funneled to Center from inside and outside of region

scanners and the newly developed body scanners are not needed at every hospital. While competition for personnel could be encouraged between different regionalized health systems, the acquisition of staff and equipment would be justified by their utilization rather than their attractiveness.

The Roemer plan does not contain extensive provisions for early intervention through screening of cases of disease in the community in locations other than primary health centers. Screening could be better accomplished at major institutions, such as schools or work establishments, where large numbers of people are concentrated. Primary prevention would also require the allocation of resources so that illnesses resulting from poor working conditions or poor health habits could be avoided altogether. Prospective studies that follow respondents over time indicate that good health practices, such as avoidance of smoking and drinking and taking regular hours for sleep, meals, and exercise, result in longer life. A California study showed that good health habits resulted in seven extra years of life for middle-aged men who were compared with others of the same social class and health status but whose health-related behavior was different (Public Health Service, 1976: 14).

Thus there is an indisputable discrepancy between the resources used for health care in the United States and the unmet needs of the population as it undergoes changes. What, then, are the implications of this assertion for the sociology of health care? To analyze how an institution operates, it is important to determine who benefits and who does not. Then it is necessary to see whether different forms of organization would produce different results. One aspect to be considered is to what extent an institution receives adequate support from the society. The level of technological development is usually related to the financial structure, for the availability of investment encourages development.

Enormous financial resources are already devoted to paying for health services in the United States, and the technological developments in the field have been nothing less than extraordinary. But there is a need to match the economic and technical resources available with a new social organization and division of labor. In the health care field, this may mean dealing with the patient's psychosocial as well as medical needs.

In America, the tasks of health care, whether broadly or narrowly conceived, have been the responsibility of the medical profession. Not only has medicine controlled the technical side of health care, but it has determined the means of payment for services. In the *fee-for-service* system, the rate is determined by the provider of care, having been given a state-sanctioned monopoly through licensing. Licensing of physicians by the state made no provision for regulating the economic transaction between the patient and doctor. The medical profession itself set the task of preventing the exploitation of illness on the part of the practitioner through the lengthy period of education and training in which certain values were to be imparted. These values were to limit the potential for the physician to turn his practice into an entrepreneurial adventure. Moreover, local medical societies were to enforce an ethical code to punish those who took advantage of the patient's lack of knowledge. In a society that supports private enterprise, state regulation of fees would probably be regarded as a restraint of trade. As a result, the medical profession was left to control the relationship with the patient in all its aspects. The justification for this arrangement was that the doctor is hired by, and works for, the patient, and that inferior doctors would be driven from the marketplace by more competent ones. Competition was based on the assumption of a far more limited demand for medical services than exists today. The constancy and magnitude of the demand, as generated by government funding and private third-party payers such as Blue Cross and Blue Shield, have created opportunities for excellent incomes and abundant work for even the most incompetent and inadequately trained physicians.

The continued increase in the demand for health care services has made medicine an extremely attractive occupation. In fact, "the present physician/population ratio of 182 per 100,000 has increased from 149 in 1950 as a result of a 64 percent increase in the number of physicians without a commensurate increase in population" (Public Health Service, 1976: 21–22). Even with such an increase, the cost of health care steadily rises rather than declines.

Clearly classical market explanations assuming that supply and demand affects price do not apply to health care under the kind of control exercised by the medical profession. While more people use physicians, the explanation for the increase in costs in the past twenty years comes from the acquisition of additional techniques of diagnosis and treatment and the consequent creation of an enormous variety of allied health-worker roles to perform these tasks. There are now more than 200 different health occupations employing 4.4 million people (Public Health Service, 1976: 21). Unlike other industries, where investment in equipment either replaces labor or lowers the unit cost of the product, thereby leading to greater profits through lowered expenses or lowered prices, health care produces increasing costs in both categories. New knowledge and techniques create new procedures and routines, even when the latter's higher costs lead to further uneven distribution of services.

The financing of health care through private third-party payers or the federal government (Medicare, Medicaid) has only helped to increase prices, since there are no incentives implemented by physicians for efficiency or limits to the patient's willingness to receive a service because it is often not paid for directly. Eventually the costs that are passed along to third-party payers come out of increased insurance premiums for policyholders, increased taxes for citizens, and fringe benefits for workers in place of further wage increases.

The availability of health care is not merely determined by its cost. The development of the current system is based on the historical emergence of medicine as the dominant profession in this field throughout modern industrial societies. Yet there are differences in the ways health care (including but not limited to the physician) is paid for in different societies. The doctor-patient relationship is socially defined according to these different arrangements. However, this relationship is also structured by how people are supposed to act when they are sick. Both views are important in understanding how society deals with matters of illness and health.

REFERENCES

Blum, R. H. 1960. *The Management of the Doctor-Patient Relationship*. New York: McGraw-Hill.

Brody, J. E. 1976. "Incompetent surgery is found not isolated." *New York Times*, January 27: 1, 24.

Burkey, Richard. 1978. *Ethnic and Racial Groups: The Dynamics of Dominance*. Menlo Park, Calif.: Cummings.

Casee, E. T. 1975. "Therapeutic behavior, hospital culture and communication." Pp. 224–34 in Caroline Cox and Adrianne Mead, eds., *A Sociology of Medical Practice*. London: Collier-MacMillan.

Ebert, Robert H. 1977. "Medical Education in the United States." *Daedalus* 106 (Winter): 171–84.

Emerson, J. 1973. "Negotiating the serious import of humor." Pp. 269–80 in Arnold Birenbaum and Edward Sagarin, eds., *People in Places: The Sociology of the Familiar*. New York: Praeger Publishers.

Glazier, W. 1973. "The task of medicine." *Scientific American* (April): 13–17.

Keusch, G. T. 1975. "Malnutrition and infection: Deadly allies." *Natural History* (November): 27–33.

Koos, Earl L. 1954. *The Health of Regionville*. New York: Columbia University Press.

Kubler-Ross, Elizabeth. 1969. *On Death and Dying*. New York: Macmillan.

Langer, W. L. 1977. "What caused the explosion?" *New York Review* 28 (April): 3–4.

Lyons. R. 1977. "Refusal of many to heed government health advice is linked to growing distrust of authority." *New York Times*, June 12: p. 55.

McKeown, Thomas. 1976. *The Modern Rise of Population*. New York: Academic Press.

Pellman, D. R. 1976. "Learning to live with dying." *New York Times Magazine*, December 5th: 44*ff*.

Public Health Service. 1976. *Forward Plan for Health: FY 1978–82*. Washington, D.C.: Department of Health, Education, and Welfare.

———. 1978. *Health United States: 1976–77*. Washington, D.C.: Department of Health, Education, and Welfare.

Quint, J. C. 1965. "Institutionalized practices of information control." *Psychiatry* 28: 119–32.

Reinhold, R. 1977. "New population trends transforming U.S." *New York Times*, February 6: 1, 42.

Roemer, M. I. 1973. "An ideal health care system for America." Pp. 77–93 in Anselm Strauss, ed., *Where Medicine Fails*. New Brunswick, N.J.: Transaction Books.

Sadusk. 1959. "Breakdown in doctor-patient relationship is shown by malpractice suits, says psychologists in C.M.M. study." *Bulletin of the American College of Surgery* 44: 137–40.

Sidel, Victor W., and Ruth Sidel. 1978. *A Healthy State: An International Perspective on the Crisis in United States Medical Care*. New York; Pantheon.

State of New York. 1976. Report of the special advisory panel on medical malpractice. Albany: State of New York.

3

Social Theories about Patient-Practitioner Relationships

Human life is group life. Individuals cannot live without the protection and support that groups provide. Group membership results in certain obligations that members owe to the collectivity. Being members of groups also helps us to impose order on the social environment.

Individuals are categorized according to their membership in particular groups or organizations and according to their positions within different groups. These positions, or statuses, are fundamental ways of giving and receiving social identities. Social categories result from recognition of the importance of such common characteristics as age, sex, occupation, or neighborhood. People can be defined as friends or enemies, potential business partners or conjugal mates, or simply as acquaintances.

Recognition of the meaning of membership and its expectations is part of being a fully competent member of society. We see ourselves as others see us. This reflexiveness makes group living possible because it allows us to participate in particular social situations. Conformity is not just a result of wanting to fit in but depends on the fit between a particular person and what is expected of a member; it is also a result of the fit between the expectations held about what characteristics a participant will have and a particular situation (Goffman, 1963: 2). These expectations about social life are acquired relatively early in life, and interaction between human beings is facilitated by these shared understandings.

Some social relationships are built on the interdependence between categories of positions. Many positions or statuses involve doing things for others. Social categories represent a division of mutually dependent activities: Teachers require students, mothers require children, and baseball managers require players. Titles are given to participants to provide clear indications of the socially assigned identities and indicate the *terms* of the relationship; that is, who is to do what, where, when, and how.

Finally, all relationships have *stages*, constituting a natural history of the association between people (Goffman, 1971: 192–93). These stages are similar to the life cycle, with a beginning, middle, and end, and movement through the stages is dependent on many factors that exist both outside the relationship and internal to it. First, in patient-practitioner relationships, a variety of conditions can influence their development. Second, as a special social unit, the expectations that are jointly held by sick people and healers will be different than those held in teacher-student, parent-child, or player-manager relationships. Many health care practitioners learn this through vocational experience that has been full of conflict. Since social relationships can affect whether sick people get well, it is necessary to examine social relationships in the study of social aspects of health care.

Theory about health care practitioner-patient relationships developed out of the sociological interest in the dynamics of modern industrial society. Two problems that emerged from the work of nineteenth-century European sociologists Emile Durkheim and Max Weber generated this interest: (1) How is social order maintained in modern society with its detailed division of labor, emphasis on efficiency, and lack of opportunity for people to feel part of something larger than their own self-interested pursuits? and (2) How does the emergence of the role of the professional in society depend on these characteristics of society? A third question related to the growth of the professions is whether applied knowledge could be a new form of power and whether the professions would seek to monopolize or share their knowledge. Control over knowledge in the production and distribution of goods and services, as well as the coordination of labor power, was a major interest of Karl Marx, who is considered to be one of the early contributors to theoretical sociology. Similar problems have been raised about the field of health care and other human services (Reader and Goss, 1959; Hughes, 1959).

This chapter will examine how different sociological theorists have considered the health care practitioner-patient relationship. While the ideas expressed here can be applied to all relationships between healers and the sick, they are derived from observations of physicians who practice medicine within the established health care system in American society. We will not consider relationships between faith healers, herbalists, or chiropractors and patients. The established health care system includes many other health care workers besides physicians, such as paramedical personnel, but they are not as directly responsible as physicians for diagnosis and treatment of patients, nor do they have as much control over their work setting. The doctor-patient relationship is the most significant point of contact in the established health care system.

TALCOTT PARSONS: THE "SICK ROLE"

One of the earliest efforts to understand the social and psychological dynamics of doctor-patient relationships was ingeniously developed by the late Talcott Parsons (1951: 428–79). Starting from the perspective that illness disrupts social life, Parsons moves to the idea that a sick person can be excused from fulfilling obligations. Any member of society can use illness as an acceptable excuse for not meeting his or her obligations. Therefore, it is necessary to regulate and validate illness claims. Hence the rise of the health care expert to determine whether a person is ill or is suffering from some psychological disturbance without an organic basis. Medicine has been assigned the responsibility by society to diagnose and treat people who are not physically ill but who are unable to perform full-time social roles.

Illness is disruptive because people are interdependent in work or family life, and members may begin to suspect the motives of another for failing to meet obligations, leading to interpersonal conflict. The sick role legitimately permits people to be excused temporarily from responsibilities, but it also tempts them to misuse it.

> The fact that the relevance of illness is not confined to the nonmotivated purely situational aspect of social action greatly increases its significance for the social system. It becomes not merely an "external" danger to be "warded off" but an integral part of the social equilibrium itself. Illness may be treated as a mode of response to social pressures, among other things, as one way of evading social responsibilities. [Parsons, 1951: 431]

An institutionalized set of procedures has emerged for dealing with this potential problem. American society, like all societies, has encouraged the development of occupational role specialists in health care. Medicine has been delegated a monopoly over this area because the knowledge required to perform these tasks must be acquired through contact with other physicians who educate and train future doctors. This solution is based upon cultural values associated with secular, rationalistic, and naturalistic understanding of illness and its treatment. This view is in opposition to the supernatural interventions found in spiritualism, Christian Science, or magic. While there are many nonscientific aspects to the doctor-patient relationship, the *grounds* for medical intervention are based on the use of empirically validated technology.

In terms of the social relationship between doctor and patient, the latter initiates the contact, but the control of the interaction almost immediately shifts to the former. The physician determines whether a person can be allowed to play the sick role before any help or treatment is provided. The diagnosis serves to legitimate or validate the illness perceived by the patient. Validation is necessary in order for a person to be able to receive an "exemption from normal social responsibilities, which of course is relative to the nature and severity of the illness." Seeking an exemption is "not only a right of the sick person but an obligation upon him" (Parsons, 1951: 436–37). People who refuse to see a doctor are regarded by others as rule violators as much as the malingerer. The sick person is usually not held accountable for his or her illness, and a refusal to seek care is suspicious to others. Even in cases of venereal disease, people are expected to seek help. A person who is sick is not only expected to see a doctor but to cooperate with him in order to get well.

Since performers of sick roles receive a great deal of attention—from professionals, friends, or family—the new problem of motivation emerges: how to make care effective without making it too comfortable. Once a person is beyond the initial stage of diagnosis, he or she might consciously or unconsciously want to continue this stage. While the physician is expected to solve the patient's problem, he must also attempt to deal with the potential residual effects of playing the sick role, such as making it prolonged or permanent, involving others in responsibility for the condition, or redefining the illness as a justification for social support. Other patients may deny the extent of their incapacities or deny that death is near, demonstrating great fear of dependency. Moreover, the patient has little knowledge by which to judge the performance of the physician.

Emotional stress is experienced by doctors as part of their work, brought about by the objective uncertainty of their knowledge and its application. The techniques validated on one population may not work on another. Medical intervention in previous cases may have been based on having seen only the most severe cases, and the course of a disease may be self-limiting, not invariably requiring treatment. Physicians are expected by others to intervene where illness exists, even when successfully proven treatment procedures do not exist.

Emotional stress may also result from intimate contact with an attractive patient or from the information received about that person's life. The opportunities to alter the relationship and make them more personal abound, and doctors as well as patients may take advantage of this for many reasons. Because of this, examining rooms are separated from offices, setting apart the specific medical purpose of undressing; physicians often have a nurse present during physical examinations; and first names are avoided. The importance of maintaining objectivity or distance is sometimes found in the unwillingness of doctors to treat members of their own family because they might overlook something in the hope of not finding the symptom of a disease.

Parsons sees the ordinary physician as being almost as involved with the feelings of patients as the psychiatrist, the one specialty in medicine that deals with emotions. That feelings play an important part in the doctor-patient relationship cannot be denied. Patients require reassurance and a clear understanding of what is wrong, and they often get another opinion when they are dissatisfied with the information or the treatment they receive. As a result, some diagnostic work is repeated unnecessarily. Despite the feelings that are likely to arise when people play the sick role, Parsons claims that built-in constraints can prevent this kind of behavior from emerging. Here the use of social categories can clearly initiate and sustain an important social relationship. Taking the sick role limits the uncertainty that patients have about their illness.

> . . . the role of being sick as an institutionalized role may be said to constitute a set of conditions necessary to enable the physician to bring his competence to bear on the situation. It is not only that the patient has a need to be helped, but that this need is institutionally categorized, that the nature and implications of this need are socially recognized, and the kind of help, the appropriate general pattern

of action in relation to the source of help, are defined. It is not only the sick person's own condition and personal reactions to what should be done about it which are involved, but he is placed in an institutionally defined framework which mobilizes others in his situation in support of the same patterns which are imputed to him, which is such an important feature of his role. The fact that others than the patient himself often define that he is sick, or sick enough for certain measures to be taken, is significant. [Parsons, 1951: 475]

The sick role may be a way that dissatisfied individuals channel their anger, particularly where group support is unavailable or where their dissatisfaction, if publicly expressed, would meet with extreme disapproval or hostility. Furthermore, by taking on the sick role, one gives up the claim that there are other causes for a person's problems, such as discrimination, injustice or political repression. When political dissent, for example, is defined as mental illness, as in the case of the Soviet Union and other countries (and even in a few instances in the United States, as with the poet Ezra Pound), then authorities do not have to take it seriously.

The sick thus become a statistical status class and are deprived of the possibility of forming a solidarity collectivity. Furthermore, to be sick is by definition to be in an undesirable state, so that it simply does not "make sense" to assert a claim that the way to deal with the frustrating aspects of the social system is "for everybody to get sick." [Parsons, 1951: 477]

Two thoughts are merged in Parsons's concept of the sick role: (1) the potential for deviance whenever the sick role is claimed, and the societal requirement that certain occupational role specialists make the decision rather than leaving it in the hands of the individual; and (2) the way in which some people are permitted or even encouraged to play the sick role, allowing members of society to engage in some deviant behavior rather than allowing more serious social conflicts.

It is extremely difficult to disprove any of these assertions. Parsons does not identify the different ways in which the sick role could be performed according to different types of illness and disease. Rather, he sees sickness as acute and temporary, when it could easily involve permanent impairment, as in the case of a handicapping condition such as polio or a pervasive developmental disability such as mental retardation.

Some illnesses affect different aspects of life more than others. A person recovering from a heart attack may be able to do some paperwork at home before he is ready to commute to work, whereas the person who suffers from arthritis may have to change jobs. A person employed as an engineer would have less difficulty returning to work wheelchair-bound compared with the construction worker. The various career contingencies of the role are ignored in Parsons' concentration on acute rather than chronic illness.

The model of illness that Parsons uses to develop his theory of the doctor-patient relationship is familiar, being similar to that used by the medical profession, as presented in Chapter 2. Based on success in treating infectious disease, illness in this scheme is shortterm, easy to diagnose, and with relatively little consequence beyond a period of confinement to a hospital bed. In addition, the emotional or nonrational aspects of the relationship are seen from the perspective of the working physician. Feelings are seen as impediments to the technical treatment of the patient and the successful performance of the temporary although deviant role of being sick. Return to full-time social roles results from following doctors' orders rather than from opportunities sought by both physician and patient to work together toward cure or amelioration.

True to this model of illness, Parsons intersects the process of becoming sick at the point of entry of the doctor. Some critics of the concept of the sick role have called attention to the ways in which the patient's informal social support system, made up of family, friends, and neighbors, can shape the performance of the patient (Gallagher, 1976: 213). Whether a patient will follow the doctor's orders depends on views held on medical practice by the groups to which patients belong, the availability at home of help with the treatment regimen, and the meaning bestowed on missing certain individual or group activities (Bloom, 1963: 33–38). The failure to conform may result from the patient's interest in maintaining a certain self-image rather than from a motivated violation of the treatment regimen. The person who leaves a hospital bed against medical advice to attend the wedding of a friend exemplifies a strong interest in maintaining other role commitments besides the sick role.

Several critics have also pointed out that focusing on the doctor-patient relationship ignores the complex social organization of health care and its division of labor and technology. These factors that are built into the health care system can have an enormous influence on treatment (Gallagher, 1976: 213), particularly where the physician's contact with the patient is mediated by a variety of paramedical personnel (Gerson, 1976: 222). Even when doctors and patients agree, the relationship exists within a context that can subvert their shared goals. "At every point in the career of the relationship between physician and patient the context of negotiation between them is constrained—often subordinated—to the larger scale organizational arrangements which surround the relationship" (Gerson, 1976: 222).

While this criticism implies that Parsons fails to see the conflict and trade-offs between doctors and patients, it does not claim that the relationship is symmetrical, with power equally shared. In his reconsideration of the sick role and the unique moral authority of the physician, Parsons reinforces his concept of the asymmetrical character of the relationship, comparing it to that between teacher and student.

> The most general basis of the superiority of health agency personnel generally, and physicians in particular, seems to me to rest in their having been endowed with special responsibilities for the health of persons defined as ill or as suffering threats to their future health, who have come under their jurisdiction, that is, who have become in some sense patients of the individual physician or of the health care organization in which he performs a role. This is to say in very general terms that the physician has been institutionally certified to be worthy of entrusting responsibility to in the field of the care of health, the prevention of illness, the mitigation of its severity and disabling consequences, and its cure insofar as it is feasible. [Parsons, 1975: 266–67]

The professional has authority by virtue of ability, knowledge, willingness to assume responsibility (i.e., "a sacred trust"), and a lifelong care commitment. Parsons sees this hierarchical difference as specific to the business at hand. However, others have noted that physicians accumulate many advantages and privileges that affect interaction with patients, demanding compliance in areas that are not directly related to health care (Ehrenreich and Ehrenreich, 1974: 26–40). The superior position doctors have in the prestige hierarchy and in earning power can often make patients feel that they are being slighted or asked to show deference above and beyond ordinary respect. Paramedical workers have often noted that doctors can slight the contributions made by others to health care. In summary, there is a tendency for the doctor to expand his authority into areas that are not always related to the main tasks of prevention, diagnosis, treatment, and the reduction of human suffering.

Parsons's major concerns are with the ways in which the adaptive and integrative capacities of society are affected by illness. In looking at society as a social system, he assumes that there is interdependence between the various parts and raises the question: What are the various ways in which social order and survival of a society occur, despite many human activities and desires that can alter and disrupt that system? Almost all unexpected behavior, then, is regarded as a threat to the social system. Many sociologists are critical of this view of nonnormative behavior because it sees any deviation, whether voluntary or involuntary, collective or individualized, as a threat to the integration of society and, conversely, any mechanisms of social control as promoting these conditions of stability. By examining health and illness in this way, one may come to the unwarranted conclusion that existing institutions have an inherent right to exist because they produce social order. Accordingly, some interpretations of Parsons suggest that advocates of change are teaching people how to destroy social order rather than to build better institutions.

DAVID MECHANIC: DISEASE AND ADAPTIVE BEHAVIOR

David Mechanic approaches the doctor-patient relationship from a social psychologic perspective, focusing on the adaptive behavior of individuals. Starting from the idea that human behavior is best understood as activity undertaken in order to control immediate environments and life situations, he examines reactions to illness in the same way (Mechanic, 1968: 2). He avoids many of the problems addressed by Parsons concerning the equilibrium of society and its adaptive and integrative tasks. However, his most recent work retains the same theoretical orientation but draws most broadly on empirical materials from epidemiology and health services delivery research (Mechanic, 1978).

Everyone must make sense out of one's position in the social environment, and those who become ill must do this more immediately. Similarly, those who provide care are also concerned with their own needs. Thus social interaction is initiated when people seek to deal with their lack of fit with the social environment.

> In short, illness behavior and reactions to the ill are aspects of a coping dialogue in which the various participants are often actively striving to meet their responsibilities, to control their environment, and to make their everyday circumstances more tolerable and predictable. [Mechanic, 1968: 2]

The sociological examination of illness and disease cannot be performed outside the context of the struggles that go on in the social environment. If a community has certain resources available, it may define illness and react to it differently than if those resources were not there. For example, before the establishment of the People's Republic of China and the development of a national public health program, the Chinese defined schistosomiasis (a terrible disease caused by a blood fluke or microscopic worm that inhabits the blood vessels of the liver and intestines) as inevitable. New definitions were possible only when resources were allocated to fight it. A massive campaign was carried out in the Chinese countryside in which the environmental supports for the blood fluke were destroyed (Horn, 1969: 94).

Human beings seek to maintain favorable definitions of themselves, derived from the reactions received from others. Therefore, any failure to maintain health will call into question the continued flow of social approval received from others. Deviance, because it can affect one's self-image, concerns all members of society, regardless of the consequences of illness to disrupt the internal order of society or its capacity to survive. Mechanic starts from the subjective aspect of social life and defines health and illness in terms of the consequences for the individual: "The concept of disease usually refers to some deviation from normal functioning which has undesirable consequences, because it produces personal discomfort or adversely affects the individual's future health status" (Mechanic, 1968: 15)

Much of health-related behavior is an effort to cope with this problem, making manageable what had been unmanageable. A person may or may not seek help from the physician. His or her methods of coping are derived from what has been learned in interaction with members of his or her social class, ethnic group, and religious congregation. Playing the sick role vis-à-vis the doctor may be the result of the failure of these informal but significant sources of help. Seeking professional advice and services may also result from the encouragement provided by these groups. In any case, "the concepts of *normality* and *deviation from normality* are implicit in both lay and medical evaluations of disease" (italics in original) (Mechanic, 1968: 28).

Starting from the assumption that the views held by the doctor and the patient will not be identical, one can anticipate that both will negotiate a great deal. Patients debate what is wrong rather than accept the sick role and adhere to the implicit rules or norms of it. Doctors attempt to work with the views held by the patient about health and illness so long as they are not harmful to the patient's future health. These assumptions suggest that the sociologist could find a negotiation process rather than a one-sided and clear-cut diagnosis.

The idea of deviation from normality becomes the starting point for looking at the social aspects of illness, including the performance of the sick role. Since there is little consensus on what criteria should be used to define normality, even in physical and certainly in behavioral or psychological states, a variety of research questions can be raised: Is there an objective standard against which all cases can be compared? What are the most frequently defined deviations from normality? How do others react to certain physical features or behaviors of the person? Mechanic does not prefer one definition of normality over the others, but he uses these differing perspectives as variables that can affect the doctor-patient relationship.

The negotiation of the diagnosis can go in many directions. Since the focus is on deviation from normality, the question still remains: How do certain behaviors or features of the person become defined as illness rather than as crime or immorality? The answer depends not only on the expressions the putative deviant presents to others but also on what motives are ascribed to the person. In other words, the behavior or characteristics are either regarded as harmful or harmless and either the person's fault or not. Usually this "deviation becomes visible to people in the community when they recognize a person's inability or reluctance to respond in a particular expected way (in terms of normative expectations)" (Mechanic, 1965: 275).

A person is defined as sick when no evil motive can be imputed or, at times, when the act is viewed as inexplicable according to the others' understanding of human behavior. A rich person arrested for shoplifting may be defined as sick, whereas the poor person will be regarded as a petty criminal. The person who is regarded as physically ill usually has visible signs of disease and is not considered responsible for it. In contrast, the person who deliberately becomes exposed to disease or engages in self-mutilation to avoid military service is not allowed to play the sick role without also being labeled as crazy, disturbed, or an evader of a moral duty.

One interesting implication of Mechanic's theorizing about the doctor-patient relationship is that it affords great opportunity to focus on the career of the sick person prior to contact with the medical profession. It is also possible to see how nonmedical definitions of health and illness are important in understanding the health and illness behavior of patients, both in seeking medical attention and in complying with doctor's orders.

Mechanic could go further in his thinking about the negotiated character of the doctor-patient relationship, allowing us to view the patient and the practitioner as engaged not only in a struggle for the maintenance of favorable definitions of self but also control over the definition of the situation. How the authority of the physician is maintained, modified, or dissolved in face-to-face interaction with patients is an important unanswered question. Similarly, Mechanic does not deal with the theoretically important issue of how medicine became the dominant profession in health care, and whether it is possible for other health care practitioners to gain a greater share of power and control over their own work.

ELIOT FREIDSON: PROFESSIONAL CONTROL

Sociologists have long been interested in the growth of the professions in modern society, but few sociologists have focused on the social organization of professions as much as Eliot Freidson. He finds that control over one's work situation through a monopoly over that practice is the central characteristic of professions. Therefore, this advantage in social power may be just as important to a profession as having a unique and effective set of techniques to help others. The possibility is considered that control may be acquired prior to recognition of techniques.

Freidson's interest in doctoring is in the nontechnical aspects of medical work, consisting of interpersonal and organizational situations. Strategies are always developed in institutional contexts. Mechanic starts with patients and their problems, whereas Freidson begins with the situation of medical workers and their work.

The approach that Freidson adopts is one developed in the sociology of work, mainly by his teacher E. C. Hughes. Workers of any type always try to gain control over their work, including not only the immediate environment but the acquisition, dissemination, and application of knowledge (Freidson, 1970a: 97). This assumption is useful in generating questions about the doctor-patient relationship. The medical profession not only determines *who* is sick but what physiological characteristics constitute a disease. Medicine is a comprehensive institutionalization of the role of the healer in confirming the right of the patient to not meet full-time role obligations. Moreover, social action is generated on the basis of this social process.

> Only among human animals is there language and meaning. In human society, naming something an illness has consequences independent of the biological state of the organism. Consider two men in different societies, both with the same debilitating infection: in one case, the man is said to be ill, put to bed, and taken care of by others; in the other case, he is said to be lazy, and he is abused by others. The course and outcome of the disease may be the same biologically in both cases, but the social interplay between the sick man and others is significantly different. [Freidson, 1970b: 209]

Sociologists study the irrational and the rational aspects of the doctor-patient relationship. What human beings believe about others and themselves is important information, whether the illness in question has a biological or physical origin, or whether the techniques for identification and treatment are perfected. Freidson, along with Parsons and Mechanic, accepts the view that illness is a form of social deviance, but he focuses on the constructed character of sickness. The deviance from normality is "*thought* to have a biophysical cause and to require biophysical treatment" (italics in original) (1970b: 212). Yet even if a biophysical cause can be determined and a course of treatment specified, the character of social life makes for certain predictable responses according to what people believe about the disease, themselves, and others. These responses may vary according to the age of the sick person, the disruption of family life and aspirations, the visibility of the illness, its permanency, and so forth. Therefore, the study of deviance requires examination of the official and unofficial reactions to deviance as well as the person so labeled (Freidson, 1970b: 216).

Freidson categorizes illness according to various social implications, but he makes it clear that these classifications are not absolute, since shared meanings change. The most important feature of his classification scheme is that it enables one to see how the definition of the sick person is socially influenced.

Two considerations will help to determine the societal reaction to deviance: "(1) the imputation of responsibility to the person being labeled (with all that responsibility implies for imputed motivation), and (2) the degree of seriousness imputed to his offense (with all that implies for adopting a new role)" (1970b: 230). The person who acquires the sick role will generally be regarded as not being responsible. In other words, it is involuntary deviance, as analyzed by Erving Goffman in his book on the management of spoiled identity, *Stigma* (1963).

The stigmatized person is regarded as different from others in an undesirable way. This differentness is disruptive of ordinary social interaction for several reasons. First, conventional interaction may be affected from the initial uncertainty as to what a disabled person will demand from others. If there is a crippled man at a party, will a woman invite him to dance, hoping to compensate for his "natural" shyness? Second, disability is rarely acquired in a conscious way, so the normal person is still interacting with an intellectually competent person in most instances. Moreover, since the disability was unintentionally acquired, the normal person cannot hold the stigmatized person accountable. Third, the question of how the handicapped regard his or her situation and how others perceive his or her adaptations to it produces further uncertainty. Does the normal person see the handicapped individual as psychically scarred? Can the normal person still take for granted those beliefs once held in common with the now handicapped one? Will the disabled person think that the normal person regards him or her as being a different personality because of the disability?

Becoming stigmatized assigns a special burden to the person as a result of exclusion from opportunities to perform competently as an ordinary member of society. Freidson now conceives of the sick role as involving three kinds of legitimacy, making the person performing the role more or less acceptable to others.

> (1) *conditional legitimacy,* the deviant being temporarily exempted from normal obligations and gaining some extra privileges on the condition that he seeks the help necessary to rid himself of his deviance; (2) *unconditional legitimacy,* the deviant being exempted permanently from normal obligations and obtaining additional privileges in view of the hopeless character imputed to his deviance; and (3) *illegitimacy,* the deviant being exempted from some normal obligations by virtue of deviance for which he is not technically responsible but gaining few if any privileges and taking on some especially handicapping new obligations. [italics in original] [1970b: 236]

The type of legitimacy variable is crossclassified by Freidson according to the degree of seriousness to create six possible ways of performing the sick role. Table 2 describes these outcomes. The scheme is useful because it encompasses the entire social construction of illness, making it possible to show how redefinitions can move a minor, conditionally legitimate illness such as a "cold" to a more serious and even handicapping condition. Presenting the stages of illness sequentially increases our power to explain

Table 2 Types of Deviance for Which the Individual is Not Held Responsible, by Imputed Legitimacy and Seriousness (Contemporary American Middle-Class Societal Reaction)

Imputed seriousness	Illegitimate (stigmatized)	Conditionally legitimate	Unconditionally legitimate
Minor deviation	Cell 1. "Stammer" Partial suspension of some ordinary obligations; few or no new privileges; adoption of a few new obligations.	Cell 2. "A Cold" Temporary suspension of few ordinary obligations; temporary enhancement of ordinary privileges. Obligation to get well.	Cell 3. "Pockmarks" No special change in obligations or privileges.
Serious deviation	Cell 4. "Epilepsy" Suspension of some ordinary obligations; adoption of new obligations; few or no new privileges.	Cell 5. "Pneumonia" Temporary release from ordinary obligations; addition to ordinary privileges. Obligation to cooperate and seek help in treatment.	Cell 6. "Cancer" Permanent suspension of many ordinary obligations; marked addition to privileges.

Source: Eliot Freidson, *The Profession of Medicine: A Study of the Sociology of Applied Knowledge*, p. 239.

how the agencies of control react to this type of biophysically imputed deviance. The foundation of this reaction will be located in the beliefs about the patient and constraints that exist in the health care professions.

Freidson carefully builds a case for the social construction of illness by citing instances of overdiagnosis and overprescribing by physicians in a number of controlled studies. These findings demonstrate that the expectations for physicians to locate illness are built into the doctor-patient relationship, producing pressures to identify illness, give patients relief from symptoms and uncertainty, and maintain one's practice (and the accustomed rate of remuneration). In a field study of a prepaid group practice, Freidson claims that medicine has a bias toward defining a phenomenon as illness, with great contempt shown for colleagues who fail to treat the more serious of suspected ailments (1975: 131).

The care provided by the physician reinforces the hopes of patients that something can be done for their maladies. Faith can effect the patient beneficially, quite independent of a particular therapy. Freidson cites several studies by Arthur K. Shapiro on the placebo effect in medicine, evidence of the intersubjective nature of clinical practice: "The practicing physician is likely to believe in the therapy he uses; in believing, he influences the patient to respond favorably and influences himself to see improvement if not cure" (1970b: 268–69).

The applied knowledge of medicine is often based on the unsystematically collected information available to practitioners. What doctors know about a disease is often the result of how ordinary people interpret their condition. The actual incidence and manifestation of illness depends strongly on the variety of cases seen, a result of the layman's conception of illness, and whether it warrants medical attention. It is reasonable to expect that these conceptions of illness are patterned according to ethnic differences in the interpretations of symptoms and how they are presented to physicians. The routes by which people become patients can vary by the degree of overlap with the professional forms for defining illness and the linkages that exist within the lay referral system. In some instances, the person who has some discomfort or other symptoms will deal with them without medical intervention, and in others, he or she will be "led or pushed down the path toward special management, and it becomes organized into a special role" (1970b: 300).

Becoming a patient is only the beginning of contact with the health care system. The patient is transformed into what Goffman calls "a serviceable object" (1961: 379). Work roles in hospitals or medical group practices are coordinated and organized into specific time and space frameworks. The need to maintain schedules for staff requires that patients be treated at the pace set by the health care team. Therefore, a number of nonmedical but supposedly necessary administrative considerations may enter into the treatment process. The use of forceps and anesthesia in childbirth, for example, may result from tight scheduling of delivery room time rather than being medically indicated. Such practices speed up the delivery of babies even when there are some risks to the infant and mother.

One interesting feature of Freidson's theorizing on the doctor-patient relationship is that he does not assume that there is agreement between the perspective and interests of patients and physicians; nor does he assume unalterable conflict between these two groups. This question remains open to observation: "interaction in treatment should be seen as a kind of negotiation as well as a kind of conflict" (1970b: 322). The medical profession applies knowledge to produce a successful outcome. In doing so, doctors attempt to shape the patients' behaviors and perspectives.

Different types of illness and different types of patients also influence the relationship between doctor and patient, making for a sharing of power. Building on the work of Szasz and Hollander (1956), but also noting their limitations, Freidson shows that a variety of relationships are possible for the performers of the two roles. These range from activity-passivity, as in the case of a person in a coma or undergoing surgery, to one of mutual participation, where the patient can and does communicate. In turn, the physician attempts to persuade or convince the patient in the latter case rather than acting directly or providing guidance.

Freidson retains the concept of deviance as essential in any analysis of the doctor-patient relationship. Yet, unlike Parsons, he avoids the psychological and affective consequences of illness. He also focuses more than either Parsons or Mechanic on the application of knowledge as a social process that encourages conformity. Freidson imputes rationality to the patient: the person knows that applied knowledge is good, so there is no need to argue or express doubt. He avoids questions related to the politics of health care, involving the allocation of scarce resources used by both role partners. Quite apart from the obvious—that patients are concerned about what is happening to their bodies and doctors are simply doing a job—there are more complex contradictions built into the relationship (Gerson, 1976).

Understanding these paradoxical features of the doctor-patient relationship requires an assumption that people grow from their efforts to adapt to their environment when fair exchanges occur. In the doctor-patient exchange, the physician gains remuneration for his services as well as prestige if treatment is successful, while the patients gain or lose their health. The patient is restored, but he or she cannot grow intellectually from the experience, except in the case of mutual participation. (Psychoanalysis as an intellectual endeavor rather than as treatment may be an exception to this statement.) While this outcome may not be perceived as alienating or frustrating by the patient, it is a built-in limit to personal growth through the doctor-patient exchange. Merton and Barber note there is also resentment toward professionals who "live off" other people's troubles.

> Yet the interests built into the professional role have a dual character: they require him to give the best possible service to his clients, to remove or ameliorate their troubles so far as he can, and at the same time the continuing problems of clients provide him with his livelihood. [1976: 27]

While Freidson acknowledges the accumulated advantages that doctors have in their relationship with patients, he rarely addresses questions concerning the accumulated resentments and frustrations incurred by patients. This relationship can be seen from the point of view of acutely aware patients, conscious of their powerlessness and lack of involvement in their own care.

WAITZKIN AND WATERMAN: EXPLOITATION AND ILLNESS

Howard B. Waitzkin and Barbara Waterman provide the most direct critique of health care in American society. Starting from a socialist perspective on society and health care, they view the treatment received by patients as affected by the context of monopoly capitalism. The patient's health status depends on the amount of care he or she can purchase, the profits expected and realized by those who control the health care delivery system, and the information control systems implemented by the medical profession to keep patients from learning how to take care of themselves or make informed decisions about treatment.

The analysis of the exploitation of illness in capitalist society begins by asking whether a humane health care system basically in the hands of private enterprise is possible. The major interest presented in the study of health care as an institution is to see how it encourages the society to reproduce itself according to its own image. The health care system is similar to the educational system in that it provides support services for the economy by ensuring an adequate labor force. On a political level, allowing people to play the sick role fosters social stabilization, and providing unequal care for the rich and the poor motivates people to protect what they have. Those who are allowed to play the sick role on a more or less permanent basis are a potential human resource, providing cheap labor when needed. In addition, there are direct economic consequences of producing illness in the form of stable profits for drug companies and the other producers of technology used in diagnosis and treatment (1974: 34).

Waitzkin and Waterman look for evidence of social conflict that can lead to social change as well as examining how the adoption of the sick role can redirect dissent into socially acceptable forms. The recent activities of the physically handicapped in fighting against discrimination in employment and housing can be accounted for by the development of a number of factors that bring them into closer contact with each other, permit them greater mobility, and increase their willingness to take risks.

Unlike other theorists, Waitzkin and Waterman do not conceive of the sick role as potentially disruptive to social relationships. They see the sick role as a societally preferred option for the dissenters or oppressed, which prevents the politically active and collectively oriented voluntary deviants from changing their position in relation to other groups. Therefore, according to Waitzkin and Waterman, deviance does not arise from the sick role in the social construction of illness, as Freidson would have it, but *precedes* its adoption by the person. The sick role becomes a thing in itself, a seductive trap for those who might use their anger for social change: "The sick role provides a controllable form of deviance which mitigates potentially disruptive conflicts between personality needs and the social system's role demands" (1974: 38).

The analysis would be more effective if Waitzkin and Waterman asked questions about the consequences of the availability of the sick role, formulating a situation where this option was unavailable. In other words, what would happen if the sick role were not a viable role? Alternatively, what would happen if unrestricted access to the sick role existed and physicians and other health care workers left it up to the individual? Instead, they focus on the interchange between personality needs and social system requirements.

> When conflict arises between personality needs and role demands, the sick role provides one mechanism by which this conflict can be resolved. The sick role allows the individual to deviate from normal role demands and, by the attention and nurturance one is likely to receive, to satisfy certain personality needs. These outcomes represent secondary gain *to the individual.* While the sick role allows a limited degree of deviance, however, it is a form of deviance which can be carefully controlled without major social disruption. By providing a controllable,

> nondisruptive mode of deviance when conflicts arise between personality needs and role demands, the sick role helps preserve social stability and thus offers secondary gain *to the social system* [italics in original]. [1974: 41]

Waitzkin and Waterman support these assertions by extensive references to the manipulation of the sick role among welfare recipients in order to get extra benefits, in mental hospitals, totalitarian states, prisons, military service, and draft deferments. Many of the cases cited are of people living under a great deal of surveillance by authorities and peers. The adoption of the sick role may be a way to avoid direct social conflict between opposing groups, but it also may be a way to carry on that conflict. Under conditions of close supervision, where freedom of movement is restricted, feigning illness or lining up for sick call is one way to communicate with others to form a political alliance or strike a bargain. Being sick is a way of protecting one's ego when the surroundings become too close. In Goffman's world of staff and inmates, it is a way of surviving through working the system (1961: 173–320). It is also a way to create privacy. To be alone or to be away from familiar surroundings may be difficult. Considering all these possibilities, playing the sick role encourages voluntary, active political dissent and potential institutional change in tight quarters, permits a respite from institutionalization, and allows the person a sense of limited control. Thus the struggle for human dignity may be carried on when a dominant group has an overwhelming monopoly of power.

In less supervised settings, the acquisition of the sick role also permits greater contact with others who are similarly situated, and this may encourage new cultural and political formations. Many of the voluntary associations of parents of the handicapped or among the physically disabled themselves started this way. Group support often requires admitting that one is different.

Playing the sick role also helps to restore belief in society's rules. In many instances, people contract diseases despite their careful conformity to the current rules for maintaining health. Receiving health care services helps to restore belief in the rules by interpreting this divergence from normality.

Finally, Waitzkin and Waterman can be criticized for exploring extreme situations, such as the armed forces, prisons, and mental institutions. They avoid the experiences that are closer to the daily interactions of patients and physicians. The various struggles to get help, to participate in one's own care, and to make choices among various medical procedures can be found at this point. In particular, the chronically ill and their families understand the full range of suffering that goes beyond the pain of illness. Patients can be treated abruptly when they have justifiable complaints about their care, a fine but less extreme location for the collection of data on the exploitation of illness.

In their discussion of the restrictions on medical information and communication, Waitzkin and Waterman note significant effects. Patients become both more docile and more irritated in their relationship with providers of health services: "The physician's ability to control and manipulate information creates a basic asymmetry in the doctor-patient relationship. Professional dominance is grounded in a stratified distribution of technical knowledge" (1974: 75).

The physician's domination is partially based on keeping the patient ignorant of the progress and procedures used in his or her care, and this prevents the patient from attempting to make any independent assessment. There are several reasons for this practice, including the lack of desire to be bearers of bad news, their own unwillingness to admit uncertainty, the use of the patient's uncertainty to gain cooperation, and the medical mystique surrounding the physician's special area of competence and knowledge. Patients, it is assumed, will not understand, and if they did, they would be powerless to aid themselves. Ironically, Waitzkin and Waterman review several recent studies that show that making information available to patients encourages compliance, since many of the anxiety-provoking consequences of uncertainty are eliminated (1974: 80).

What is missing from this discussion on restricted communication are the efforts engaged in by patients, both overtly and covertly, to acquire information from health care practitioners or glean it from observing what procedures are being performed. To simply say that patients are subject to restricted communication does not reveal that they want more information, nor does it examine the satisfactions they may receive from having enough information. Their lack of control over the technical processes of health care and information about what can be done for them does not make them feel less needy or less angry. It is possible to locate these feelings more directly than simply being passive in the presence of physicians.

The social theories of patient-practitioner relationships show how the behavior of each role partner can influence the prevention or treatment of disease. If a person's health status can be influenced by the underlying structure of social behavior, then it follows that the responsibilities of health care experts also extend to monitoring their own behavior. Their activities involve direct contact with patients and, indirectly, to maintaining medical standards. However, the lay person may or may not benefit from the contact, and the expert may or may not act in accordance with professional ethics. The doctor-patient relationship is influenced by a variety of factors related to the social organization of medicine and its financial structure, rather than by concerns for the patient. Consequently, the capacity of a profession to engage in self-regulation and peer review is often more of a myth than a reality.

Unlike the merchant and customer, where each one is out to protect his interest, doctors are supposed to act in the public interest. The general impression today is that they have neglected this aspect of their task.

The mandate for self-regulation was given to medicine in the first quarter of the twentieth century, following a campaign to restrict unlicensed practice. Since then, the profession has become the dominant one in health care, providing almost all of the experts and major decision makers. The basis for this control results from perfecting certain dramatic technological advances, the modern emphasis on self-development, and the use of information and procedures created by various specialists. These factors help to account for the preeminence of medicine, but they also generate, paradoxically, further developments that call into question the central role of the physician.

REFERENCES

Ehrenreich J., and B. Ehrenreich. 1974. "Health care and social control." *Social Policy* (May/June): 26–40.

Freidson, Eliot. 1970a. *Professional Dominance: The Social Structure of Medical Care.* New York: Atherton Press.

———. 1970b. *The Profession of Medicine: A Study of the Sociology of Applied Knowledge.* New York: Dodd, Mead.

———. 1975. *Doctoring Together: A Study of Professional Social Control.* New York: Elsevier.

Gallagher, E. B. 1976. "Lines of reconstruction and extension in the Parsonian Sociology of illness." *Social Science and Medicine* 10 (May): 207–18.

Gerson, E. M. 1976. "The social character of illness: Deviance or politics?" *Social Science and Medicine* 10 (May): 219–24.

Goffman, Erving. 1961. "The underlife of public institution: A study of ways of making out in a mental hospital." Pp. 173–320 in *Asylums: Essays on the Social Situation of Mental Patients and Other Inmates.* Garden City, N.Y.: Anchor Books.

———. 1963. *Stigma: Notes on the Management of Spoiled Identities.* Englewood Cliffs, N.J.: Prentice-Hall.

———. 1971. *Relations in Public: Micro Studies in the Public Order.* New York: Basic Books.

Horn, Joshua. 1969. *Away With All Pests! An English Surgeon in People's China: 1954–1969.* New York: Monthly Review Press.

Hughes, E. C. 1959. "The study of occupations." Pp. 442–58 in Robert K. Merton, Leonard Broom, and Leonard S. Cottrell, Jr., eds., *Sociology Today: Problems and Prospects.* New York: Basic Books.

Mechanic, David. 1968, *Medical Sociology: A Selective View.* First ed. New York: The Free Press.

———. 1978. *Medical Sociology: A Comprehensive Text.* Second ed. New York: The Free Press.

Merton, R. K., and E. Barber, 1976. "Sociological ambivalence." Pp. 3–31 in Robert K. Merton, ed., *Sociological Ambivalence and Other Essays.* New York: The Free Press.

Parsons, Talcott. 1951. *The Social System.* Glencoe, Ill.: The Free Press.

———. 1975. "The sick role and the role of the physician reconsidered." *Milbank Memorial Find Quarterly* (Summer): 257–77.

Reader, G. G., and M. E. W. Goss. 1959. "The sociology of medicine." Pp. 229–46 in Robert K. Merton, Leonard Broom, and Leonard S. Cottrell, Jr., eds., *Sociology Today: Problems and Prospects.* New York: Basic Books.

Szasz, T. S., and M. H. Hollander. 1956. "A contribution to the philosophy of medicine." *American Medical Association Archives of Internal Medicine* 97: 585–92.

Waitzkin, Howard B., and Barbara Waterman. 1974. *The Exploitation of Illness in Capitalist Society.* Indianapolis: Bobbs-Merrill, Studies in Sociology.

Part Two

THE SOCIAL STRUCTURE OF HEALTH SERVICES

4

The Profession of Medicine

Increasingly in modern society, necessary tasks are accomplished through the use of experts who give advice and expect that advice to be followed. Relationships with experts are based on the belief in the efficacy of the provider's technology. Moreover, this technology is not a well-kept private secret but is shared by those with similar social identities (Larson, 1977: 14–15).

Only in this century has the medical profession emerged as the socially defined repository of expertise necessary for prevention, treatment, and amelioration of disease and illness. The current organization and delivery of health and medical care in the United States and elsewhere developed over a long period of small and sudden changes, reflecting developments in society generally and in science and technology specifically. The institutional development of medicine and knowledge of disease is a tale of theoretical and practical advances in environmental control based on close observation and reasoned hypothesizing. In addition, the elimination of famines from some parts of the world, mainly where industrialization advanced most rapidly in the nineteenth century, made people more capable of withstanding infection. Medicine became more effective as a service when it had access to this secret ally—good nutrition. And so, ironically, treatments became the central foci of health care, even when preventive measures made it possible (McKeown, 1965).

The forms of organization and delivery of health care reveal the built-in limitations to the use of resources. Human needs are usually met through some institutionalized procedure, making it possible not only for people to stay alive but to feel secure or learn how to perform necessary tasks. When resources are allocated according to one set of priorities, other priorities may not be met. Priorities are based on having control over how others define their rights and responsibilities, a capacity to get others to do things independent of whether or not they want to (Weber II, 1968: 926). Power, then, involves definitions of social reality as well as sheer coercion or intimidation (Weber, III 1968: 941–52).

In some societies, healing is performed by practitioners of magic, designated religious personnel, and the scientifically based expert. What distinguishes the magician from the scientifically based expert has more to do with the way the role of the expert is conceived by others and tied into a special enterprise set apart from other human endeavors. In modern secular societies, the scientific expert usually has society's approval. The expert is regarded as part of an established and organized procedure for taking care of problems. In other words, the expert is part of a recognized field with predictable patterns of use.

In health care, these patterns are widely believed to be appropriate ways of dealing with illness and accident. When a person says, "I'm not feeling well," another person will often automatically say, "Why don't you see a doctor?" Where there is societal approval for a way of dealing with a problem, the way becomes institutionalized and legitimated, with most people believing in the skills of the practitioners and the duty of those with problems to seek their help.

An institution is defined as an organized way of providing some important service. Once the legitimacy of an institution is established as the primary provider of important services, as in matters of life and death, criminality, or safety, it can control those who will be allowed to perform these tasks. In contemporary society, the professions have gained control over their work environment and the requirements of entry into their fields; they have established ways of categorizing the problematic aspects of daily life and routine procedures for dealing with them. The professions have convinced society at large that they are capable of coping with the uncertainties of living. In an industrial society, which is based on a highly refined division of labor, they perform many coordinating and social control activities by determining such questions as who is capable of working, who may own what property, the contractual obligations between consumers and suppliers or between management and labor, and how to build transportation networks or edifices that permit safe and easy access (Hughes, 1967: 1–14).

The expert in contemporary society seeks to apply knowledge, not merely to understand the ways of the natural and social world. The role of the expert is made up of expectations about the way individuals with special social identifications (doctors, lawyers, engineers, clergy) will probably act in specific situations and in contact with others who also have some special social identification (patients, clients, parishioners). But there are also expectations held about what should be the proper beliefs and attitudes expressed by experts. Thus society expects that specific manners of expression will go along with the specific procedures performed by the expert. We might expect that lawyers be aggressive, doctors thorough, engineers precise, and clergy moral.

Social interaction would be unmanageable if it were not guided by role expectations. Social life becomes more predictable as a result of the development of shared situational expectations among individuals with special social identifications. These exchanges link performers, so roles can be discussed as a unit of social interdependency. The idea that the expert needs a client does not imply that the relationship is equal. Nor does this mean that because the client needs an expert, the relationship bestows greater prestige, power, or privilege on the giver of advice or performer of procedures. That experts acquire these properties may be a result of the justifications created to legitimate the relationship rather than a result of something within the relationship itself (Birenbaum, 1978).

Roles are often paired so that members of society not only hold these expectations about others but also can develop them about themselves, capable of playing reciprocal roles even prior to experience. Thus, for example, physicians will act in a special way in the presence of others seeking care. In general, trust is extended to physicians when the request is made that a patient undress in order to be examined, while a similar request made by a lawyer to a client would be regarded as out of order. In following any course of action, such as seeking health care or legal counsel, we generally take into account the particular social position of others and the situational context.

What are the components of an expert's role? All roles have an instrumental side, oriented to getting certain things done, and an expressive side, representing the needs and preferences of collective life. Instrumental activities are means to achieving ends, while expressive activities are ends in themselves. Also an activity may be both instrumental and expressive at the same time. As ideas, these ways of looking at roles are useful because they help to identify tensions that are built into successful and competent performance.

Physicians may be resented by patients not because of the quality of their work but because such experts live off the existence of others' problems (Merton and Barber, 1976). The more the service provider focuses on dealing with the troubles of patients, rather than preventing or preparing the patient to avoid trouble, the more resentment can exist. Patients also express dissatisfaction with the health care expert when unexpected illnesses are uncovered, or, alternatively, when the patient suspects that he is ill and either nothing is discovered or no treatment is provided. Finally, any long-term service-receiving relationship is resented by both giver and receiver, since no resolution of the problem appears in sight. This would be particularly true for the chronically ill and disabled, or for people who have entered long-term psychotherapy. Sometimes it appears to both parties that the relationship has become an end in itself.

The role of the expert, then, is made up of expectations. In the case of the physician, cure, prevention, and easing the burden of injury or disease can be seen as activities prized by society. The pursuit of these goals is respected by most members of the society even when the ways of accomplishing them are criticized. Reaching these goals requires the development of means or procedures, usually in the form of applying knowledge. The range of available procedures constitutes *technology*, making treatment available or potentially available. Technology in this context consists not only of what is in use, but what could be used, a distinction that raises questions about why certain practices are not introduced and others are maintained. Finally, the application of knowledge requires that it become standardized into *techniques* so that any performer of the role will possess a minimal level of competency and be able to accomplish the major tasks of health care (Perrow, 1965).

The medical expert became recognized as an important provider of support services in a society where labor's availability was becoming increasingly important. When production on farms or in factories was based on a goal of selling in a remote market place and where transportation was needed for long-distance shipping, efficiency became important. Moreover, breaking down the work process into detailed and specialized labor also meant that later stages in production could not be accomplished unless earlier tasks were completed. Under these conditions, having the worker away from his or her job, or, for that matter, the entrepreneur away from his or her place of business, was a liability. The division of labor, specialization, and the commercial way of life became recognized as an end in itself (Ure, 1861). By the late eighteenth century, belief in the rightness of these ways of organizing production and distribution was so strong that Benjamin Franklin could say in *Poor Richard's Almanac:*

> Remember, that *time* is money. He that can earn ten shillings a day by his labour, and goes abroad, or sits idle, one half of that day, though he spends but sixpence during his diversion or idleness, ought not to reckon *that* the only expense; he has really spent or rather thrown away, five shillings besides. [As quoted by Max Weber, *The Protestant Ethic and the Spirit of Capitalism,* 1958: 48.]

During the early period of industrial capitalist development, the physician was more effective in the area of public health than in diagnosis and treatment. The growth of industries and the commercialization of agriculture brought about substantial changes in living patterns. Even prior to this increase in factory work, the cities of Western Europe began to grow as new opportunities in trade appeared. Since city dwellers could not raise their own food, new agricultural techniques were introduced and the available arable land was used to meet these demands. As a result, people were often driven off their small plots by fraud, force, or hunger, and they began to roam the countryside looking for work or were pushed and pulled toward the factories. Laws prevented people from resettling in the country without means of support, and many were driven elsewhere to look for employment and/or subsistence from churches and the state-sponsored poorhouses. Some found themselves living in abject poverty, conditions that breed disease and dispair (Moore, 1966).

Many of the poor from the countryside found themselves working for low wages in the cities and living in overcrowded housing without adequate light and means of sanitation. Critical to their health was an adequate supply of food, a decent means of sanitation, and a pure supply of water. Some diseases were the direct result of inadequate diets, deficient in protein or vitamins. These deficiencies further weakened the poor, so they could not resist infections.

Some supporters of the new system of production argued that poverty was the only way to get people to work (and hence justified low wages), but it also provided the perfect environment for the spread of disease. Public health measures in Europe and the United States came about as a result of fear of contagion, since the propertied class could not remain completely apart from the poor.

> By the mid-nineteenth century, it was recognized that epidemic diseases were promoted by social conditions, especially poverty and crowding, but that wealthy were not immune to them. These "egalitarian" diseases stimulated interest in disease control; it was recognized that prevention was possible through isolation (quarantine) and sanitation and not only through the ministrations of physicians and surgeons. [Greifinger and Sidel, 1976: 10]

Efforts to improve sanitation and the water supply often meant making sure that sewage did not contaminate water used for drinking, cooking, or even washing. Water was free in the country, but in the city the poor had to buy it. Henry Mayhew, an important English social critic in the nineteenth century, reported that the London poor often took their water from the ditches that ran alongside their tenements. In the midst of a cholera epidemic, which left 13,000 dead in London and 20,000 in the rest of England, Mayhew ventured forth on his famous walk through the "morbid districts and deadly cantons" of the capital of world trade in the most advanced industrial nation, the very center of national pride and power:

> We then journeyed on to London-street, down which the tidal ditch continues its course. In No. 1 of this street the cholera first appeared seventeen years ago, and spread up it with fearful virulence; but this year it appeared at the opposite end, and ran down it with like severity. As we passed along the reeking banks of the sewer the sun shown upon a narrow slip of the water. In the bright light it appeared the colour of strong green tea, and positively looked as solid as black marble in the shadow—indeed it was more like watery mud than muddy water; and yet we were assured this was the only water the wretched inhabitants had to drink. As we gazed in horror at it, we saw drains and sewers emptying their filthy contents into it; we saw a whole tier of doorless privies in the open road, common to men and women, built over it; we heard bucket after bucket of filth splash into it, and the limbs of the vagrant boys bathing in it seemed by pure force of contrast, white as Parian Marble. . . .
>
> In this wretched place we were taken to a house where an infant lay dead of the cholera. We asked if they *really did* drink the water? The answer was, "They were obliged to drink the ditch, without they could beg a pailful or thieve a pailful of water." But have you spoken to your landlord about having it laid on for you? "Yes, sir; and he says he will do it, and do it, but we know him better than to believe him." [As quoted by Eileen Yeo and Edward P. Thompson, *The Unknown Mayhew*, New York: Schocken, 1971: 21, first printed in the *Morning Chronicle*, September 24, 1849, and later reprinted in Viscount Ingestre, ed., *Meliora* (1852)]

THE DOCTOR: EXPERT AND RESPECTED FIGURE

In the late nineteenth century, public health measures were instituted in cities. Sewers were closed and relatively pure drinking water was provided.

The greater availability of food to the work force also enabled individuals to resist infection. The difficulties in getting healthy recruits or conscripts for the Crimean War convinced the lawmakers in England to limit the working day for women and children. While government leaders recognized human resources as something to be protected, union leaders saw a special value in the movement to shorten the working day so that more time could be found to organize and to engage in self-improvement. The very struggle toward shorter hours gave workers a tremendous sense of self-respect (Thompson, 1963: 340).

At the same time, major discoveries in biology enabled physicians to learn more about diseases and to discover ways of preventing and treating them. As a result, the general population became convinced that medicine could cure people in large numbers. New knowledge became widely distributed among *all* who practiced medicine, a far cry from the time when only a few "wizards" were recognized.

The knowledge derived from the germ theory of disease in the nineteenth century. When Pasteur was able to immunize sheep in the fields of France against the deadly anthrax disease, he made believers out of many who were skeptical of his claims. The immunized sheep rose to the shepherds' call, while the nonimmunized died. Even more dramatic was his success in isolating the virus that produced rabies in dogs and hydrophobia in humans. In 1885, Pasteur saved the life of a child who had been bitten by an infected dog by inoculating him with a weakened form of the virus (de Kruif, 1926). The applicability of the germ theory reduced the dangers of certain death to a mortality rate of less than one percent.

Lord Lister, the great English physician, revolutionized surgery by applying Pasteur's discoveries in sterilizing instruments and operating rooms with carbolic acids. The prevention of infection in surgery increased the recovery rates enormously. The technical application of the germ theory was further enhanced by the invention and utilization of ether as an anesthetic. Now surgery could be more easily taught, with more time available to impart knowledge to others (Shyrock, 1936).

The invention of the X-ray machine in 1895 made it possible for the physician not only to diagnose more precisely but also to check up on the healing process and evaluate procedures. Applied knowledge grew dramatically, and a scientific literature was developed and made available to all physicians and their students. More important, this knowledge was used to develop standard procedures, which were communicated through lecture and demonstration to new members of the field.

At the end of the nineteenth century physicians were becoming more in demand, and more people were entering medicine. The number of medical schools increased, particularly in the United States. However, some physicians connected with well-established medical schools at major universities decried the training received by graduates of some of these "diploma mills" and called for state licensing. Critics were particularly appalled by the often unsubstantiated claims of success in treating certain diseases for which no standard cure or treatment existed. They wanted to ensure that every medical school graduate had the same standard training and held to the same ethical standards (Rothstein, 1972).

Some critics of contemporary medicine claim that in gaining a monopoly over health care services physicians have destroyed the good with the bad. That is, many alternative health care practitioners had operated with reasonable models of health and illness that were based on ecological theories of the fit between the individual and the natural environment. Even Pasteur had seen the germ theory of disease in this context.

Nevertheless, before licensing became widespread in the United States, many physicians were strictly entrepreneurs who sought to expand their incomes so long as there was a demand for their services. This was also true for many nonmedical healers, and it may still be true today in such practices as chiropractic (Roebuck and Hunter, 1974). Licensing may not alter the private-enterprise character of medicine, but it does make regulation potentially possible.

Physicians who make unsupported claims can be compared to practitioners of traditional medicine in other societies, as in India, where one doctor claims to be better than the other on the basis of some unique talent. Where such claims are made, there are usually sharp differences in the *type* of knowledge applied in practice from that found in scientifically based medicine. Charles Leslie contrasts what he calls *technical* and *tacit knowledge:*

> Technical knowledge is highly teachable. It can be explicated in textbooks and manuals and organized into courses or other units of study arranged in sequences of increasing complexity and inclusiveness. Thus, it can be standardized, and it can be externalized in the manipulation of tools, machines, laboratory equipment, and abstract figures such as graphs, charts, and equations. Tacit knowledge cannot be explicated with the effectiveness of technical knowledge; it must be learned by imitating the example of a master. This is one source of the moral bond between teacher and student, and the legitimate foundation for the ritualization of professional training. Because a profession is an art as well as a skill, the best instructors are practitioners as well as teachers. And because they communicate the tacit knowledge of the profession by example, they have need of ceremony. Tacit knowledge lends mystery to a profession and enhances its authority. [1972: 50]

Leslie captures the difference between a standardized set of knowledge and implicit skills that can be taught as a way of solving problems. He also suggests that there is a symbolic side to the role of being a physician. This aspect of the role has to do with the ways in which performers define themselves and are defined by others, with their place in society, and the larger social functions that may be performed by diagnosing and curing individuals. The very act of naming reduces uncertainty for the person who suspects that he is ill, because it defines the unexpected and clears doubts, although it may also increase fear and apprehension.

When a disease or accident occurs, people may question why it happened to them. The doctor helps to explain the course of illness and recovery, putting this event within the same explanatory framework as less eventful occurrences. In this way, a patient's motivation to conform is reaffirmed despite an unexpected, inexplicable event.

The physician may also be an inspirational role model. The role of the physician is well suited to perhaps undeserved hero worship. But the praise once offered to doctors as guardians of the common good and the savers of life is somewhat muted now. In large organizations, the physician has become an official, bound by the same set of rules that limit the patient's freedom of action. The regulations concerning conduct and the exchange of service for fees set the terms of the relationship. Patients often complain that doctors fail to show compassion to the sick. Where the flow of patients depends less on patient referral than in the past, formality and distance may replace a warm, casual approach.

The physician who is able to communicate despite these bureaucratic restrictions is respected because he or she shows that one can be technically correct and approachable at the same time. In many ways, the physician as the compassionate expert has become a culture hero, defining "the ingredients of typical situations, depicting appropriate behavior and accompanying motivations and interpretations" (Myerhoff and Larson, 1965: 188). Medicine has increasingly taken over for the police and the courts in such areas as the treatment of drug addicts, alcoholism, delinquency, and vagrancy. But the advice that physicians give is more in what they do than say.

This status has been acquired as much by what physicians have not been in the past as what they have been. First, national public opinion surveys show that physicians have high prestige, outdistanced only by Supreme Court justices. In contrast, a powerful person such as a factory owner who employs about 100 people was ranked thirty-first (Sennett and Cobb, 1973: 22). Professionals, according to Sennett and Cobb, may be considered special by the general population because they are free of the constraints of power: They do not take orders from others, nor do they have to boss people around unnecessarily. This special position is changing as medicine increasingly becomes part of large organizations, where physicians may coordinate a detailed division of labor.

Second, the physician has great responsibility in identifying physical accidents, insults of birth, and life stress: when a defective child is born; when people cannot take care of themselves and need some brief asylum from the larger society; when others, in seeking relief from the knowledge that they are failures, retreat from their full-time obligations into playing the sick role. These situations allow the physician to validate biological and personality differences and at the same time maintain belief in society's conforming motives.

Clearly, the authority exercised by the physician is moral as well as technical (Siegler and Osmond, 1973). This moral authority does not end the assignment of labels to those who are permanently damaged. Conformity is encouraged by showing others what could happen if they do not take care of themselves or if they drop out of productive roles. In the past, the physician was involved in staging public spectacles of ridicule in which the mad and the poor were put on display, reminding conforming members of society that they were comparatively well off (Foucault, 1965: 68). The public trials of the witches in Salem were also a lesson to conforming members of the town to create and adopt new rules of behavior (Erickson, 1966).

Third, the moral authority of the physician is not only found in defining and isolating those who are different in physical makeup and actions, but in setting rules of correct behavior. These activities involve the physician in guiding the patient in how to recover from illness and how to stay well. The physical effects of drinking, smoking, and drug use are shown by United States Public Health Service doctors to be dangerous to health. The physician has great authority in this area and can deny a hospital bed to a patient who is not following his orders.

The special status of physicians as disinterested parties not directly in control of their patients' lives, in contrast to one's employer, for example, make them ideal agents in giving directives for living. The convergence of the technical and the moral authority of medicine came about in the early twentieth century in the United States. The elite physicians based at university medical schools pressed for both state licensing of physicians and uniformity in training. Under the impetus of the recommendations of the Flexner Report, an analysis of medical education by Abraham Flexner, released in 1910, major transformations were made to ensure minimal standards of competency: "With uniform training, every licensed physician could be expected to have a basic technical education more or less equivalent to every other's and distinct from that of any other kind of healer" (Freidson, 1970: 21).

State licensing of physicians was encouraged by Flexner, a social worker, because he recognized the physician's social functions in an industrial society. Flexner was most concerned about the conditions of the laboring poor concentrated in the large industrial and manufacturing cities of the Eastern seaboard and the Midwest. The major source of this labor supply was from massive immigration to the United States from Eastern and Southern Europe. Overcrowding and inadequate ventilation and sunlight lead to high rates of tuberculosis and other diseases. Furthermore, socialists and anarchists in America were making headway in convincing these newly proletarianized peasants and artisans that they did not have to tolerate these conditions.

Flexner saw medicine as one way of making life somewhat easier for the poor. He envisioned that the licensed physician would become a public servant, sacrificing income to serve humanity. Proper medical education would train the physician to be oriented to the community, providing medical care free of charge or at moderate cost to those who could not afford it. As a political and social reformer at a time of great labor unrest marked by long and bitter strikes, Flexner was well aware that it was important to make workers feel that they were part of the American mainstream. Providing health services to the needy was one way to do this, while at the same time it ensured a healthy labor force.

THE CHARACTERISTICS OF A PROFESSION

The doctor is admired not only because of his or her freedom from having to give and take orders but also for his or her autonomy from commercial concerns. The physician can practice while realizing steady and handsome compensation. Even if employed by an organization, the salary will put a physician in the highest one or two percent of the population. While this income is subject to some uncertainty, depending on a ready market, few doctors suffer from unemployment. Insurance plans to pay for hospital services were introduced during the Great Depression, when many patients could not afford the fees charged for these services. Since then, growing participation in such plans as Blue Cross and Blue Shield and other forms of medical insurance has expanded and made the physician's income secure.

Even when the physician is completely salaried or paid on a strict capitation basis (where care is provided for a given number of individuals rather than only those in need), the prestige given to the physician is far greater than in most other occupations. In England or the Soviet Union, where national health services are free, the doctor's income may be higher than that of factory workers, but it is not as high as in the United States. Compared to occupations with the same length of training, such as college professors, the average net income of physicians in the United States may be four or more times as great. Where professionals are salaried, the differences are not so extreme.

These limits to income do not restrict competition for entry into medical school in the Soviet Union or England. Some graduates of English educational and training programs find it extremely difficult to obtain positions in hospitals as specialists (or consultants, as they are called in England). Often they emigrate to other English-speaking countries, especially the United States, where earning potential is high if they can pass the equivalency examinations. Specialists in England could work as general practitioners, but many prefer to leave the country rather than work in positions for which they are overtrained.

The intrinsically interesting work of health care is made even more attractive to the physician by having control over the work setting. Even in hospitals with a nonmedical chief administrator, physicians can invoke medical authority to achieve change in many nonmedical procedures relative to patients. Even when salaried, physicians collectively negotiate with administrators of programs, as in England, over the number of patients to be seen in a day or over the medically desirable load of patients for a general practitioner. This capacity to be free from restrictions also extends to patients. A physician can tell a patient that he or she is not being cooperative, for example (Freidson, 1970). This characteristic is in an ideal sense limited to the technical side of medical practice. However, the line between the technical and the social side of medicine is not always clearly drawn.

Professional autonomy does not end at the workplace. Physicians also have control over the criteria for admission to their profession. They exercise this control through their associations, the best known in the United States being the American Medical Association. The state medical societies affiliated with the AMA control membership on the boards of licensing. The boards determine eligibility to take the medical examination and the validity of complaints against licensed physicians.

The AMA not only attempts to restrict the practices of licensed physicians so that they do not make unsubstantiated claims for cures or nostrums, but it also guards against nonmedical health care practitioners making similar claims. Furthermore, it regulates the education, training, and utilization of nonmedical health care personnel such as nurses and pharmacists.

Lengthy periods of education and training are the major means by which the physicians are expected to acquire values of service. In addition, physicians are sworn to uphold a code of ethics and are expected to exercise peer control by reporting the incompetent or exploitative practitioner to licensing authorities. However, as will be shown in Chapter 5, this kind of enforcement rarely takes place.

Autonomy at the workplace is accompanied by the efforts of professional associations to control the major aspects of the health care institutions. Local medical societies in the United States determine who has admitting rights at hospitals, an important feature of the private practice of medicine. Physicians who disagree with the policies of the AMA have found themselves refused membership in local societies, thereby losing their right to admit patients to hospitals (Freidson, 1970: 29).

The domination of health care organizations by physicians is illustrated by the ways in which they control information about the patient's condition. Rarely are nurses and other paramedical personnel permitted to discuss illnesses with patients. Even when technical information such as the name of the medication is sought, nurses will often advise patients to ask the doctor (Houston and Pasaman, 1972). Nurses were once not permitted to make obvious diagnoses even of the most limited kinds.

In the United States, the capacity of the medical profession to control its own work extends far beyond the strictly medical aspects of applying techniques and evaluating and maintaining standards for training. The medical profession also controls nonmedical conditions, such as the form of compensation for services rendered, the number of physicians, and the education and duties to be performed by paramedical personnel. Interestingly, dentistry is the only profession equal to medicine in controlling training.

How did this come to be? Akers and Quinney (1968) compared five health professions according to organizational activities, length of education, extent of contract among members, and percent of practitioners who belonged to professional associations. They found that medicine and dentistry were far better organized than optometry, pharmacy, and chiropractic. Findings of this kind are difficult to use for firm conclusions because the time order of the variables is not precisely fixed. In other words, medicine and dentistry may be more effectively organized because they have more autonomy. Given the great variety and essentially nonmedical tasks over which medicine has gained control, it would appear that it is extremely powerful. Not only has medicine maintained its autonomy, but it has extended its scope to new areas, acquiring jurisdiction over new services, such as those for family planning, old age, and low morale, which were previously untreated (Ehrenreich and Ehrenreich, 1974: 30).

A critical area of control for physicians is the capacity to set fees for service. Even in the United States, where third-party payers reimburse patients or pay the bill directly, the doctor still has the right to set fees above what is available from the insurance plan. The right to bill the patient extends even to ancillary physicians, who provide indirect services called for by the attending physician. Anesthesiologists, radiologists, and pathologists are entitled to submit separate bills so long as the attending physicians call for their services. The focus of concern of the AMA is the doctor-patient relationship and control over it. Some physicians teach or do research, but the AMA does not object to their being salaried.

The argument is made that the doctor-patient relationship is best preserved for the benefit of the patient when the patient is directly employing the doctor, rather than the doctor being employed by an administrator in a group practice or a hospital. Standards might be lowered, according to this reasoning, if a nonmedical person could tell the doctor what to do. Administrators might get the doctor to skimp on work and save money for the employer. Essentially, this justification is a sociological argument for keeping the fee-for-service relationship. Similar arguments made about the absence of peer review in solo practices and the tendency to relax standards are curiously ignored by the defenders of the fee-for-service system (Freidson, 1970: 32). In addition, the continued use of a fee-for-service system through Medicaid payments has led to financial exploitation of the taxpayer and the patient. The state and local medical associations have been reluctant to become involved in regulating physicians who overtreat Medicaid patients, however.

Still, the question remains: Do standards of care deteriorate if physicians are salaried rather than self-employed? This can be answered by looking at prepaid medicine in two contexts: the United States, where such prepaid group practices are still unusual, and the National Health Service in England, where the state runs and pays for all care. England will be examined first because of the extensive experience that has been available since World War II in what is sometimes called in the United States "socialized medicine."

ENGLAND'S NATIONAL HEALTH SERVICE

The Labour Party government initiated the national health service in 1948 to provide welfare services for the entire population. All health care was either free or had minimal fees. The program was financed from tax monies and administered by the Ministry of Health. While some private physicians still practice and some employers have insurance plans, state-supported health care is widely accepted in England. The British Medical Association still controls technical matters, such as the criteria of admission to medical school, the curriculum, and licensing. There are regularly scheduled negotiations between the BMA and the Ministry of Health to settle such matters as patient load and salary.

Other factors enter into examining the effectiveness of the National Health Service to deliver care. Historically, medicine developed along two paths in England, with general practitioners working exclusively in community practice and specialists or consultants involved in hospital practice, where they controlled a number of beds devoted to treating cases in their speciality. General practitioners could only refer patients and did not admit patients to hospital, but left this task in the hands of consultants.

The National Health Service has made an effort to distribute doctors equally throughout the population. The same is true of hospitals and the consultants who practice in them. The quality of medicine practiced in the community was and still is affected by the sharp separation between general practitioners and consultants. General practitioners must acquire new knowledge on their own rather than through extensive contact with consultants.

The quality of care is directly affected by the way patients are assigned to general practitioners under the National Health Service. General practitioners are paid on a capitation basis and are responsible for a fixed number of patients each year. While there are no advantages to performing extra and unnecessary procedures under this system of payment, general practitioners are also expected to pay for office expenses out of their fees. This arrangement provides them with no incentive to acquire new equipment because this cuts their income, and they cannot expand their practice by taking on additional patients.

The enforcement of the terms of the contract is not completely in the hands of physicians. Patients can file complaints through service committees, which are connected to the 134 district councils that oversee care, according to a regional or catchment area system. Payments can be withheld for failure to perform according to contract. Patients also have the right to change physicians.

The National Health Service makes somewhat less use of the hospital as a source of care than do doctors or patients in the United States. One interesting point of comparison between England and the United States is in the number of hospital beds available per hundred people in the population. According to 1963 figures, there were 9.1 beds per 100 in England as compared to 10.5 per 100 in the United States. The yearly rate of admission to hospitals in England was 88 per 1,000 population, compared with 130 per 1,000 in the United States. Interestingly, the English patient spends an average of 15 days in a hospital bed, compared with 8 days for the American (Anderson, 1972). There is general satisfaction with the National Health Service among English users; thirty years after its inception, 84 percent of the British are satisfied with the present program, despite it being sorely underfinanced (Apple, 1978).

What inferences can be drawn from this difference? Are Americans healthier than the English? Are English doctors uninterested in their patients? First, nurse-midwife services are available in England, and most births take place in the home. This difference would raise the number of days hospitalized because the short-term maternity stay would not enter into these figures. Second, the traditional separation between general practitioner and hospital-based consultant means that some continuity of care is lost. With the case admitted to the hospital, consultants may repeat diagnostic workups on patients. Third, it is possible that general practitioners refer only the most serious cases to the hospital, knowing that only the most seriously ill will be admitted. Unlike a fee-for-service system, unnecessary hospitalization would not occur, since performing more procedures will not increase income for the general practitioner (Mechanic, 1968).

PREPAID GROUP PRACTICE

In the United States, the two major privately sponsored medical care programs are the Health Insurance Program of Greater New York and Kaiser-Permanante in California. In both, a group of doctors, who can provide all medical specialties and services, contracts with a number of patients who will be cared for, no matter how frequently or infrequently they use the service. Some scattered evidence suggests that while patients do use the program for minor ailments or injuries that could be taken care of at home, they also tend to come in for more preventive tests and do not let symptoms of serious illnesses go unreported. Furthermore, more frequent use of paranatal care seems to have a payoff in lower rates of infant mortality. Few patients complain that they have little control over doctors because they are not paying for the service directly. If anything, patients are more demanding of services, particularly diagnostic tests (Freidson, 1975), since all services are already paid for. A prepaid plan in Seattle now makes the primary care or general practice physician financially responsible for all services to which patients are referred, giving the doctor the monetary incentive to keep costs down (Reinhold, 1980).

Despite the claims made by associations of physicians that the doctor-patient relationship will be interfered with if the fee-for-service system is replaced, questions arise as to whether self-serving reasons are involved and whether the dominance of medicine by physicians has led to a self-regulating profession in the public interest.

Recent social legislation sought to provide minimal standards of care for the elderly and the poor who were not able to purchase medical care through third-party payers or directly. At the same time, the effort was made to preserve the autonomy and control of the doctor-patient relationship in the hands of physicians. In addition, the recent increase in the number of doctors in the United States has made peer regulation more difficult. Chapter 5 will discuss how the social and technical changes in modern health care influence the capacity of the state and local medical societies to regulate members of the profession.

REFERENCES

Akers, R. L., and R. Quinney. 1968. "Differential organization of health professions." *American Sociological Review* 33 (February): 104–121.

Anderson, Odin. 1972. *Health Care: Can There be Equity? The United States, Sweden and England.* New York: Wiley Interscience.

Apple, R. W. 1978. "Britain's 30-year health service: Hope gives way to resignation." *New York Times,* July 6: A1,2.

Birenbaum, Arnold. 1978. "Status and role." Pp. 128–39 in Edward Sagarin, ed., *Sociology: The Basic Concepts.* New York: Holt, Rinhart, and Winston.

deKruif, Paul. 1926. *The Microbe Hunters.* New York: Harcourt. Brace and World.

Erickson, Kai T. 1966. *The Wayward Puritans: A Study in the Sociology of Deviance.* New York: John Wiley.

Flexner, Abraham. 1910. *Medical Education in the United States and Canada.* New York: Carnegie Foundation for the Advancement of Teaching, Bulletin 4.

Foucault, Michel. 1965. *Madness and Civilization.* New York: Pantheon.

Freidson, Eliot. 1970. *The Profession of Medicine: A Study of the Sociology of Applied Knowledge.* New York: Dodd, Mead.

———. 1975. *Doctoring Together: A Study of Professional Social Control.* New York: Elsevier.

Greifinger R., and V. Sidel. 1976. "American medicine: Charity begins at home." *Environment* 18: 7–18.

Houston, C. S., and W. E. Pasaman. 1972. "Patient Perceptions of Hospital Care." *Hospitals* 46 (April): 79–74.

Hughes, Everett C. 1967. "Professions." Pp. 1–14 in Kenneth S. Lynn, ed., *The Professions in America.* Boston: Beacon Press.

Larson, Margali Safatti. 1977. *The Rise of Professionalism: A Sociological Analysis.* Berkeley: University of California Press.

Leslie, C. 1972. "The professionalization of Ayurvedic and Unan's medicine." Pp. 39–54 in Eliot Freidson and Judith Lorber, ed., *Medical Men and Their Work: A Sociological Reader.* Chicago: Aldine.

McKeown, Thomas. 1965. *Medicine in Modern Society.* London: Allen and Unwin.

Mechanic, David. 1968. "Some notes on medical care systems: Contrasts in medical organization between the United States and Great Britain." Pp. 325–64 in *Medical Sociology: A Selective View.* New York: The Free Press.

Merton, R. K., and E. Barber. 1976. "Sociological Ambivalence." Pp. 3–31 in Robert K. Merton, *Sociological Ambivalence and Other Essays.* New York: Free Press.

Moore, Barrington. 1966. *The Social Origins of Dictatorship and Democracy: Lord and Peasant in the Making of the Modern World.* Boston: Beacon Press.

Myerhoff, B., and W. R. Larson. 1965. "The doctor as culture hero: The routinization of charisma." *Human Organization* 24 (3): 188–91.

Perrow, C. 1965. "Hospitals: Technology, structure, and goals." Pp. 910–71 in James G. March, ed., *Handbook of Organizations.* Chicago: Rand McNally.

Roebuck, J., and R. B. Hunter. 1974. "Medical quackery as deviant behavior," pp. 300–311 in Clifton D. Bryant, *Deviant Behavior: Occupational and Organizational Bases.* Chicago: Rand McNally.

Rothstein, William. 1972. *American Physicians in the Nineteenth Century.* Baltimore: Johns Hopkins University Press.

Reinhold, R. 1980. "Doctors cut costs in Seattle plan." *New York Times,* February 12, pp. c1, 2.

Sennett, Richard, and Jonathan Cobb. 1973. *The Hidden Injuries of Class.* New York: Vintage.

Shyrock, Richard. 1936. *The Development of Modern Medicine.* London: Oxford.

Siegler, M., and H. Osmond. 1973. "Aesculopian authority." *The Hastings Center Studies* 1 (2): 41–52.

Thompson, Edward P. 1963. *The Making of the English Working Class.* New York: Vintage.

Ure, Andrew. 1861. *The Philosophy of Manufactures.* London: H. G. Bohn.
Weber, Max. 1958. *The Protestant Ethic and the Spirit of Capitalism.* Translated by Talcott Parons. New York: Scribners.
———. 1968. *Economy and Society.* 3 Vol. Guenther Roth and Claus Wittich, eds. New York: Bedminster Press.
Yeo, Eileen, and Edward P. Thomspon. 1971. *The Unknown Mayhew.* New York: Schocken Books.

5

Social Control and Deviance in Medicine

Social control, an aspect of modern sociology that has been attracting increasing scholarly attention, is a perspective on social life based on many sound assumptions, the main one being that during the course of the day all of us do many things that we would prefer not to do, or resist doing such things that sorely tempt us.* Social control operates not only to prevent deviant behavior but to contain it through identification of disapproved acts. When people get together and talk about their absent friends, when they ridicule rivals, or when they use sarcasm to bring a potentially rebellious member of their group back into line, they are practicing social control. These activities set the deviant apart from conforming members of groups and reaffirm the rules of membership.

Social control operates through law, and through authority figures on whom we are dependent, such as parents. In the field of health care, standards are maintained by state agencies that regulate professional medical conduct or the behavior of other health care practitioners. These state bureaus or offices can discipline those found guilty of professional misconduct.

The regulation of health care practitioners is primarily in the hands of state boards of licensing and the various watchdog committees of the American Medical Association. The medical profession is largely self-governing, and it sets standards for training, skills, and duties of others in the field of health care. One of the AMA's tasks is to guard the rights of physicians. Efforts by other health care practitioners to increase their responsibilities are often met with hostility by the AMA, except where the tasks are specifically turned over to others by physicians (as in the case of dentists, nurses, and others).

---

*An earlier version of this chapter appeared as "Medicine, social change, and deviant behavior," in Edward Sagarin, ed., *Deviance and Social Change, Sage Annual Reviews of Studies in Deviance* 1 (1977): 139–54.

The study of deviance in medicine has been guided by this orientation. Some sociological literature has focused on practices that deceive patients, such as spurious nostrums, devices, and treatment (Roebuck and Hunter, 1974: 302–6). Marginal practitioners, both in and outside of organized medicine, are sometimes viewed as exotic creatures (Cowie and Roebuck, 1975). Chiropractic has been subject to many attacks, some with careful documentation (*Consumer Reports*, 1975: 542–48, 606–10). With an estimated 5 million people in the United States and Canada using chiropractors, the battle continues (Yesalis et al., 1980; Silver, 1980). Recently the National Institutes of Health funded a Toronto study of the effectiveness of spinal manipulation on back problems (Blumenthal, 1979). Chiropractors are now eligible to be reimbursed for services rendered to Medicaid patients.

Some sociologists who have focused on deviant behavior in medicine have explained its presence as resulting from the failure of some physicians to acquire the right set of values. (Dansereau, 1974: 88–89). This interpretation ignores the unethical behavior that is found not only in solo practices, but in the cooperative enterprises of some who operate legitimate health facilities.

The purpose of examining social control and deviance in medicine is to show how medicine and health care have changed and how the new forms of deviance have outrun the mechanisms of social control. Many changes are related to the financing of health care, the increased demand for services, the growth in the utilization of new technical procedures, and new advances in knowledge. These conditions, which help to shape the field of health care, have also made possible new forms of unethical practices.

While physicians are licensed by the state, physicians sit in judgment, both formally and informally, on their peers. This capacity to be self-regulating demonstrates that medicine has enormous control over the entire field of health care. This capacity to command others also means that many physicians can be relatively unconcerned about the practices of their fellow physicians. In New York State, "of the 1,191 complaints about physicians received by the State Health Department's Office of Professional Medical Conduct during a recent 16 month period, only 31 came from other doctors, and only 37 came from medical societies" (Rensberger, 1977: B3).

THE ORGANIZATION OF MEDICINE

At one time, the medical doctor was similar to the small businessman or a craftsman who owned his own shop. He not only worked alone, but he could work anywhere, since his tools were portable and his medicines were often of his own preparation. Babies were delivered at home, and appendectomies were performed on kitchen tables. With the growth of technology in medicine came the need to acquire more equipment and to rely more on the services provided by nurses, pharmacists, and technicians. Medical practice no longer followed the small-business model, and the forms of deviance associated with it, known as quackery, have been joined by new forms that have become part of the medical routine.

This chapter will focus on how two kinds of deviant behavior are related to these changes in the organization of health care: (1) the overutilization of services encouraged by certain new ways of paying for health services, and (2) medical neglect or negligence resulting from higher rates of intervention through surgery and medication, leading to disorders that were not there before treatment. These illnesses or conditions that result from medical intervention are called *iatrogenic* disorders, and some critics of contemporary health care consider them to be far worse than other diseases (Illich, 1975).

Some might argue that instances of fraud, abuse, inappropriate personal conduct, and incompetence may simply increase one's sense of outrage or fear of doctors. This discussion of deviance will be linked to an examination of the procedures and resources available to the medical profession and state regulatory agencies to prevent and punish deviant behavior. Finally, some current and future developments in the area of social control in medicine will be discussed. It is within the medical profession itself that some of the most important criticisms and insights concerning current needs for reforms have been emerging. It is important to understand why this is happening.

Fraud and abuse by physicians and other health care personnel serving the poor have increased tremendously since the introduction of the federally funded Medicaid program. At one time, physicians whose practices were made up of mainly poor patients were seen as saints or martyrs. *The Last Angry Man*, a popular novel by Gerald Green, extolled the devotion of a doctor who cared for the poor. Even today, in the People's Republic of China, Dr. Norman Bethune, a Canadian surgeon who served with the Red Army, is used as a model of sacrifice and the internationalist spirit. In the past in the United States, many physicians would reduce their fees for the poor, and they donated time and services to charity patients in free clinics.

The Johnson Administration witnessed the passing of the necessity of some physicians to serve the poor with less remuneration than other physicians. In 1965, Congress passed a law establishing a new program of health insurance for people 65 years old or over. This major piece of social legislation was called Medicare, Title 18 of the Social Security Amendments Act of 1965 (Public Law 89–97). A second part of the law provided health insurance for all who could not afford to pay for health care, known as Medicaid. The patients who are covered under this program are not just the very poor but anyone who is "medically indigent," including people who are working as well as those receiving public assistance. Physicians are paid on a fee-for-service basis set by the federal and state administrators of the program. The fees are somewhat lower than those charged by other doctors in the area, and some physicians who own or operate "shared health facilities" that serve Medicaid often use various fraudulent techniques to improve their incomes.

The medical profession has not taken an active interest in correcting these unethical and illegal practices. Abuses of the Medicaid program were reported as early as 1973 in a Pulitzer Prize-winning series of articles in the *New York Daily News*. A Senate Subcommittee report on these fraudulent and abusive practices followed (1976). While the administrators of the Medicaid program set the fees in order to keep costs down, no provisions were made to limit the number of procedures that could be performed by any single physician, nor did they have appropriate funds to hire personnel to monitor the quality of the care or check whether patients were actually in need of care.

The planners of the program did not want to interfere with medical organization or restrict participating physicians from increasing the size of their practices. Nor did they want to limit their incomes. To encourage participation by physicians, the program administrators trusted physicians not to exploit the situation. Most professionals will at some time be subjected to temptations to violate their ethical code, it is clear, however, that some types of practices constrain the physician to violate their ethical code more frequently than others. Similarly, when conditions change, rule-violating behavior will be reduced or take different forms.

Each role in health care is subject to different opportunities to deviate from the social code of a hospital or professional association, depending on its size, extent of contact between various occupational specialists in the division of labor, prestige of an occupation, observability of performance, and contact with colleagues. Despite this variability, professionals are expected to act ethically no matter whom they treat, who pays the bill, or how they are paid.

In a case of a chiropractor convicted of Medicaid fraud (Lubasch, 1976: 30), a Federal District Court Judge, Charles L. Brieant, Jr., ruefully suggested that while the defendent was a fine practitioner the evidence showed him to be guilty of theft. The judge outlined the basic sociological problem:

> Those greater minds than ours who contrived this Medicaid legislation created a very easy and obvious means to steal public funds. Why did they do this? I think the answer is two-fold.
>
> First, legislators thought that physicians were above that sort of thing because of the respect they receive from the community and because of the standing they have, that they would not do any such thing.
>
> I think also that the Government believed they did not want bureaucrats intervening between the physician and his patients solely to prevent fraud. Their expectations were not fulfilled, and you are not alone among those who engaged in fraud and there is no excuse for it. [Lubasch, 1976: 30]

MEDICAID MEDICINE

Government intervention in the form of Medicaid, financed under Title 19 of the Social Security Act, was hailed by Lyndon B. Johnson as the best way to "assure the availability of and accessibility to the best health care for all Americans regardless of age, geography, or economic status." (Staff Report, 1976: 1). Instead, Medicaid has led to the formation of a two-class medical care system, segregating the poor even more than in the past. Moreover, it has permitted the proliferation of health care practices that generate substantial incomes and abusive and fraudulent practices. Instead of being organized to serve society, Medicaid practices often serve the practitioner. As one dentist told investigators, "the way the system is structured the trick is to see as many patients as possible as quickly as possible. Visits must be brief. Accordingly, it is uneconomical to give good care" (Staff Report, 1976: 18).

The deviance produced by "Medicaid mills" has its own culture and unique nomenclature. These organized practices in health care provide students of deviant behavior with a glimpse into corporate white-collar crime, which is usually off limits to academic observers (Wheeler 1976: 531). Also, the nomenclature blurs the distinctly illegal character of the activities, making it possible to compartmentalize deeds that run counter to professional ethics.

> "Ping-ponging" is the expression given to the most common mill abuse, the referral of patients from one practitioner to another within the facility, even though medically there is no need.
>
> "Ganging" refers to the practice of billing for multiple service to members of the same family on the same day.
>
> "Upgrading" is the practice of billing for a service more extensive than that actually provided.
>
> "Steering" is the direction of a patient to a particular pharmacy by a physician or anyone else in the medical center. [Staff Report, 1976: 18–19]

Investigators for the Senate Subcommittee on Long-Term Care presented 200 instances of patients in New York City with minor physical complaints who were overtreated in 70 percent of the cases. However, such conventional practices as taking the temperature and measuring blood pressure were omitted. Examinations of ears or eyes and mouths were performed in a most careless manner. A throat was examined by shining a flashlight from a distance of five feet from the patient and (of course) without using a tongue depressor (Staff Report, 1976: 44).

The growth of these abuses and fraudulent practices was encouraged by the application of the fee-for-service model at a somewhat lower than customary rate of reimbursement. It has also been possible under Medicaid reimbursement to employ various paramedical personnel, whose services are billed separately. The more services performed by optometrists, podiatrists, chiropractors, and others, the greater the volume of profit to the Medicaid employer.

The AMA was reluctant to abandon the fee-for-service system in the Medicare and Medicaid programs for fear of establishing a precedent for prepaid health service on a national (or nationalized) basis for the entire population. While the AMA and others bitterly opposed Medicare before it was made into law, they responded favorably after passage, and there was no organized boycott of patients (Colombotos, 1969: 1).

Since the rate of reimbursement from Medicaid is lower than rates set in private insurance plans or even Medicare (which sets rates according to customary fees), some physicians have refused to take indigent patients, whereas others have concentrated on their care. Medicine for the poor is in the hands of a few high-volume billers, where "7 percent of the doctors practicing in New York City's Medicaid program earned 50 percent of the total paid to all doctors" (Staff Report, 1976: 14).

The volume of billing found in a practice seems to be related to financial arrangements. In states where reimbursement procedures can take up to six months (as in New York), financial corporations or factoring firms have acted as collection agents for the practitioners. In exchange for immediate payment, practitioners charge anywhere from 12 to 24 percent of the face value of the invoices. It has also been pointed out by participating physicians that the actual interest rate is closer to 48 percent per year, since the factoring firm may receive reimbursement in half the time expected. The use of financial corporations encouraged practitioners to increase their volume to make up for the difference in lost income. Medicaid mills using factoring firms tended to have twice the income of other practices. The volume and expenses in small practices, however, does not make factoring profitable.

Shared health facilities that specialize in Medicaid patients also engage in other practices, which, if not clearly illegal, are regarded as unethical. Owners of shared health facilities are found to lease office space in exchange for a percentage of gross income, and they share fees between two or more physicians for reimbursement for the services rendered by one physician alone. The AMA regards "rebates on prescription and appliances, the ownership of clinics or laboratories by joint stock companies composed in part or in whole by physicians, and the percentage lease renting of pharmacy space for a pharmacy owned by a physician or physicians as clearly unethical" (Staff Report, 1976: 67). Enforcements of these rulings of the judicial council of the AMA are up to the local or state medical societies. During 1966–76, the Medical Society of the County of New York did not expel a single physician for abuse of Medicare or Medicaid, and it referred only 14 complaints to the professional conduct offices of the State Departments of Health and Education (Staff Report, 1976: 197).

While these practices encourage overbilling in order to maintain high volume in reimbursement, physicians who engage in unethical practices are not subject to formal sanctions from the agency devoted to maintaining them. Because of the lack of budget for hiring field auditors and investigators, enforcement by appropriate state and city agencies is weak and irregular. And Medicaid-practice owners are well aware of these limited sanctions. Fines are charged against future billing, and they encourage further abuses and fraud in order to recoup earnings lost (Staff Report, 1976: 145). Physicians are also aware that certain practices such as billing for nonexistent patient visits (or nonexistent patients) involve greater risks than simply overbilling for an actual visit. These tactics depend on knowledge of the limits of enforcement and the risks involved, producing a Dickensian parody of professional behavior.

> You never put through for a patient you didn't see. The patient might have been on vacation or in the hospital. That's the only way that they can hang you. I'm not that stupid. It is stupid to write bills on patients you didn't see on dates you

> weren't in your office. Other things (kinds of fraud) are all right. But if you put down anything strange, you'd better set a date or a note explaining it. Those are the things to look for. [Staff Report, 1976: 59].

The organization of medical care for the poor makes it almost impossible for informal peer pressure to enforce the standards of practice effectively. First, the work of physicians in Medicaid practices is insulated from peer review by the nature of their inhouse referral system, which involves few of the standard medical specialists except those required in order to receive reimbursement. Many medical practitioners who do not have affiliations with medical schools or voluntary hospitals deal mainly with proprietary hospitals that do not set high standards for attending physicians. Therefore, the work of Medicaid physicians cannot be observed, nor can they learn from more highly qualified practitioners. Second, many physicians in these practices are either from foreign medical schools or have just finished residency requirements. As such, they are subject to financial pressures that encourage them to seek immediate income opportunities, resulting in further exclusion from peer review.

Patients themselves provide little effective pressure on Medicaid practitioners. Being unfamiliar with medical terminology, the poor can often be manipulated into unnecessary tests, X-rays, and procedures. The poor seem to be getting form without substance in health care. It comes as no surprise then, that since the inception of the Medicaid laws in 1964, the patterns of utilization for the poor and the better off have been reversed so that the former were using physicians' services at a somewhat higher rate than the rest of the population. However, better off people were still more likely to take preventive steps such as taking Pap tests, eye tests, and glaucoma examinations (U.S. Department of Health, Education, and Welfare, 1976: 18). Patients are also not regarded by Medicaid practitioners as effective witnesses against them if their billing is subject to auditing. Since consumers in these cases do not pay for services and cannot exhaust their benefits, there are few incentives for them to become knowledgeable consumers of health care.

The extension of health services to the poor under Medicaid legislation can be regarded as simply the wasteful practices of welfare state legislation, or it can be seen as the result of economic practices that have increased the marketing capacities of providers of services and purveyors of drugs and equipment. As in other industries, they seek to avoid declining profits. To meet these needs, more stable and larger markets are sought for products and services (Braverman, 1974: 265). Since the medical marketplace, like other marketplaces, is uncertain, providers often seek to *induce* or manufacture a stable demand that can support their needs.

Also higher profits are sought by providers of risk capital in those sectors of health care that have not developed fully institutionalized relationships with patients and third-party payers. As in other industries, new forms of production are built upon the employment of marginal operatives, unprotected and unrestrained by more traditional practices and protective associations such as unions.

Higher-status physicians linked to voluntary hospitals or medical schools would be loath to risk their reputations and participate in the marginal operations disparagingly regarded as Medicaid mills. While more reputable physicians do not participate in these practices, they tolerate their existence. County and state medical societies are composed of physicians from regions where Medicaid mills flourish; state licensing boards are made up of these same physicians. It is important to examine whether physicians can regulate incompetency or inappropriate behavior among peers.

MEDICAL NEGLECT AND NEGLIGENCE

Codes of ethics are created by professions to remind practitioners of what they can and cannot do. However, they are more effective in preserving the independence of the professional practitioner than in removing those who behave inappropriately or are technically incompetent. In fact, the increase in the number of malpractice suits in the United States in the last decade and the rapid rise in the cost of malpractice insurance may be partially a result of the failure to regulate the medical profession effectively.

State regulatory boards have been reluctant to revoke the licenses of physicians and thereby deny their livelihood. In 1975, Dr. Robert G. Derbyshire of the New Mexico Board of Medical Examiners and Dr. Roger O. Egeberg of the Department of Health, Education, and Welfare estimated that 16,000 physicians were incompetent or unfit out of a total of 320,000 licensed physicians in the United States (Rensberger, 1976: 20). While 5 percent of all physicians are deemed incompetent or unfit, only an average of 66 licenses are revoked each year. During the period 1969–73, twenty states took no disciplinary action at all. Moreover, regulatory boards such as the New York Board for Professional Medical Conduct are often understaffed and cannot pursue many investigations.

Many state regulatory boards have been limited largely to dealing with cases of misconduct that involve criminal convictions. The New York State legislature, in response to the malpractice crisis, introduced new grounds for defining professional misconduct, including "practicing the profession fraudulently, beyond its authorized scope, with gross incompetence, with gross negligence or incompetence on more than one occasion" (State of New York, 1976: 150). In addition, the new laws create intermediate penalities, such as temporary suspension of licenses, censure, suspension and retraining, and fines (State of New York, 1976: 149). While this new range of sanctions seems more fitting to the new criteria for investigation and discipline, there is no evidence of an increase in more vigorous pursuits of inappropriately behaving or incompetently performing physicians. Even formal study of mortality in hospitals where malpractice is discovered does not lead to disciplinary action (*New York Times*, 1976).

How can this lack of enforcement be accounted for? Some clues may be found in the organizational routine of the profession, which encourages the development of networks of colleagues who exchange services and often confer on cases. Those practitioners whose work is regarded as substandard may not be utilized by the colleague network and are subject to what Eliot Freidson refers to as a "personal boycott" (1970: 191). As a result of these informal sanctions, practitioners snubbed in one sector of the field will often move beyond the observability of those who invoked these sanctions. Instead of maintaining contact and seeking to upgrade the performance of the delinquent physician, the upright performers of these roles seek to protect their own reputations and their right to practice independently. As Freidson indicates, several mutually exclusive circles may exist in the same region.

> The consequence is that a "single" inclusive profession can contain within it and even encourage markedly different ethical and technical practices, limited in a very superficial way by the common core of training required for licensing and by writings of the leaders of the profession. Insofar as the local practitioner population is large enough, the segregated networks are at least partly ordered by prestige, and only the higher levels are linked in with (and contribute to) the national and international associations representing various formal aspects of the profession. [1970: 199]

Rather than conceptualizing the medical profession as a company of equals, Freidson suggests that various castes may exist, unified only in that they provide medical services and have the same title. A number of interesting questions can be raised: Do physicians who begin their careers serving the poor in Medicaid mills, without admitting rights to voluntary hospitals or medical school faculty appointments, remain in that position throughout their careers, no matter how well they do financially? Do physicians cast out of the elite institutions join those who service the lower orders? Can negative reputations be overcome?

REACTIONS TO DEVIANCE

Physicians who observe instances of abuse, fraud, incompetence, unethical exploitation, neglect, and negligence are not reluctant to warn their colleagues. However, correction and instances of public castigation are rare, except where personal misconduct such as drug addiction is involved. Relations may never be severed in a formal way because one never knows when fellow professionals may meet again or whether the same accusations will be made to the accuser. There seems to be no group support for invoking formal punishments, and internal exile seems to be used, thus avoiding conflict or unpleasant scenes (Rensberger, 1977: B30).

The person who is not subject to formal sanctions may retain an image of uncertainty and ambiguity when there is no alternative to the informal system of reassignment, resignation, and relocation in another city. And there is no formal system for upgrading competency at this time. Rarely are efforts made to improve the skills of the physician subject to informal sanctions.

The steps necessary for retraining and improvement of performance could be initiated by the upright physician. Moreover, both upright and delinquent physicians could separate the deviant acts from the actor himself, providing an opportunity to ceremonialize the occasion and restore belief in the professional who is being questioned, rather than crystallizing the deviance into an organized career.

Dealing with Medicaid abuse and fraud requires both professional and state intervention. However, the interpersonal forms of control suggested in the previous discussion would not be fitting, since the deviance has become an "institutionalized evasion" of professional, technical, and ethical standards (Merton, 1957: 317). This form of deviant behavior may require the public implementation and enforcement of values in medicine that direct a physician to public service above all other considerations (Freidson, 1975: 127). Such steps would be difficult to undertake unless supported by public service oriented physicians wishing to end the separation of care for the poor from services from those who are better off.

Evidence suggests that sufficient numbers of physicians whose access to a livelihood is not restricted by the professional associations are committed to reform. As of 1974, only 60 percent of physicians were involved in office-based practices, with the rest in hospital-based practices (22.1 percent), teaching, administration, and research (Silver, 1976: 47). These differences are crucial in understanding where movement for reform is coming from within medicine.

If the structure of health services generates its own deviance, then it can generate its own reaction to deviance. The demands for reform in the organization and delivery of health care may well result from structured discrepancies between "culturally induced personal aspirations and patterned differentials in access to the opportunity structure for moving toward those aspirations by institutionalized means" (Merton, 1976: 125). Social movements, as Dubin (1959) has noted, constitute a special form of deviance when people seek to develop new institutionalized means to achieve culturally approved goals.

Reforms to improve the level of competency of the medical profession and reduce the patterned fraud and abuse in Medicaid practices could result from the social changes that have encouraged these forms of deviant behavior. First, the high volume of demand for health services, increased utilization of technology, and the more refined division of labor can be used to justify the institutionalization of new regulatory practices, because older forms of regulation are not adequate. Second, computer technology can be utilized to determine the rates of deviance and identify its differential location in the health care delivery system. Finally, there are sufficient numbers of physicians involved in planning who are concerned with issues related to quality of care as well as distribution.

Such "corporate rationalizers," as identified by Robert Alford (1972: 143), form a network of medical systems specialists who recognize the need for the reallocation of resources. The structured constraints toward social control are as evident in these conditions produced by social change as the deviant behavior it has produced. The two processes, as always, are connected through the social structure.

Although many of the unethical and incompetent behaviors discussed here are not standard, the current mechanisms of social control are ineffective. While peer regulation through collegial contact may be effective to prevent certain kinds of deviant behavior, other kinds fall outside the scope of the group norms of medicine. In other words, rules may simply not exist for which these practices are violations.

That the leaders of any institutionalized sphere are aware of the extent to which actual role performers live up to normative expectations should come as no surprise, given their location in the group (Merton, 1957: 342). However, the degree of supervision that can be engaged in by leaders is "itself limited by the norms of the group" (Merton, 1957: 343). Close supervision would be a violation in itself of the spirit of collegiality. Yet even when the norms do not restrict supervision, enforcement is limited by the increased segmentation of the field. Informal means of social control are most effective when there is a great deal of face-to-face contact. The elites in medicine are not always linked to the deviants through an organization that permits them to exercise control officially. Effective enforcement cannot be promoted unless this kind of reorganization takes place.

Are there inducements within the field of health care to encourage members to seek more effective enforcement? The greatest inducement would be to maintain full control over the means of health care, a right that physicians in many other countries do not have where national health services exist. It is ironic that the original resistance to state regulation of Medicare and Medicaid by the AMA has permitted the growth of routine deviation in the field and has set the groundwork for even more control than was originally anticipated. This constraint toward more social control could help to reform much of the current structure of organized health care in the United States.

The financing of health care is now organized around a combination of private and public insurance programs. In New York State, for example, "Medicare and Medicaid provide 41 percent of the income of hospitals, Blue Cross provides another 22 percent, and other direct public funds or private insurance funds account for an additional 27 percent so that 90 percent of hospital income is derived from third party payers" (State of New York, 1976: 15).

The ultimate bill payers are consumers and taxpayers. Despite increasing disaster coverage for Americans through insurance programs, out-of-pocket or direct payments have increased in all age brackets during the past twenty years. Health care consumers are saying that paying the doctor hurts, and they are beginning to complain through malpractice litigation and support for national health insurance programs. At the same time, many consumers would like to maintain the high standards found usually in medical centers with medical school and university affiliations. In addition, there are fears that the doctor-patient relationship will be altered by changes in the way medical services are required.

To deal with the question of whether the practitioner-patient relationship can be made more effective, the strategies used by patients must be examined. Since the patients are strangers in the hospital or clinic, their concerns about their own welfare are paramount.

REFERENCES

Alford R. 1972. "The political economy of health care: Dynamics without change." *Politics and Society* (Winter): 1–38.

Blumenthal R. 1979. "Chiropractics drawing increasing scientific interest." *New York Times*, October 8, p. B8.

Braverman, Harry. 1974. *Labor and Monopoly Capital: The Degradation of Work in the Twentieth Century*. New York: Monthly Review Press.

Consumer Reports (September 1975): 542–48. "Chiropractors: Healers or quacks?" Pt. I.

Consumer Reports (October 1975): 606–10. "Chiropractors: Healers or quacks?" Pt. II.

Cowie, James, and Julian B. Roebuck. 1975. *An Ethnography of a Chiropractic Clinic: Definitions of a Deviant Situation*. New York: Free Press.

Colombotos, J. 1973. "Physicians and medicare: A before-after study of the effects of legislation on attitudes." *American Sociological Review* 34: 1–17.

Dansereau, H. K. 1974. "Unethical behavior: Professional deviance." Pp. 75–89 in C. D. Bryant, ed., *Deviant Behavior: Occupational and Organizational Bases*. Chicago: Rand McNally.

Department of Health, Education, and Welfare. 1976. *Forward Plan for Health: FY 1978–82*. Washington, D.C.: Department of Health, Education, and Welfare.

Dubin, R. 1959. "Deviant behavior and social structure: Continuities in social theory." *American Sociological Review* 24: 147–64.

Freidson, Eliot. 1970. *The Profession of Medicine: A Study in the Sociology of Applied Knowledge*. New York: Dodd, Mean.

———. 1975. "The social control of the professions: Toward ethical reform in a 'delinquent community.' " *Program of General and Continuing Education in the Humanities Seminar Reports* 3: 121–27.

Illich, Ivan. 1975. *Medical Nemesis*. London: Calder & Boyers.

Lubasch, A. H. 1976. "Chiropracter given 4-year prison term." *New York Times*, September 9, p. 30.

Merton, Robert K. 1957. "Continuities in the theory of reference groups and social structure." Pp. 281–386 in *Social Theory and Social Strucutre*. Rev. and enlarged ed. Glencoe, Ill.: The Free Press.

———. 1976. "Structural analysis in sociology." Pp. 109–44 in *Sociological Ambivalence and Other Essays*. New York: The Free Press.

New York Times, October 5, 1976, p. 20. "A Study of malpractice deaths reported ended without action."

Rensberger, B. 1976. "Unfit doctors create worry in profession." *New York Times*, January 26, pp. 1 and 20.

———. 1976. "Thousands a year killed by faulty prescriptions." *New York Times*, January 28, pp. 1 and 17.

———. 1977. "Albany report cites medical cover-up." *New York Times*, May 12: B 12.

Roebuck, B. J., and R. B. Hunter. 1974. "Medical quackery as deviant behavior." Pp. 300–311 in C. D. Bryant, ed., *Deviant Behavior: Occupational and Organizational Bases*. Chicago: Rand McNally.

Staff Report, Subcommittee on Long-Term Care of the Special Committee on Aging, United States Senate. 1976. "Fraud and abuse among practitioners participating in the Medicaid program." Washington, D.C.: U. S. Government Printing Office.

Silver, George. 1976. *A Spy in the House of Medicine.* Germantown, Md.: Aspen Systems.
———. 1980. "Chiropractic: Professional controversy and public policy." *American Journal of Public Health* 70 (April): 348–50.
State of New York. 1976. "Report of the special advisory panel on medical malpractice." Albany, N.Y.: State of New York.
Wheeler, S. 1976. "Trends and problems in the sociological study of crime." *Social Problems* 23: 525–34.
Yesalis, C. E. III, *et al.* 1980. "Does chiropractic utilization substitute for less available medical services?" *American Journal of Public Health* 70 (April): 415–17.

6

Patients and Practitioners

Health care is directly influenced by those who provide it and by those who receive it. In this chapter, health care will be examined according to the kind of experiences that occur again and again when people become ill and seek professional help. Illness behavior takes into account a great range of conditions. And it would be short-sighted to ignore various social determinants of a person's health that are beyond the concerns of currently established health care delivery systems.

A person's health may be dramatically affected by his or her position in society. Even at birth, there are greater risks for infants born to poor young black women out of wedlock than to married white women in their twenties (Kessner, 1973). The type of work one performs has a direct effect on health and longevity, a finding that can be traced back as far as the eighteenth century (Knowles, 1977). Personal habits such as smoking, exercise, and eating have been shown to affect the life expectancy patterns of men (Belloc and Breslow, 1973).

Many major diseases can be prevented by changing work and living environments or through serious health education programs that clearly present the facts about drinking, smoking, and diet. At present, very little of the health budget in the United States is spent on disease prevention and control measures, health education, or environmental-health research. The allocation for these important aspects of health care amounts to only 3.25 percent of total health expenditures (Knowles, 1977: 65).

To explain why such a small proportion of total health expenditures goes toward prevention, we must look at health care within the context of what Americans believe about themselves and their health and examine what people have learned to value or prefer in their relations with others or in their images of themselves. For example, when people ignore the advice of government officials in favor of safety restraints in cars or against the use of saccharin as a sugar substitute, it may be because of firmly held beliefs that it is up to the individual to choose to take the risks involved (Lyons, 1977).

What this point of view fails to take into account is the burden the individual places on others by becoming ill or injured.

Americans' strong belief in individual rights fits well into the larger notion that the best way to take care of the needs of all people is through the free enterprise system. This system is based on the free and unrestricted acquisition of private property (legally protected) and the right of those who wish to work for others to buy and sell their labor in the marketplace. One can characterize this point of view as competitive individualism (Slater, 1970). Independence is valued because it is a sign of one's capacity to compete. Staying healthy and energetic is one way to appear independent, and it maintains one's competitive edge. Being attractive is not strictly an end in itself but a means of gaining success through influence over other people. In a country where buying and selling is the way in which goods and services are exchanged, a great deal of contact occurs between strangers, and first impressions become important.

Horace Miner, in his funny but sophisticated parody of an anthropological description of the American household, points out how much emphasis is placed on grooming and health.

> While much of the people's time is devoted to economic pursuits, a large part of the fruits of these labors and a considerable portion of the day are spent in ritual activity. The focus of this activity is the human body. . . .
>
> The fundamental belief underlying the whole system appears to be that the human body is ugly and that its natural tendency is to debility and disease. Incarcerated in such a body, man's only hope is to avert these characteristics through the use of the powerful influences of ritual and ceremony. Every household has one or more shrines devoted to this purpose. . . .
>
> The focal point of the shrine is a box or chest which is built into the wall. In this chest are kept the many charms and magical potions without which no native believes he could live. These preparations are secured from a variety of specialized practitioners. The most powerful of these are the medicine men, whose assistance must be rewarded with substantial gifts. However, the medicine men do not provide the curative potions for their clients, but decide what the ingredients should be and then write them down in an ancient and secret language. This writing is understood only by the medicine men and by the herbalists who, for another gift, provide the required charm.
>
> The charm is not disposed of after it has served its purpose but is placed in the charmbox of the household shrine. . . .
>
> The daily body ritual performed by everyone includes a mouth-rite. . . . In addition to the private mouth-rite, the people seek out a holy-mouth-man once or twice a year. [1956: 503–7]

Prevention requires long-range planning, whereas the health view of Americans is short-range, based on their individualistic, pragmatic, and technological orientations to the physical and social world, which includes their own health. What people expect from health care practitioners is derived in part from the values that they want to maintain and what they have experienced in the past. David Mechanic, in summarizing studies of health care consumers, notes the common elements:

> They seek to have a personal physician or a comparable source of care that is readily accessible to them and convenient to use. They want and expect their care to be competent, but they are equally concerned that those who provide it have an interest in them as people. They expect also that an adequate system of more specialized services will exist, if they should need them, and that they can obtain these services at a price that does not threaten them economically. [1972: 2]

Despite the simplicity in this statement, Americans are complicated in their behavior when it comes to using health care organizations such as private-practice physicians, clinics, and hospitals. And as in most other forms of social life, there are class-related differences in responding to the same symptoms. Whether to take a symptom seriously and seek professional help may depend on what rules exist among membership groups, such as families or neighborhoods. Furthermore, different ethnic groups seek alternative health care practitioners before turning to the established system. Finally, people who are better off may be risking less economically when they take a day off to see the doctor than those who are poor, who may not be covered by health insurance and may lose a day's pay, if not their job, if they are absent.

Illness behavior may vary by ethnicity. Zola studied patients at a Boston eye, ear, nose, and throat clinic and found that Irish and Italian patients from the same socioeconomic background with the same disorders presented different symptoms. Irish patients were more likely to locate pain in the parts of the body that were most appropriate to the clinical services provided. However, they were less likely than Italians to admit to pain. Italians were also more willing to admit that the symptoms they experienced made them irritable, affecting how they got along with other people (Zola, 1966). This initial point of contact between patient and practitioner may have serious consequences. If a person does not express symptoms clearly so that health care practitioners can understand or interpret them, a complete examination may never be given and certain diagnostic procedures may be overlooked.

Communication related to pain has been studied by physiologists and psychologists after physicians had noted different levels of pain tolerance (see Beecher, 1946, 1959, 1966). Interest in ethnic differences in response to pain stemmed from Zborowski's work on male patients in a New York City Veteran's Administration Hospital. He found that Italian, Jewish, Irish, and "Old American" patients responded differently to the same type of back injuries. (Old Americans were white Protestants of English, Scottish, or Welsh backgrounds.) Jewish and Italian patients were much more vocal and emotional in their complains about pain than were Old Americans and Irish. Both Italians and Jews sought to gain attention from their families because they were ill, although Italian men tried to conceal weakness in front of their families. Whereas the economic effects of their absence on the family's well-being gave great concern to Jews, this was not a major factor among Italians. The latter worried less when given pain-killing medication and expressed great confidence in their doctors, but the Jews felt that the medication only took care of the symptoms and did not deal with the cause of their complaint.

So what does the ethnic factor indicate? On the whole, Jews were more skeptical about the physician's competency, an intellectual style often associated with minority-group status. Zborowski also found that the more education and more prestigious the occupation of the patient, Jewish or Italian, the more likely the response to pain would resemble that of the Old American. As might have been expected, native born Jews and Italians were more assimilated than the foreign born (1952: 16–30), but a more detailed statistical analysis does not show these differences disappearing when education and socioeconomic status are controlled (Zborowski, 1969: 248). Laboratory studies confirm some of the findings on the culturally acquired differences in response to pain (Sternbach and Tursky, 1965; Tursky and Sternbach, 1967, as cited in Zborowski, 1969: 249–50). Other observers have also found ethnic differences in response to pain (Winsberg, 1969: 105–14), and there is virtually no challenge to such findings among scientists.

In a community study of knowledge of disease and prevention, attitudes toward medical care, and response to illness, Suchman (1964: 319–31) found ethnic and class variation. The more exclusive the social contacts of the ethnic group and the more group solidarity shown, the more alienated the group members were from the larger society. Therefore, they were less likely to accept the objectives and methods of the formal medical care system (1964: 323). In this comparison of black, Puerto Rican, Jewish, white Catholic, white Protestant, and Irish respondents, those whose contacts were mainly from the same group had more popular or nonscientific health orientation. Ethnic differences decreased greatly when social-class membership was controlled.

Group membership is sometimes a barrier to seeking professional health care among respondents with high dependence on traditional institutions such as the family and church. Therefore, assuming the sick role is difficult when it means being cut off from the sources of reward found in these institutions. This study suggests that social ties may be as important in encouraging or discouraging participation in the professional health care world as values or beliefs about health.

Culture provides recipes for living when people are well, and similar responses are available to follow when people are sick. As children, individuals learn to respond to stress situations that affect their parents, and they may unwittingly model their behavior accordingly. At the same time, the reduction of incidences of acute disease reduces opportunities to play the sick role in childhood actively (Osmond, 1980). Rather than having to invent new responses to stress situations, the ethnic group culture provides a proven set of responses. Illness behavior that is remote from the model held by health care practitioners concerning how patients should act often appear irrational or unpredictable, but nevertheless it is one way to survive difficulties. Some of these difficulties produced by the onset of diseases are related to the anxieties people experience about their future and those of their loved ones. Other anxiety-producing difficulties have to do with the limits to individual freedom and self-determination that illness creates.

BECOMING A PATIENT

If we use Mechanic's definition of illness as deviation from normal limits, then certain behaviors will occur to encourage adaptation. Once symptoms are identified by a person, many questions will be raised about his or her future. Even on a commonplace level, people may wonder about a condition: How serious is this illness? Will I miss going to that party I am looking forward to? Will I lose out on that chance for promotion? Questions of a more ultimate concern may also emerge: Will I live? Will anyone ever marry me? Will I walk again?

The career of the patient begins when he or she starts to use available information to deal with illness. A person with a headache turns to the aspirin bottle. If the pain persists or becomes unbearable, he or she may seek medical intervention. Yet many serious diseases begin with the presence of some symptom that can be identified as transitory. Sometimes people notice that they can no longer do routine tasks, such as threading a needle. The parents of polio victims saw the first signs of that dreaded disease as merely the onset of a cold or some other ordinary illness, such as a stiff neck (Davis, 1963: 21). A warning stage followed where parents became aware that the illness might be far worse. The cues came from a number of sources, including additional symptoms, the child's behavior, knowledge of other cases of polio in the community, and the doctor's tentative diagnosis (Davis, 1963: 25–26).

This beginning stage of the career of polio victims and their families can be characterized by structured uncertainty because of the limited possibilities that exist for interpreting these signs of disease. Only a small number of outcomes are possible. In a different way, parents of mentally retarded children experience a similar career sequence. The absence of neurological development, such as not sitting up at around six months, or the presence of physical stigmata, indicate that their child might be different. Despite these signs, "few parents at this point believed their children were mentally retarded. Since the discrepancies were manifested by the absence of achievement, rather than the presence of specifiable symptoms of illness, many mothers considered them to be transitory aspects of maturation" (Birenbaum, 1971: 18). Here the will to believe and the desire not to know determine the form and content of the lay diagnosis.

The uncertainty experienced by the families of polio victims or mentally retarded children raises many questions that can be resolved by the further development of symptoms, recovery, or neurological development. Parents' suspicions can be easily resolved in this way; sometimes further suspicions may appear. Continued contact with and advice from health care personnel produces new considerations for the patient or guardian. Patients may feel, with or without justification, that those who provide health care services have not told them everything. They may become suspicious when the physician spends a great deal of time performing a particular diagnostic procedure, for example.

Some patients infer from such behavior that they are not being told the full extent of their illness, its seriousness, or the likelihood of serious permanent impairment. They often derive this secondary information from a physician's behavior: from topics avoided in conversation, from physical responses such as heavy perspiration or the avoidance of eye contact, or by answering the patient's questions with questions, getting the patient to provide his or her own answers. Finally, patients can tell when they are not being told everything when they observe others observing them intensely. This may be particularly evident in teaching hospitals when rounds are conducted to show uncommon diseases or the effects of new or unusual procedures.

From the point of view of the professional, the patient needs help, usually through the application of a proven procedure. As a patient, one may agree, even lightly referring to "taking in the old machine for a tune up." However, when doctors become patients, even with their superior knowledge of procedures, they may suspect all is not right and often express the same feelings as lay people.

Knowledge is the basis of the relationship between practitioner and patient, and knowledge is applied through techniques of diagnosis and treatment. Receiving health services is a unique social situation, (Goffman, 1961: 346) and patient compliance is important in arriving at a successful treatment of the problem. Sometimes compliance is induced for other reasons. Health care practitioners often do not let the patient know when they do not know what needs to be done or that something has gone wrong (although the sophistication of patients, increased record keeping, and the specter of malpractice may alter this characterization). The reputation of the doctor and the hospital depends on keeping such information from patients. In order to maintain confidence, the patient must be treated with respect, and some common patient reactions such as puzzlement and bewilderment have to be dealt with indirectly.

The goals of service are still primary, despite the need to attend to the impressions made on patients. Moreover, medical services are usually offered by one physician to many patients, and care often involves a team of professionals, making the use of time and place a crucial factor in getting things done. Organizational goals, usually expressed in the form of productivity or maximized use of facilities can become more important than a particular patient's need to receive an explanation for why a procedure is being performed. Sometimes patients receive the wrong procedure as a result of these organizational goals.

From the perspective of patients or their guardians, contact with physicians and paramedical personnel sometimes makes them feel that they are not being treated as people. This point of contact reduces the patients' sense of control over their own lives. The patient sometimes is treated like a serviceable object under the justification that in order to care for many patients in the same setting, time and space must be used efficiently. The condition presents a dilemma to all who work in health care professions. As the cost of care rises, patients may be less willing to tolerate unexplained practices. Goffman aptly articulates the need to consider the human side of medical work, a task that practitioners often fail to perform.

> The server has contact with two basic entities: a client and the client's malfunctioning object. Clients are presumably self-determining beings, entities in the social world that must be treated with appropriate regard and ritual. The possessed object is part of another world, to be construed within a technical, not a ritual, perspective. The success of the serving depends on the server keeping these two different kinds of entities separate while giving each its due [1961: 329]

THE PATIENT IN THE ORGANIZED WORLD OF HEALTH CARE

Starting with Goffman's acute observation, the patient who comes into the organized world of health care is both a product to be changed or altered (i.e., made better) and a member of the organization. Health care organizations cannot exist without patients, thus patients become the lower-level personnel in the organization. The longer the patient stays in a hospital, the more this characteristic is apparent, as in the case of mental patients (Goffman, 1961) or those in a rehabilitation hospital (Roth, 1963).

Objections can be raised to viewing the patient as almost an employee. The patient pays for the services received, either directly or indirectly. The payers in a strictly business relationship would seem to have the upper hand, telling the seller of a product or service when, where, and how they want delivery. Yet patients cannot tell professionals how to proceed, even where they can set the terms of the service, as in the case of a national health service that employs physicians.

When patients pay for a consultation with a physician, it appears that they are employing the provider of services. Yet patients do not own the office or the tools or machinery used. Even when groups of patients contract with physicians to provide all medical services required, as in the case of Hospital Insurance Plan of Greater New York, Kaiser-Permanente of California, or the new congressionally sanctioned Health Maintenance Organizations, the group practice provides equipment and facilities.

In general, physicians practice in hospitals that are voluntary and nonprofit, meaning that others do not live off their labor, realizing income without work. Administrators cannot earn more by getting greater productivity out of the medical staff.

By and large hospitals are overseen by a board of directors or trustees made up of unpaid but supposedly public-spirited members of the community. They are usually influential in the business world, and are capable of raising money for the hospital. Hospitals can acquire wealth by increasing their assets, but individuals cannot gain from the disposition of the assets.

Patients can be compared to students insofar as students pay fees and, in most instances, draw no financial remuneration for their participation in university life. As in the case of students' contact with faculty, the patient has far less power than the doctor or other health care personnel. Control over the situation remains in the hands of the health care personnel because of the uncertainty faced by the patients about their illnesses. Two propositions from the literature on organizations neatly summarize how power is maintained:

> *Information control.* The more exclusively an individual controls information about areas of uncertainty in an organization, the greater his power to control others' behavior.
>
> The greater the consequences the resolution of an uncertainty has for an individual, or the larger the network of individuals affected by the resolution of an uncertainty, the greater the power of whoever controls information about that area of uncertainty. [Collins, 1975: 310]

Organizations are created to solve problems that cannot be solved on one's own or through informal groups such as families. Usually they are initiated to serve some cultural value or belief, and resources are allocated for this purpose. Some organizations have developed standard procedures for turning out a product and for creating a uniform commodity. One may be able to tell the difference between Coke and Pepsi, but it is difficult to tell which area of the country a can of Coke came from or whether the same ounce of Pepsi drunk in a glass came from one can or another. Service organizations have a variety of complex tasks to perform, and they often depend on using the client to determine how a problem is to be solved. Communication between client and practitioner is based on giving and acquiring information.

Health care organizations are created to solve the problems of patients, but since information is controlled by professionals, patients often do not know what they must do in order to be cooperative. Sometimes the physician's uncertainty is kept from the patient in order not to appear incompetent and to maintain a favorable impression. Patients have been found to terminate relationships with physicians when the doctors are perceived as being inadequate, incompetent, or less skilled when compared to other physicians (Hayes-Bautista, 1976: 12; Kasteler et al., 1976: 328–39).

The solutions of health care organizations are fairly predictable, including the type of procedures performed, who is to perform them, and the amount of time and space required. Staff time and the use of space (e.g., hospital beds, operating rooms, emergency services) are major problems that must be managed by the administration. Similarly, in group practices, the overuse of laboratory staff time can become a problem when many tests are ordered, some of which are not medically indicated (Freidson, 1975: 61).

Standardized technical procedures may exist, for example in dealing with the problem of prevention of smallpox through immunization. Other tasks require investigative work to determine one ailment from many others where symptoms are similar, as in the case of lupus, a disease of the immunization system of the body. Uncertainty and unpredictability prevail: The long-term outlook for the patient with lupus is highly unpredictable; therapy may work in some cases and fail in others.

Certainly, preventive health care through immunization procedures lends itself to scheduling, either through massive campaigns to get everyone inoculated (as took place in the case of swine flu) or through regular visits to health care organizations for inoculations, usually given early in life. Nevertheless, medicine is hardly unanimous in approving these costly efforts that afford so little protection.

Some problems treated by health care organizations are not predictable, either because the patient does not know when he or she will need treatment, as in the case of an automobile accident, or how long the treatment will take, as in the case of recovery from an amputation of a leg. Under these conditions, the use of staff time and the management of space becomes more complicated. At such times, patients' cooperation is usually required. Patients can feel powerlessness when expected information is not forthcoming, and thus treatment can be undermined.

Organizations develop plans for dealing with the expected, using, for example, experiences based on different times of day or night, on weather, or on neighborhood. Emergency rooms of city hospitals treat a great number of gunshot and knife wounds on summer evenings. For the practitioner, emergencies often become routine. Standardized procedures exist for treating emergencies, such as cardiac arrest or acute appendicitis, and techniques are available to assess the performance of the task. Utilization of procedures can be reviewed through examination of tissue removed in operations, determining whether the surgery was justified, or through examining the adequacy of prescribing a particular drug to a patient with certain symptoms. Standing review committees made up of physicians and other professionals perform these tasks in most hospitals.

Certain facilities and organizations have been developed within hospitals for dealing with the volume of unpredictable cases. Some emergency-rooms cases do not require immediate attention, and a special position may be created to deal with this problem. The triage nurse sorts out patients who need immediate care, those who can wait, and those who can be seen at another time in an appropriate ambulatory or outpatient clinic. Some of these decisions are easily made, as when a stabbing victim is brought in by ambulance. However, the more ambiguous the case, the more difficult the decision and the greater the uncertainty over whether the person needs treatment. One can become fearful of being indifferent for a patient's complaints or not taking a complaint seriously. The following story is related about a triage nurse at Bellevue Hospital in New York City, perhaps the most famous emergency room in the United States.

> "I remember this tremendously fat woman who was brought in just before my tour was finished," the nurse related. "She complained of chest pains. She was three times my size, and there were no aides around at the time to help me undress her. So I struggled with her, and I hated it because she must have fallen into some dog feces.
>
> "I kept saying to myself, there's nothing wrong with her. I'm going through all this for nothing. And I said to her, 'Oh, lady, I wish you were thinner'; and I knew that I wouldn't want any daughters of mine ever doing what I was doing.
>
> "The woman was given a cardiogram, and then she began to turn blue. She died

quietly. There was nothing I or anyone else could have done to save her, but I cried for days afterward." [Sullivan, 1977: B4]

Fred Davis, in his study of the families of polio victims, observed that information control is exercised by physicians on the child's prognosis long after clinical certainty has been established: ". . . uncertainty, a *real* factor in the early diagnosis and treatment of the paralyzed child, came more and more to serve the purely managerial ends of the treatment personnel in their interaction with parents" (Davis, 1972: 243)

Davis suggests several plausible reasons for the discrepancy between what is known by health care personnel and what is told. First, telling parents that their children would be crippled for life would often involve an extreme emotional reaction to which physicians would have to immediately respond. Second, since the outcome was initially uncertain, parents continued to believe that full recovery was possible, often passing up useful rehabilitation procedures and therapy. Finally, getting the parents to accept the outcome, one which almost always radically redefines the family and the child, is a task that physicians would prefer to avoid (1972: 243–44).

Davis also examines the differences in presenting a prognosis when doctors are self-employed and are based in the community compared with doctors who work at a hospital. While community-based physicians are often encouraged to see a family through the bad news of learning that their child will be disabled, they also avoid expressing uncertainty even when they are clinically unsure or because they want to maintain a good reputation among neighborhood clientele. Referrals to specialized clinics for diagnosis may be based on the family physician or pediatrician's desire to give information in a direct manner, but not in a way that would affect the personal relationship with the family (Davis, 1972: 246).

Similar themes are found in other families experiencing crises. Attendance of mothers at developmental disability clinics helped them to understand their children's mental retardation and get a definite medical opinion. As a result, mothers could reevaluate their expectations for the child while acquiring a naturalistic explanation of the origin of the disability.

> Respondent: . . . and of course, I didn't know what to do. I had never come in contact with any retarded children at all. I mean, I'd see somebody on the street and I—I didn't look. I—you know. But it was—I took her from doctor to doctor, and frankly, they don't know either. So . . .
>
> Interviewer: What did the doctors say—the ones you went to?
>
> Respondent: Ah, they said, well, from what they could see according to her development, according to her age, she seemed retarded. But still, they said let's see what happens. Sometimes after a year, you know . . . I went to a meeting, and I spoke to somebody, you know, who knew. And he said go down to Flower and Fifth (Avenue Hospital). That's the place to. I said, I have never heard of it. I says. And as far as that, Columbia (Presbyterian Hospital) is better. And they said no, go there. And I saw the difference once I went there, you know.
>
> Interviewer: What do you mean, you saw the difference?

> Respondent: Well, they really knew. I mean they knew what they were looking for. You know at that time she didn't walk, you know. Her feet were like this. And when I took her to the Orthopedic Department—because at Columbia, you know, you get a workup, individually—and there a few doctors looked at her and said, you know, I think she has club feet. [Birenbaum, 1969: 380]

INFORMATION AND COMPLIANCE

The sociological study of information control in organizations reveals a great deal about the situation of patients in the organized world of health care, and it establishes that sharing information can improve the rate of compliance of patients with treatment regimens. This is particularly evident in the behavior of patients with regard to taking medication for illness where there are no visible symptoms or where symptoms are sporadic. Learning how to tell patients what to do is a skill that may be just as important as diagnosis or treatment.

Communication in health care has become the concern of many professionals, not just of doctors. Recently, the Millis Report (1975), a study of pharmacy, recommended that pharmacists learn how to instruct patients in the use of medications. To accomplish this goal, pharmacists were recommended to take courses in the social and behavioral sciences. There is good reason for this: Studies of compliance with treatment regimens involving medication reveal a startling low rate of success in getting patients to follow doctors' orders. In one study, no more than half and as little as one-quarter of the patients were even taking the drugs prescribed (Haggerty and Roghman, 1972). And this situation is aggravated when one takes into account whether other instructions relating to the drugs were obeyed; for example, frequency, time, and accompanying food or drink.

Whereas great progress has been made in health care technology, social skills are necessary to get patients to follow treatment regimens. Simple technology exists for the control of rheumatic fever through oral penicillin treatment, and urine analysis indicates whether patients actually took the drug. In one controlled study, 36 percent of 136 patients took this medication one-fourth of the prescribed time or less (Gordis, Markowitz, and Lilienfeld, 1969a: 173). In the same study (reported by Gordis et al., 1969b), compliance was more likely to occur where rheumatic heart disease was present, a more serious illness than rheumatic fever, and where activity was medically restricted. In addition, previous hospitalization for acute attack was associated with higher rates of compliance with the treatment regimen. Higher frequencies of noncompliance occurred in larger families and in those that displayed fatalistic attitudes toward life. Such findings can help identify families that need additional instruction on the use of the medication.

Communication involves responding to patients as well as directing them. In the doctor-patient relationship, one must be able to listen as well as instruct. The nostalgic image of the family doctor, often invoked when contemporary health care is criticized, represents a wish for someone who will encourage the patient to communicate. Leon Eisenberg, a psychiatrist, expresses the importance of this. Ideally, the following expectations suggested by Eisenberg will improve the quality of health care.

> The doctor's task ought still to be to educate the patient about the meaning of the illness and the methods for its remedy, after he has learned the patient's conception of its cause and how it might be treated. The process is one of exchange of information, the goal is the demystification of medical procedures, so that the patient is able to make his own decisions and thereby assume responsibility for acting. [1977: 237]

What actually goes on between doctor and patient is often not very rewarding or encouraging to the patient. In a study of the procedures used by medical students to gather information about children's symptoms, the analysis of the information by students and their supervisors to obtain the diagnosis, and the application of remedies appropriate for the respected diagnoses, observations were made and judged by a panel of pediatricians. Data were collected from direct observations of history taking and physical examinations, interviews, and a review of the child's hospital record (Duff, Rowe, and Anderson, 1972).

Referral notes from physicians, public health nurses, or agencies accompanied the twenty-five children who were examined. Medical students were able to evaluate in advance whether the case was of potential interest to them. Six students thought they would learn something from the visit, three were neutral, and in sixteen instances, students concluded that the child was of minimal interest to them. Ten of these 16 were children who subsequently presented symptoms of "developmental, behavioral or social problems as the primary basis for their complaints, and the students felt that such patients did not prepare them for treating diseases in the future" (1972: 841). The other six cases were seen by students to be "intake visits" for the specialty clinics, e.g., allergy, cardiology. These interviews were resented because students felt that they were not learning anything from them.

The first encounter between students and the parents can hardly be said to encourage cooperation; nor did students do better in making the children feel comfortable.

> At the beginning of the history taking session, 16 students (64%) introduced themselves; the others started the encounter with questions, usually about the chief complaint. In all instances, regardless of the topic being discussed, children were present throughout the visit. In spite of the fact that 16 children were more than three years of age and had at least some ability to communicate verbally, only two students directed some questions or other forms of attention to the child before starting the physical examination. [1972: 841]

The panel of pediatrician-observers categorized the problems presented as 12 percent physical, 26 percent psychosocial, and 52 percent a combination of the two. Twenty-three students were observed turning aside 156 questions or leading comments by parents; in twenty-seven instances eleven students injected their own value judgments in evaluating the parents' comments. Observations and interviews revealed that students and families agreed in five cases on what were the main problems of the child. Physical examinations went smoothly in nine cases, all where students made efforts to prepare the child before beginning procedures.

The importance of gaining the cooperation of the parents as well as the child was indicated by the assessments made of the problems presented. Problems were assigned from a medical management standpoint to four categories: simple (20%), moderately complicated (20%), very complicated (24%), and extremely complicated (36%). Eighty percent of the problems were seen as complicated, mainly medical problems that were worsened by the neglect or failure of parents to note or monitor the child's chronic condition (e.g., anemia), secondary illnesses (e.g., pneumonia), or somatic and behavioral complaints (e.g., destructive behavior) by a child whose mother was divorced.

It is clear from this study that the quality of communication between doctor and parents of patients was unsatisfactory. Clinical visits resulted in major contributions to problem solving in six instances (24%), according to the authors' evaluation of the clinic contribution; minor contributions were made in only five cases (20%); and no significant contribution was made in fourteen cases (56%). Only four student-family pairs agreed in post-clinic interviews that the management was satisfactory; seven pairs agreed the management was unsatisfactory; the remaining fourteen had various combinations of feelings or no opinion. The authors conclude that except in cases where symptoms were obvious (e.g., heart murmurs, congenital deformity), presenting easily diagnosed and readily managed problems (24%), there was little effort or interest evinced by clinic personnel. "As a result, many common problems of children were neglected; and we infer that the teaching of professionals was correspondingly defective" (1972: 846).

The significance of this study should not be downplayed because it was conducted on medical students and their supervisors. A number of studies of patient satisfaction with doctor-patient interaction report that the failure to meet certain implicitly held expectations will lead to dissatisfaction. Few of these studies indicate whether dissatisfaction significantly affects compliance with treatment regimens.

One aspect of doctor-patient interaction is the reception of clear information and the comprehension of that information as to the illness diagnosed. In a study of a clinic population in a Cleveland hospital, investigators found that only four in ten patients understood the nature of the illness when the physician's diagnosis was used as the criterion. Only 44 percent were aware of the prognosis for their illness, with patients suffering from acute conditions more aware of their problems in general than those suffering from chronic conditions (Sussman et al., 1967). Interestingly, patients tended to blame themselves for failures to understand instructions from physicians or descriptions of their condition.

In general, patients thought they were receiving good care and complained only when they thought they were not receiving sufficient attention.

> There is, however, one element in the area of patient experience which does matter, and that is *time spent with the physician.* Patients who spend less than 15

> minutes with the physician are much more likely to be dissatisfied with the clinic than those who spend more time, and the differences are statistically significant. [italics in original] [1967: 68]

Patients also expect certain kinds of questions to be asked in the consultation with physicians that would enable them to articulate their major concerns (Korsch, Gozzi, and Francis, 1968). The patients' compliance with medical advice increased when physicians took the time to explain the cause of an illness (Francis, Korsch, and Morris, 1969), and parents were more likely to regard contact with pediatricians rewarding and satisfying when they received praise for the care they gave to the child (Freeman et al., 1971: 298–311).

Do changes in procedures encourage patients to present concerns that are ordinarily ignored in office visits? Korsch and her associates attempted to increase the amount of time spent with each mother coming in for routine purposes with a well child by adding contact with a nurse. The time spent was increased from an average of ten minutes for the physician to twenty-one minutes for the nurse. This increase in time did not qualitatively alter the nature of the interaction, since the nurse placed the same emphasis on the components of the visit. Increasing the time for interaction between patient and practitioner without increasing the skills of the practitioner gives the appearance of quality care without its substance. Interestingly, the research interviews elicited areas of psychosocial concern and behavior problems, rarely expressed by mothers to the physician or nurse (1971: 483–88).

Few studies examine the ways in which physicians transmit their expectations and motivate their patients. In a notable exception, Svarstad asked why physicians sometimes fail to achieve the patients' conformity with medication advice. There was systematic observation of 153 adult patients interacting with 8 full-time physicians, a review of medical records and pharmacy files, followup interviews with the patients about a week after their clinic visits, and validation of the patients' reported behavior by means of a "bottle check" (Svarstad, 1976: 223). Thus Svarstad focused on three aspects of the physician's role performance: (1) the nature of physician's instruction to the patient, including the clarity of instructions, the availability of written instructions, the consistency between verbal and written instructions, and physician information about the name and purpose of the drug; (2) the efforts made to motivate the patient through friendliness, justification, and the invocation of medical authority; and (3) monitoring the patient's use of previously prescribed drugs (Svarstad, 1976).

The results of this study indicate that combinations of high instructional effort with friendly or authoritative communication is associated with conformity with medical service.

> Under the conditions of high, moderate and low effort to motivate, the rates of behavioral conformity were 80 percent, 41 percent, and 13 percent, respectively. The relationship between physician effort to motivate and patient behavior was even more evident when the amount of physician instruction was taken into account. Under high instruction, patient conformity ranged from 100 percent (high effort) to 11 percent (low effort). In contrast, patient conformity ranged from

> 60 percent (high effort) to 13 percent (low effort) under the condition of low physician instruction. [Svarstad, 1976: 234]

Svarstad notes the importance of physicians' elicitation of feedback from patients in order to find out whether the patient understands or needs further clarification, instruction, or interpretation. Followup is also required to maintain patient compliance, in order to elicit complaints about the treatment plan, and indications of whether drugs were being taken or used appropriately (1976: 235). Patients often have questions or complaints but do not know whether they have the right to complain or whether they will be humiliated, reprimanded, or in some other way punished for admissions of disagreement with the doctor's advice. Communication between the patient and the doctor sometimes breaks down over the prescription, and the former may conceal his nonconformity. Errors in clinical judgment can follow, based on receiving inaccurate information from the sick. Those who develop a mistrust of physicians, on the basis of receiving an inappropriate treatment regimen, sometimes go off on their own, creating, in effect, their own treatment plan. If patients have opportunities to admit to nonconformity and there is a demonstration of responsiveness by the physician, then compliance occurs.

People who seek help from organized health care are not always aware of the expectations for their behavior. Practitioners often take for granted that patients understand their instructions, or they fail to emphasize the importance of a followup sufficiently. The quality of health care ultimately rests on these systematic efforts, exemplified in a comprehensive-care program that reduced the incidence of rheumatic fever in Baltimore children. While a 60-percent reduction in the incidence of new cases appeared in census tracts where children received this type of care, the rate remained unchanged among children living elsewhere in the city where routine care existed (Gordis, et al., 1973: 331).

The organizational framework of health care is confusing enough for patients, but it is in the process of change. Increased confusion may result despite improvement in technical effectiveness, however. Caring involves concern for the nontechnical as well as the technical aspects. Increased differentiation of tasks often leaves patients feeling that no one is looking out for them, even when they are receiving sophisticated treatment. The major changes in knowledge, technology, financing, and demand have helped to shape health care delivery, and the complicated work of curing and caring for the sick has taken on new dimensions.

REFERENCES

Beecher, Henry K. 1946. "Pain in men wounded in battle." *Bulletin of U.S. Army Medical Department* 5: 445–54.

———. 1959. *Measurement of Subjective Responses: Quantitative Effect of Drugs.* New York: Oxford University Press.

———. 1966. "Pain: The mystery solved." *Science* 151: 840–41.

Belloc, M. B., and L. Breslow. 1973. "Relationship of health practices and mortality." *Preventive Medicine* 2: 67–81.

Birenbaum, A. 1969. "Helping mothers of retarded children use specialized facilities." *The Family Coordinator* 18 (October): 379–85.

———. 1971. "The recognition and acceptance of stigma." *Sociological Symposium* 7 (Fall): 15–22.

Collins, Randall. 1975. *Conflict Sociology: Toward an Explanatory Science.* New York: Academic Press.

Davis, Fred. 1963. *Passage Through Crisis: Polio Victims and Their Families.* Indianapolis, Bobbs-Merrill.

Davis, F. 1972. "Uncertainty in medical prognosis: Clinical and functional." Pp. 239–48 in Eliot Freidson and Judith Lober, eds., *Medical Men and Their Work: A Sociological Reader.* Chicago: Aldine.

Duff, R. S., D. S. Rowe, and F. P. Anderson. 1972. "Patient care and student learning in a pediatric clinic." *Pediatrics* 50 (December): 839–46.

Eisenberg, Leon. 1977. "The search for care." *Deadalus* (Winter): 235–46.

Francis, V., B. Korsch, and J. J. Morris. 1969. "Gaps in doctor-patient communication: Patients response to medical advice." *New England Journal of Medicine* 280: 535–40.

Freeman, B., et al., 1971. "Gaps in doctor-patient communication: Doctor-patient interaction analysis." *Pediatric Research* 5: 298–311.

Goffman, Erving. 1961. "The medical model and mental hospitalization: Some notes on the vicissitudes of the tinkering trades." Pp. 321–86 in *Asylums: Essays on the Social Situation of Mental Patients and Other Inmates.* Garden City, N.Y.: Doubleday Anchor.

Gordis, L., M. Markowitz, and A. M. Lillenfeld. 1969a. "Studies in the epidemiology and preventability of rheumatic fever IV. A quantitative determination of compliance in children on oral penicillin prophylaxis." *Pediatrics* 43: 173–81.

———. 1969b. "Why patients don't follow medical advice: A study of children on long-term antistreptococcal prophylaxis." *Journal of Pediatrics* 75: 957–68.

Gordis, L. 1973. "Effectiveness of comprehensive care programs in preventing rheumatic fever." *New England Journal of Medicine* 289 (August): 331–335.

Haggerty, R. J., and K. S. Roghman. "Non-compliance and self medication." *Pediatric Clinics of North America* 19: 101–15.

Hayes-Bautista, D. E. 1976. "Termination of the patient-practitioner relationship: Divorce, patient style." *Journal of Health and Social Behavior* 17 (March): 12–21.

Kasteler, J., R. L. Lane, D. M. Olsen, and C. Thetford. 1976. "Issues underlying prevalence of 'doctor-shopping' behavior." *Journal of Health and Social Beahvior* 17 (December): 328–39.

Kessner, D. S. 1973. *Infant Death: An Analysis of Maternal Risk and Health Care.* Washington, D.C.: Institute of Medicine, National Academy of Sciences.

Knowles, Jr. 1977. "The responsibility of the individual." *Deadalus* (Winter): 57–80.

Korsch, B. M., E. K. Gozzi, and V. Francis. "Gaps in doctor-patient communication: Doctor-patient interaction and patient satisfaction." *Pediatrics* 42: 855–71.

Lyons, R. D. 1977. "Refusal of many to heed government health advice is linked to growing distrust of authority." *New York Times* June 12, p. 55.

Mechanic, David. 1972. *Public Expectations and Health Care: Essays on the Changing Organization of Health Services.* New York: Wiley Interscience.

Millis, John. 1975. *Pharmacists for the Future: The Report of the Study Commission on Pharmacy.* Ann Arbor, Mich.: Health Administration Press.

Miner, H. 1956. "Body ritual among the Nacirema." *American Anthropologist* 58: 503–7.

Osmond, H. 1980. "God and the doctor." *New England Journal of Medicine* 302 (March 6): 555–58.

Roth, Julius. 1963. *Timetables.* Indianapolis: Bobbs-Merrill.

Slater, Philip. 1970. *Pursuit of Loneliness: American Culture at the Breaking Point.* Boston: Beacon Press.

Suchman, E. 1964. "Sociomedical variations among ethnic groups." *American Journal of Sociology* 70: 319–31.

Sullivan, R. 1977. "Standing nightly triage watch on Bellevue's busy battlefield." *New York Times,* June 9: B1, 4.

Sussman, Marvin B., Eleanor K. Caplan, Marie Haug, and Marjorie R. Stern. 1967. *The Walking Patient.* Cleveland: Case Western Reserve University Press.

Svarstad, B. 1976. "Physician-patient communication and patient conformity with medical advice." Pp. 220–38 in David Mechanic et al., *The Growth of Bureaucratic Medicine: An Inquiry into the Dynamics of Patient Behavior and the Organization of Medical Care.* New York: Wiley Interscience.

Winsberg, B. 1969. "Pain response in Negro and white obstetrical patients." *Journal of Health and Social Behavior* 10: 105–14.

Zborowski, M. 1952. "Cultural components in response to pain." *Journal of Social Issues* 8: 16–30.

———. 1969. *People in Pain.* San Francisco: Jossey Bass.

Zola, I. K. 1966. "Culture and symptoms: An analysis of patients presenting complaints." *American Sociological Review* 31: 615–30.

7

The Social Organization and Division of Labor of Hospitals

Health care is the second largest share of the gross national product, and it is a major source of employment in the United States, with more than four million people providing direct or indirect health care services, and it is the most important source of new jobs. The demand for care seems endless, and the field of medicine encourages this expansion by taking on new tasks (e.g., the treatment of alcoholism), developing new technologies (e.g., body scanners), and identifying new diseases (e.g., hyperactivity in children). The number of physicians has increased, and there are now 171 physicians for every 100,000 people (American Medical Association, 1974: 120). Physicians make up only ten percent of the total number of health care positions.

The development of health care as a major employer is one of the most interesting and paradoxical stories in the sociology of work because it defies the general tendency for technology to replace labor. Technology in health care encourages more employment rather than less. More than 70 percent of all health care personnel work in general hospitals. For every hospital bed in general hospitals in the United States there are 3.1 persons or full-time equivalents. Full-time equivalents refer to one-half the hours put in on the part of students or trainees, whose labor time is counted along with paid employees (Silver, 1976: 147). Labor costs account for 70 percent of the budget of major short-term general hospitals (Steton, 1977: B18).

The increase in the number of health care employees is matched by the proliferation of jobs in the field. There are more than two hundred health care specialties identified in the Department of Labor's *Dictionary of Occupational Titles*. In the late 1960s and early 1970s, many articles in major medical journals advocated the creation of new health care practitioners or evaluated their performance. The introduction of technology has not only resulted in many new positions, such as inhalation therapists and histologic or blood technicians, but these positions require assistants and aides. Occupational therapists, radiology technologists, and social workers are free to do the more complicated work, while assistants take over the routine assignments.

These changes in the division of labor have occurred under the direction and control of physicians (Cambridge Research Institute, 1975: 328). Medicine itself has become increasingly specialized, with only 47 percent of all doctors providing primary care. There are 65 AMA-approved medical specialties, and it appears that physicians in training are avoiding primary care. As of 1973, only 37 percent of physicians in residency programs were in primary care specialties (CRI, 1975: 357). The creation of the newer middle-level specialties, such as nurse practitioner and physician's assistant, has resulted from this shortage of physicians.

This chapter will use the concepts of technology, market and financing arrangements, and social organization to account for the growth of the division of labor in health care in the United States. The division of labor in health care is the product of the dynamic interplay of new factors that are continuously being added to the health care delivery system. Before this can be fully developed, it is necessary to examine the old division of labor in health care.

THE OLD DIVISION OF LABOR

The old division of labor in health care was organized around three major positions: the physician, the nurse, and the pharmacist. The services they delivered become most highly coordinated when there are predictable tasks to perform and standardized techniques available for solving these tasks. The formation of the hospital as the work place for the doctor, nurse, and pharmacist parallels the establishment of the factory for the production of goods.

Hospitals have existed since antiquity, with some Greek temples devoted to health care dating back to the twelfth century B.C. Hospitals were established in the Middle Ages by religious orders or communities to tend to the sick who had no families or who were too poor to pay for care (Haines, 1938: 405). People with family or financial means avoided hospitals because they took care of people with contagious diseases, those who were dying, or patients of low standing in the community. Simply established to do good deeds, hospitals were conceived as charitable creations performed to please God in an imperfect and uncertain world (Rosen, 1963). Later, they became established as places to learn more about nature and ways to control it, tasks that were important to the newly emerging commercial elites of seventeenth and eighteenth century Europe and America.

In the nineteenth century, community notables, mainly business and factory owners, started hospitals to create an orderly and predictable world. Physicians gave orders to nurses on how to care for patients, and pharmacists compounded medications according to the doctor's specifications. Pharmacy was once linked to the role of grocer, since many of the prescriptions were herbal in origin, and it still maintains a community orientation.

In the hospital setting, both nursing and pharmacy were dependent on the physician to perform diagnosis and treatment. Therefore, the two roles could interact with patients only under medical direction. Furthermore, the physician did not need them in order to begin diagnosis and treatment. In many instances, doctors maintained direct contact with patients throughout the illness, particularly if patients were cared for at home by a family, which could provide necessary attention. Sometimes families specialized in caring for others when individuals had no kin or in unusual circumstances, as when a traveler became ill in a foreign place.

The links between medicine and nursing were inconsistent until certain organizational and technological developments occurred in the second half of the nineteenth century, when war made nursing a necessary component of hospital care. Nurses, under the direction of Florence Nightingale in the Crimean War and Clara Barton in the American Civil War, proved their worth in saving lives. Treating wounded at or near the battlefield could not have been undertaken without disciplined nurses who could take over some of the doctor's tasks.

Prior to this, nursing was organized by religious orders and sometimes by secular organizations of women. The new form of health care resembled military organization. Orders were to be followed in a disciplined way, and specific tasks were assigned to clearly identified positions in a division of labor. Doctors and nurses were to be guided by explicitly stated duties, set down in written rules, and these positions were hierarchically organized so that decision making and information gathering—the procedures of diagnosis and treatment—were clearly in the hands of the physicians. This hierarchical organization was evident in the respect that nurses were to pay doctors, even to the point that nurses were to stand up whenever a doctor entered a room.

Such a form of social organization is based on coordinating the efforts of various specialists. The solution to the task of dealing with hundreds or even thousands of wounded followed the procedures that have come to be known as bureaucracy. The application of bureaucracy to wartime health care was necessary, given the magnitude and constancy of the problem.

During the late nineteenth and early twentieth century, technological advances made it possible to perform more precise diagnoses and treatment and to standardize surgical procedures. The invention of the X-ray machine meant that the source of some disorders could be located, and that physicians could see bones that were broken or in the process of healing. Anesthesia made surgery more manageable, while techniques established to prevent sepsis (or the infection of wounds during and after surgery), made it possible to save lives that previously would have been lost.

The introduction of new technology quickly displaced the distinguished citizens as directors of hospitals, and physicians assumed complete control over decision making, even in nonmedical areas such as housekeeping and the purchase of supplies.

The control of hospitals by medical personnel assured them that good working facilities would be available, although monetary considerations were not absent from motivation. Surgery required the availability of an operating room and assistance in performing procedures to monitor recovery, and physicians could encourage the acquisition of new technology and costly equipment.

Until this point, hospitals served the physician not so much as a workshop for treating people but primarily as a place to learn about diseases not seen in daily practice. The central location of facilities and equipment meant that several doctors could use them when needed. The availability of a nursing staff also made daily care more predictable. A pool of paying patients could be directed to a hospital where physicians knew in advance that their orders for care would be followed. Physicians had admitting rights or access to beds for patients. The house staff, composed of interns and residents, provided low-cost labor. Physicians affiliated with a hospital would supervise the house staff and also examine and treat charity patients.

Hospitals also provided a ready market for technology because they could afford to buy devices and drugs in large supply. Inventors and discoverers of technological innovations became increasingly attuned to this predictable market. The size and constancy of the market also encouraged the development of relatively cheap and effective solutions to public health problems. Immunizations against childhood diseases and the use of sulfa and antibiotics are relatively simple and low-cost solutions because they are mass produced by autonomous continuous flow processes and require relatively little labor to administer. Even more recent technological innovations in medicine have not had such significant impacts in reducing death rates.

THE MODERN HOSPITAL

The modern hospital may be one of the most complicated organizations in existence. Hospitals not only seek to save lives and reduce suffering, but they also prepare for the future. Research on disease, the evaluation of the effectiveness of drug therapies, and the evaluation of different ways of delivering services are important goals. Furthermore, many hospitals serve as training organizations for doctors, nurses, and other health care personnel. On-the-job training through internships and residency programs not only provides cheap labor to the hospital but also requires allocation of staff time for supervision of these trainees.

A hospital depends on the delegation of responsibility for daily operations, generally by the chiefs of medical services. Directors of medical services have more specialized knowledge than the physician who is president or the director of the hospital. Therefore, decisions on medical tasks must be made through intensive consultation with experts. Because the authority of the physician in the corporate organization of the hospital is recognized, the occupant of the top office is usually a physician rather than an expert in management. Some students of organizations have characterized the modern hospital as one kind of structure in which administration or management does not set goals and supervise work performance as much as provide the resources necessary to carry out goals set by the experts (Etzioni, 1961).

Hospitals have dual lines of authority because of the way in which physicians are able to override administrative decisions, although the latter had apparently been made for the good of the entire organization (Smith, 1958). The behavior of physicians does not always follow the formal rules of hospitals, as developed by administrators (Goss, 1962, 1963). The formal rules, for example, may state that the Housekeeping Department has to clean wards and rooms at 8 A.M. every morning. This rule may be set aside unilaterally by the physician who wants to perform a procedure for a patient at that hour and does not want to be disturbed. Since attending physicians may visit patients at unpredictable times, the hospital administrator may exercise little control over the coordination of work schedules.

By virtue of their economic independence, physicians are not subject to the same controls as other health care providers. Attending physicians have admitting rights at a hospital but are not paid staff members; therefore, the administrator cannot coerce physicians to be more observant of the rules. Their rights to admit patients could be rescinded, but some hospitals depend on attending physicians to refer patients and provide other services, such as teaching and clinic involvement. Prestigious physicians are attractions for the hospital, making it easier to recruit interns and residents of high quality, acquire research funding and service grants, and even to gain the affiliation of other prestigious doctors. The reputations of a hospital and its attending physicians are mutually supportive.

The physician's capacity to overrule schedules is inherent in a hospital. Because illness can be unpredictable, a physician has the right to declare a medical emergency, although it will disrupt schedules, or even order a nurse to leave an assignment to get some needed equipment (Coser, 1958). Understandably, the paramedical staff in a hospital has to work under this dual authority, as when a nurse must be responsible to both a nursing supervisor and the physicians to whom she is assigned.

Working in this kind of power structure is difficult at best. When people receive conflicting orders, they are under crosspressures, a situation that usually leads to inactivity and failure to act decisively. In one study of informal rules, "Zawacki (1963) found that role conflict results from the dual hierarchy in hospitals and that those affected respond with hostility to physicians and passive resistance to formal rules" (Rizzo, House, and Lirtzman, 1970). Some services are more likely to have emergencies and require immediate response, such as the cardiac care unit and surgical wards.

Knowledge of the market for hospital services may not be as important in predicting output as knowing the capabilities of each individual unit. The hospital director is dependent on the information received from each chief of service, who must set the goals for their own units. The director of the hospital has little access to information outside of these lines of communication.

The hospital seeks to create advances in knowledge and technique. New knowledge constantly reshapes the tasks of diagnosis and treatment, making it difficult if not impossible for a hospital director to keep up with the current developments in each field in medicine. Since most chiefs of service want to keep up with their specialties and have the most modern equipment available, the hospital director must sort out the various requests for equipment and staff, a difficult task.

Part of the complexity of hospitals can be explained by the types of services provided. Hospitals have traditionally been categorized according to whether they service all types of patients or a special type. The *general* hospital will have more or less full range of services aimed at caring for acute cases. The *specialized* hospital will take care of one particular illness, such as psychiatric disorders or tuberculosis. Other specialized hospitals may be rehabilitative, helping patients recover from stroke or adapt to prosthetic devices. Some hospitals—now called hospices—specialize in caring for the terminally ill. Extended care facilities such as nursing homes often do not employ a full-time medical staff and do not have equipment for acute care; as such they are not considered to be hospitals even though they perform similar tasks.

Hospitals also have different sponsorships. Sometimes they are created by community organizations such as churches or clubs, or public-spirited citizens may establish a hospital for a particular city or region. Governmental units create hospitals for populations not served by others. Big city hospital systems were created to serve the poor, and the Veterans Administration hospital system was created by Congress for those who served their country in the military. The federal government also operates military hospitals for its armed forces personnel and their families. All of these hospitals are non-profit facilities. Although doctors who wish to invest in health care often start profit-making facilities, relatively few are large operations, with 70 percent of them having less than 100 beds (CRI, 1975: 300).

Hospitals in the United States have more than 1.5 million beds, located in 7,123 units (CRI, 1975: 297). Because of the reimbursement patterns by Blue Cross and other private insurance plans, and by Medicare and Medicaid, hospitals have tended to increase in size. Federal funds have also paid for construction. Nonfederal, short-term hospitals during the period 1950–73 increased their bed capacity by 80 percent (CRI, 1975: 298), whereas there has been an overall decrease in the number of hospitals by 30 percent during the same period.

Payment for patient care from these third-party payers is based on a flat rate for days hospitalized. Most specific services performed are not itemized, but reimbursement is based on the overall availability of services. Smaller hospitals have fewer services and thus receive less reimbursement. In addition, private insurance plans often do not cover procedures performed on an outpatient basis. Therefore, there has been an economic advantage to hospitals to expand their bed capacity and to hospitalize patients even when inpatient status is not required for treatment.

Size provides another economic advantage to hospital administrators and encourages growth. The establishment of a unit to handle the processing of bills is less costly when a large volume of patients is cared for than when a smaller number is serviced. The unit cost for maintaining the accounts department and other support services such as purchasing is lower in the case of larger hospitals, since the personnel are already employed, space has been set aside for their work, and electronic data processing is already in use. Even when new billing clerks have to be hired, it may not mean an increase in the number of supervisors. Other kinds of support services are also more economical to operate when hospitals are large. A critical mass of patients who need a special service are required to justify such departments as occupational therapy, physical therapy, or social work (American Hospital Association, 1974).

The organization of the hospital along bureaucratic lines may appear to result from the increase in the number of beds. Size, however, does not fully explain the development of formal organizational characteristics, such as written rules, specifically designated times and groups for policy discussions, and job descriptions at all levels. Starkweather found that complexity of organization encouraged the development of formal channels of communication, agreement on common purpose, and specifications of jobs and authority. In his study of 704 general hospitals, "size, identified independently from complexity was not found to influence formal organization mechanisms significantly" (1970: 338).

General hospitals are usually found where a concentrated population provides a sufficient number of patients requiring special services. Urbanized areas where people have relatively high incomes also generate demand for a variety of programs. Public demand for burn centers, for example, is not based strictly on the number of available cases but represents an unwillingness by communities to utilize programs at distant places even when helicopter ambulances can cut travel time. Recent public efforts to maintain obstetrics units despite low use rates brought about by the reduction in the birth rate is another illustration of how the community can affect innovation. New programs found at 480 short-term general nonfederal hospitals were explained in one study by the density of the population served by the hospital and their average income rather than by bed capacity (Veney and Kahn, 1973: 142).

One of the major influences on hospital organization and the utilization of paramedical personnel and management specialists has been the need to respond to the expectations of funding sources, particularly the private insurance companies and Medicare and Medicaid. Hiring hospital personnel often depends on keeping funding sources aware of service requirements for the patients and justifying increases in reimbursement rates. As a result, the role of the top management of hospitals has become focused more on these outside contacts than on daily operation of the facility. The role of director has been split into two functions, following corporate structure models in industry. Directors of hospitals generally agree that they need to differentiate outside activities, "expanding and segregating policy-making level at the top from lower operational activities" (Todd, 1971: 56).

Reimbursement on a flat rate has encouraged employment of paramedical personnel to do many of the things formerly done by doctors. The organization of care, when seen from the perspective of how tasks are divided and assigned, involves delegation of responsibilities that once were exclusively those of physicians. In order to keep costs down, or at least give the appearance of being cost-conscious, hospital management has been constrained to innovate by replacing physicians with cheaper professionals. Saward suggests that the division of labor is encouraged by the financing of health care and will continue to produce new delegations of tasks and responsibilities from physicians to paramedical personnel.

> Present concepts of the role of the physician, the nurse and other health professionals will change rapidly under fixed budgeting for defined populations if different delivery systems are allowed to compete. If a technical task can be done by a nurse practitioner at a third of the cost of its being done by a physician, there will be an interest in the delegation of the task. [Saward, 1971: 194]

The growth of medical technology is another major influence on the costs of health care and the increased differentiation of roles and specialization. Dr. Lewis Thomas, president of the Memorial Sloan-Kettering Cancer Center in New York City, distinguishes between three levels of technology in health care.

The first level he calls "nontechnology" because it involves support in the service of the patient rather than diagnosis or treatment. "It tides patients over through diseases that are not, by and large, understood. It is what is meant by the phrases 'caring for' and 'standing by' " (1971: 1367). For example, in fatal diseases such as multiple sclerosis medical intervention cannot alter the course significantly and there are few ways to evaluate the effectiveness of the care.

> The cost of nontechnology is very high, and getting higher all the time. It requires not only a great deal of time but also very hard effort and skill on the part of physicians; only the very best of doctors are good at coping with this kind of defeat. It involves long periods of hospitalization, lots of nursing, lots of involvement of nonmedical professionals in and out of the hospital. [1971: 1367]

An expensive form of technology represents interventions in disease processes that have already taken their toll. Thomas calls this type "halfway technology": "things that are done after the fact, in efforts to compensate for the incapacitating effects of certain diseases whose course one is unable to do very much about. It is a technology designed to make up for disease, or to postpone death" (1971: 1367). An example would be organ transplants or kidney machines, which compensate for lost functions. Because medical knowledge does not understand the mechanisms in kidney failure, coronary heart disease, or cancer, it cannot prevent or reverse processes of deterioration: "It is characteristic of this kind of technology that it costs an enormous amount of money and requires a continuing expansion of hospital facilities. There is no end to the need for new, highly trained people to run the enterprise" (1971: 1368)

Finally, there are the relatively simple, inexpensive, and easily deliverable technologies based on the understanding of disease mechanisms. These "decisive technologies" make real inroads in maintaining health and are "exemplified best by modern methods of immunization against diphtheria, pertussis and childhood virus diseases, and the contemporary use of antibiotics and chemotherapy for bacterial infections" (Thomas, 1971: 1368).

In summarizing the state of scientific knowledge in medicine between 1950 and 1975, Thomas concludes that the same roster of common diseases exists now as at the beginning of the period. Cardiovascular disease, cancer, cerebrovascular diseases, and kidney disease still accounted for 79 percent of all deaths in 1974 (1977: 40). Despite the failure to develop decisive technologies for these major causes of death, the public still expects that something be done. And the rise of halfway technologies follows this demand. Thomas (1977: 38) also points out that the same set of expectations has led to the expansion and overuse of expensive diagnostic procedures, even when they are not warranted by the symptoms. Howard Waitzkin (1979: 1260–68) shows that some of this demand is induced by manufacturers. He carefully documents the growth and development of cardiac care technology and its specialized units and finds that they are no more effective than ordinary hospital care!

The field of hospital and health care administration has grown enormously because of the need for trained people who can deal with the acquisition of financial support and internal coordination. Financial experts create systems of billing and prepare documentary evidence required by various regulatory agencies in government that fund health care. In addition, applications for government grants also require predictions of expenditures for large blocks of time. Students in business administration learn to keep track of costs and income for an organization. Hospital financing is particularly complex because of the diverse nature of the sources of income, each having its own unique requirements in order to receive reimbursement for patient care.

Hospital management involving internal coordination over the use of personnel and space is distinct from the financial structure. It involves knowledge of which health care practitioners can do what tasks, both according to their training and what they are legally permitted to do. In some states, only physicians are permitted to perform medical tasks such as prescribing, and in others, nurse practitioners and physician's associates can do this for minor illnesses under standing orders. In addition, unions that represent various groups of health care workers contract to provide specified services and prevent workers from performing certain noncontractual procedures. Sometimes these tasks are considered to be below the skills of the performer of the job, as when a nurse is asked to change the sheets on a bed. In other instances, the tasks are learned on the job, but health care practitioners sometimes refuse to do it because they are not receiving appropriate compensation.

Management specialists also create new distributions of work. Job descriptions are based upon observing what kinds of tasks are performed, whether certain categories of employees are doing too much or too little, and delegating tasks that are performed by higher-paid and trained workers to lower-paid workers. Sometimes the lower-level workers are upgraded as a result of assuming new tasks. Sometimes they performed them informally without official recognition; for example, persons in charge of housekeeping may have often kept a casual watch over the supplies available on a ward before being officially delegated the task and the title of unit manager.

Scheduling is a major function in any organization, but it is particularly crucial in a hospital. Hospitals must have 24-hour coverage, even though some times may not be busy. Use patterns tell a hospital administrator when there will be a heavy call for hospital beds, but external factors such as emergencies or disasters can influence such demand. A recession in a factory town may create layoffs, giving workers time to take care of elective surgery covered in their union benefits. Space allocation related to use of personnel is important since facilities such as hemodialysis units or operating rooms can service only so many patients during a 24-hour period. Computers can help to make up schedules, but human input is required to determine the priorities of use (Reiser, 1977).

Introducing large numbers of administrative personnel into health care has been justified as a way of freeing trained professionals to deal with the patient's problems. At one time, for example, nurses in a hospital ward either wrote or typed up their notes on patients and kept track of records. Medical clerks and secretaries now do these tasks. Nurses also spent time on housekeeping tasks, such as changing sheets and serving meals. Nurses aides now do much of the "cleaning and pressing" of patients, as nurses sometimes refer to these tasks.

More authority has been delegated to administrators, freeing the professional to focus on patient care. This acquisition of authority has increased their influence, since control of information is a major source of power. Professionals are particularly sensitive to the need to create harmonious work teams, and some become dependent on administrators for early warnings of trouble. For example, information for a surgeon on the availability of favored operating room technicians and valuable operating room time may be strategic in scheduling a particularly complicated and lengthy procedure.

NURSES

By virtue of their dual careers as producers and reproducers, women are more deeply involved in both giving and receiving health care than men, and nursing has always been socially identified as a female occupation. Even more firmly established than the expectation that the physician will be a male is the expectation that the nurse will be female. Males who become nurses (outside of certain types of work, as in mental hospitals) are often popularly regarded as weak, effeminate, or homosexual. To protect male nurses from ridicule and help them avoid uneasy situations when patients expect a female nurse, hospitals sometimes create distinct job titles for them.

Occupations in health care have a substantial overrepresentation of women, although they are underrepresented in decision-making positions (Navarro, 1975). Recently, more women have entered the work force, but they are not equally distributed in the structure of occupations. Carol Brown reports that "out of 80 major occupational categories listed in the 1970 United States Census, 7 occupations contain 43 percent of all women workers. One of these occupations is nursing" (Brown, 1975: 174).

Nursing is perhaps the most important consumer-oriented role and in terms of direct contact with patients, especially in hospitals, there are no rivals to nursing. While doctors may make the decisions about treatment procedures, nurses often carry them out. As medicine became a more hospital-centered practice, more nurses were required to carry out the physicians' orders. Interestingly, the number of nursing schools and the number of nurses who graduated from them increased between 1900 and 1929, a period in which the number of medical schools and the graduates decreased sharply (Cannings and Lazonick, 1975: 195–96).

As public health measures and increased food supplies lengthened life expectancy, and as the introduction of antibiotics limited the consequences of infectious diseases, more people were hospitalized later in life for chronic disorders. Consequently, more nurses were needed to care for hospitalized patients. Increased technical responsibilities were also delegated to nurses, requiring the development of longer educational programs, with the emphasis on degree-granting baccalaureate programs. Some observers of the profession claim that nurses are still taught to do caring rather than curing. Even with their advanced technical skills, nurses in degree-granting programs are now learning how to give emotional support rather than how to diagnose and treat patients (Bullough, 1975: 230).

Registered nurses have become directly responsible for performing many information-gathering procedures and complex treatment under the standing orders of physicians. Licensed practical nurses are also involved in gathering information, such as monitoring the patient's vital signs. Nurses' aides are responsible for performing many of the housekeeping tasks related to patient hygiene and feeding. Registered nurses are involved in supervising licensed practical nurses and nurses' aides. As a consequence, registered nurses have a great deal of responsibility, but they have little say in setting policy.

It would seem the work conditions in hospitals sharpen the sense of occupational identification for nurses, a result of increased contact among nurses when their numbers were expanded. In 1972, more than 65 percent of registered nurses were employed in hospitals, as compared to almost 49 percent in 1949. At the same time, the proportion of practical nurses employed among all nurses increased from 8 to 20 percent (Cannings and Lazonick, 1975: 202). The distribution of registered nurses in the labor force decreased from 47 to 37 percent during that 23-year period. As a result of the increased number of lower-level positions, far more women in nursing are coming from ethnic or minority-group backgrounds and lower-level income groups (Cannings and Lazonick, 1975: 206).

Nurses also have longer career lines than in the past, giving them a greater stake in taking a role in policy making. The new technical and administrative responsibilities of registered nurses (and practical nurses as well) has led to demands for higher salaries and fringe benefits, often won through collective bargaining or strikes. Thus there is an increased desire, particularly on the part of registered nurses, to remain in the labor force. The feminist movement also has provided greater justification and actual support services for combining careers, marriage, and child rearing. In 1972, 25 percent of all registered nurses were under 30, as compared to 39 percent in 1949. The rate of marriage did not change during that time, so either women were staying in the profession longer, were returning after the birth of children and early years of child rearing, or were attending school later and becoming nurses when children needed less attention at home (Cannings and Lazonick, 1975: 204). These findings indicate a greater commitment to nursing as a career rather than a prelude to marriage and family life.

The widespread utilization of nurses' aides and practical nurses makes it possible for hospital administrators to realize financial surpluses that can be used on other projects. The availability of nursing students at a hospital provides an even cheaper source of labor. Surplus revenues can be used, for example, to expand the size of the hospital, establish special units, and offer high salaries and attractive facilities to high-prestige physicians. The standardization of treatment and care for certain diseases means that more expensive workers, such as registered nurses and house-staff physicians, can spend less time with a patient, leaving routine care to the less expensive personnel. Generally, patients are billed at a uniform rate for each day in the hospital, and so long as additional nurses are not hired, any patient will pay the same daily rate.

Hospital administrators who can cut down labor costs are generally rewarded with salary increases and promotions. They are dependent on getting the nursing staff of a hospital to cooperate in any alteration of the division of labor. Hence, this is a potential source of strength for nurses who wish to have a greater impact on formal decision making in health care (Cannings and Lazonick, 1975: 186). Assuming that most nurses are committed to improving the quality of health care, in addition to increasing their incomes, job security, and fringe benefits, this could place the profession in a strategically advantageous position.

As Navarro and others assert, the position of women in health care may reflect their position in the larger society. Relations with those in superordinate positions is based on a form of structured social inequality that combines gender ranking with occupational stratification. Women appear to have the characteristics of a *caste,* a group that is clearly ranked with other groups in a status hierarchy. A member of a caste belongs to it by birth and for life, forming a community within the larger community. Unlike a true caste group, as in India, women are not forced by informal sanction to remain within the group. However, most caste groups are limited to certain occupations.

While social distance usually separates members of different castes, thus precluding solidarity, the situation of women in the health care field mediates between those above them in a status hierarchy and the consumers they serve, many of whom are women themselves, either seeking health care for their children or themselves. By virtue of this point of constant contact with other women in the same occupation and with female users of health care facilities, nurses can provide a built-in or socially structured linkage between providers and consumers. Traditionally, women have given each other advice on how to survive in a caste system. Through the various consciousness movements, women have seen themselves as a group *for* themselves and as such have become a force for social change.

HEALTH CARE TEAMS

The strategic advantage enjoyed by hospital administrations in gaining authority and influence in the field has been encouraged by the adoption of the team approach. The use of halfway technology involves the extreme interdependence of various professionals. In addition, the success of the decisive technology to prevent various contagious diseases and to combat infection has meant an increase in the life expectancy rate. As a result there is more demand for treatment of the diseases of later life that are not yet responsive to a decisive technology. The health care team is a convenient and technically superior way of developing coordinated treatment plans for patients receiving complicated therapies.

Making complicated decisions about therapy requires both enormous inputs of information about the patient's condition, behavior, and previous health history and gaining the cooperation and compliance of those involved in the treatment plan. It is assumed that professionals who help to develop the plan will be more encouraged to carry it out than those who are simply told what to do. The team creates a form of involvement as well as peer pressure.

A team can be defined in terms of the goals that are established and the means necessary to accomplish those goals. Team members must be interdependent and collaborative in their efforts. Thus a doctor cannot perform a complicated therapy procedure unless blood technicians and nurses have done their preparatory work. However, blood technicians are not considered to be members of the team, whereas nurses are, because of the type and extent of contact with the patient.

A major assumption of the idea of the health care team is that a patient's problems can be best handled by those directly involved with the patient on a regular basis. While members of the health care team are responsible to a unit manager or a team leader, decisions must often be made quickly and on the basis of full information about the patient.

> . . . organizational effectiveness is increased when decisions are located as close to the problem source as possible (example, health teams make decisions on total care), decisions are made by those with the information (example, decisions about education, patient relations and so forth are made by the teams) and administrators recognize that people are most likely to support what they help to create; "ownership" in decisions goes far toward effective implementation. [Beckhard, 1972: 305–6].

Members of the team are responsible to the team leader and to the hospital's service directors, so often multiple reporting occurs. The potential for conflicting demands being placed on team members by virtue of their accountability to two supervisors should be evident.

The team approach does not always deal with the problem of the physician having great authority and the nurses and others having very little. Nurses who were trained to obey a doctor's orders often exercised little independent judgment, nor did they question the judgment of others. Mechanic reports "in Hofling's experiment, carried out on 22 wards in two hospitals, nurses on duty were asked to give a patient an excessive dose of a medicine with which the nurse was unfamiliar" (Mechanic, 1976: 73). A phone call was made in the name of a doctor whom the nurse did not know personally. The medical order was for a drug that was available but not approved for use on the ward.

> Of the 22 nurses reported on in the study, 21 followed the order and were preparing to administer the medication (before being stopped by an observer) despite the fact that the dose was double the maximum daily dose listed on the label. [Mechanic, 1976: 73].

When the same information was presented in hypothetical form to 12 graduate nurses and 21 nursing students in a teaching context, the results were reversed (Mechanic, 1976: 73). The experiment reveals that the actual situation can encourage conformity to the orders of the higher-ranked professional, particularly under the shared belief held by most practitioners that medicines are good for patients. Willingness to respond to an order is built into the situation where the loss of time involved in reflecting on whether the order is correct and legitimate can be detrimental to the patient's health. All members of health care teams must learn to sort out the unusual from the usual, a task that becomes more difficult once routines are established.

Nursing is undergoing many changes, including increasing education, greater specification of the conditions under which a nurse has a right to refuse a doctor's orders, and increasing social solidarity among fellow members. Such developments create new structural conditions that exist independently from the actual situations in which doctors and nurses interact. Therefore, the results of Hofling's experiment might not be replicated.

Rank and Jacobson performed the same experiment with hospital nurses' compliance with medication overdose orders and did not confirm the earlier findings. A physician's order requested that nurses administer a nonlethal overdose of Valium to appropriate patients.

> It was hypothesized that when nurses were familiar with a drug and were allowed to communicate freely with their peers, they would not administer an overdose of the drug merely because a physician ordered them to do so. Sixteen of eighteen nurses tested in two major hospitals refused to administer the Valium. [Rank and Jacobson, 1977: 188]

While the authors believed that knowledge of the drug's effects or group support could account for these findings, there was no attempt to examine situations where these variables were less evident. They do consider, however, other possible contributing factors to noncompliance resulting from increased willingness of all hospital personnel to question a doctor's orders, the rising self-esteem among nurses, and the fear of malpractice suits (Rank and Jacobson, 1977: 188). Other factors include the size of the work unit, the availability of consultation with other physicians, and recent incidents of the same type that might influence the results substantially.

Routines imply that health care teams can become highly specialized work units in which roles become fixed. Sometimes rotation of assignments, such as running meetings or acting as team leader, encourages members to assume more responsibility and exercise independent judgment. By setting goals that enhance individual competency for team members, important mistakes can be avoided and health care is more effective.

Sometimes team members fall into ineffective routines because they have no opportunity to express their feelings about work or colleagues. Particularly in a situation where death and dying can be a day-to-day occurrence, having team members become more sensitive to the feelings of patients if they have an opportunity to identify their own anger, frustrations, or sorrow is very helpful. Often when people do not know when and how to express their feelings to each other, they act in unproductive or counterproductive ways. Retaliation often occurs when people have a strong sense of group membership, such as families or work teams.

Some hospitals have made experts available to help health care teams deal with this. Psychiatrists will assist groups of nurses who deal with the terminally ill. In the Hospital of Albert Einstein College of Medicine in New York, adjunctive psychiatric care is provided through inservice training programs for resident physicians, nurses, social workers, nurses' aides, and physical, occupational, and speech therapists who give terminal care. As medical technology has made possible the prolongation of life in critical care cases (intensive care, cardiac care, hemodialysis, open heart surgery, cancer chemotherapy), so too it also prolongs the act of dying, pushing into the foreground the emotions and attitudes of patients, families, and professional personnel. The Department of Psychiatry counsels professionals on their attitudes, feelings, and clinical management.

The desire to reduce the cost of medical care by preventing hospitalization has been another factor in fostering the team approach. The growth of middle-level practitioners is based upon providing outpatient or ambulatory care. With fewer cases of acute illness and more of chronic illness, there has been more concern with the management of illness. As a result, monitoring patients has become a long-term, fairly routine, ongoing task. Other tasks delegated by physicians involve primary care for children, known as well-baby visits, and the physical examination of adults where standardized procedures exist. Since physicians do not always observe the patient or the work performed by the middle-level practitioner, a team approach allows information to be shared among all members. Team meetings become the central forum for the dissemination of information and the development of a treatment plan.

THE MIDDLE-LEVEL PRACTITIONER

Middle-level health care practitioners are sometimes referred to as physician extenders. Specific titles for these positions vary, with the two most popular being physician assistant and nurse practitioner. Most training programs for physician extenders focus on preparing people to assist the physician in primary care, the first point of contact between patients and the health care delivery system.

Delegating some of the tasks of the physician to physician extenders is not new. Nurses have for many years been given routine tasks that physicians found relatively simple but time-consuming. Many of the four-year baccalaureate degree programs for student nurses are based on being able to perform such tasks as taking blood pressure, administering intravenous feedings, and reading electrocardiogram machines. In fact, if a nurse could not quickly read a vital-life-sign indicator and take immediate action, many intensive care units could not have been established. The new roles of physician extenders simply follows an established trend but creates interesting possibilities.

The time seems to be right for innovations in the delivery of service, but advocates of similar plans in the past have met with considerable opposition, sometimes from surprising sources. In 1927, a physician named Alfred Worcester wrote a book that advocated

> . . . advanced training to enable the nurse to become the doctor's assistant in medical tasks. Because nursing education and nursing service would be controlled by doctors, his plans were opposed by nursing leaders representing both the Nightingale and professional orientation. Nor did he get the support of the medical profession, since he worked at a time when doctors did not feel a great need to delegate medical tasks; he might have gotten their support today. [Glazer, 1966: 27–28]

The founders of the first training programs for physician assistants and nurse practitioners, created at Duke University Medical School in 1965, were convinced that physicians had been too highly trained to do routine medical tasks. These new roles were created in order to utilize the skills of physicians appropriately and to cut the costs of health care delivery. Since both nurse practitioners and physician assistants work with the doctor, the general title of physician associate will be used here to refer to both roles.

The training programs started at Duke were two-year courses; by 1975, there were 84 training programs for physician assistants in the United States (CRI, 1975: 371). Students usually had two to four years of college and some previous health care experience. Recruitment from former military medical corpsmen and hospital nurses took place, although the tendency was for males to be tracked in physician associate programs and women into nurse practitioner training programs because of the traditional gender associations.

The cost of training a physician associate for one year is as much as a year of medical school. However, the overall length of training is less than for a physician (CRI, 1975: 376). In addition, salaries are much lower for physician associates than the mean income of $50,000 per year for M.D.s as reported in 1976 (Silver, 1976: 97). The availability of physician associates could help somewhat to lower the cost of care, provided that the billing for their services is not at the same rate as that of physicians.

From the point of view of the physician, the extender programs represent either a potential competitor or a new way to expand one's practice. A 75 percent increase in the number of patients in a single practice has been reported. And, no reduction in the quality of care was found in this physician's practice when a physician associate was employed (Cihlar, 1975: 54).

In some cases, physician associates have been utilized to provide care in isolated or impoverished areas of the country where few physicians are found. However, working under the condition of low availability of physicians does not provide the necessary consultation required to provide adequate medical care. Most physician associates work in private group practices or clinics where close contact with physicians is possible. Only 13 percent of physician assistants and nurse practitioners were found working in areas where medical care was scarce (Miles, 1975: 556).

In some practices and clinics, physician associates not only provide primary care but also treat minor illnesses, make visits to nursing homes, and monitor the recovery of patients discharged from a hospital and placed on a regimen of care and therapy at home. The last two are activities that physicians often claim they do not have the time for or do not regard as an efficient use of their time.

The development of new middle-level health care roles has created some legal problems, because many tasks are usually restricted to licensed physicians.

> Twenty-nine states have now amended their laws to provide for physician assistants. Seven states allow physicians to delegate tasks to their assistants so long as the assistant functions under the physician's supervision and control, although a question remains whether supervision has to be on the premises or can be exercised at a distance, via telephone for example. Twenty-two states, instead of leaving control of assistants to supervising physicians, have set up regulatory boards to establish rules and regulations about the education and employment requirements of physician assistants. [CRI, 1975: 378]

The emergence of the new practitioner roles has been one of the most complex social phenomena in the division of labor and organization of health care in the past decade. Many interesting issues emerge in relation to these new roles, such as the reaction by patients to receiving services from physician associates, the occupational identities created, and the response of medical and paramedical personnel.

A new division of labor is emerging in which physicians may have to share responsibility for health care with the new practitioners rather than simply delegating tasks. The changing nature of the population and its concomitant health care needs requires a shift in decision-making power to the team.

Chronic illness care and prevention of illness or its worst manifestations require the systematic monitoring of therapies and followup—tasks that can best be performed by a team. New health care practitioners must have opportunities to shape decision making and gain some control over their own work situation.

Despite the development of a team approach, many health care workers, including doctors, have found the need to form and join unions. These organizations defend the interests of various workers vis-à-vis management. Often they are concerned with maintaining or improving the member's standard of living or with their quality of work. Questions concerning the impact of unionization on health care services will be explored in Chapter 8.

REFERENCES

American Hospital Association. 1974. *Hospital Statistics.* Chicago: The American Hospital Association.

American Medical Association. 1974. *Socioeconomic Issues of Health: 1974 Edition.* Chicago: AMA, Center for Health Services Research.

Beckhard, R. 1972. "Organizational issues in the team delivery of comprehensive health care." *Milbank Memorial Fund Quarterly* 50 (July): 287–316.

Brown, C. 1975. "Women workers in the health service industry." *International Journal of Health Services* 5: 173–84.

Bullough, B. 1975. "Barriers to the nurse practitioner movement: Problems of women in a woman's field." *International Journal of Health Services* 5: 225–33.

[CRI] Cambridge Research Institute. 1975. *Trends Affecting U.S. Health Care System.* Washington: U.S. Government Printing Office.

Cannings, K., and W. Lazonick. 1975. "The development of the nursing labor force in the United States." *International Journal of Health Services* 5: 185–216.

Cihlar, C. 1975. "Stephen L. Joyner, P.A.," *Hospitals,* 1 June: 54.

Coser, R. 1958. "Authority and decision-making in a hospital: A Comparative Analysis." *American Sociological Review* 23: 56–63.

Etzioni, Amitai. 1961. *A Comparative Analysis of Complex Organizations: On Power, Involvement and Their Correlates.* Glencoe, Ill.: The Free Press.

Glazer, W. 1966. "Nursing leadership and policy." Pp. 1–59 in Fred Davis, ed., *The Nursing Profession: Five Sociological Essays.* New York: John Wiley.

Goss, M. E. W. 1962. "Administration and the physician." *American Journal of Public Health* 52: 183–91.

———. 1963. "Patterns of bureaucracy among hospital staff physicians." Pp. 170–94 in Eliot Freidson, ed., *The Hospital in Modern Society.* New York: The Free Press.

Haines, A. J. 1933. "Nursing." *Encyclopedia of the Social Sciences* 6: 405–11.

Mechanic, David. 1976. "The design of human service systems: Implications from organizational theory." Pp. 58–79 in *The Growth of Bureaucratic Medicine: An Inquiry into the Dynamics of Patient Behavior and the Organization of Medical Care.* New York: Wiley Interscience.

Miles, D. 1975. "Physician's assistants: The evidence is not in." *New England Journal of Medicine* 293 (September): 555–56.

Navarro, V. 1975. "Women as producers of service in the health sector of the United States." *Proceedings of the International Conference on Women in Health.* Washington, D.C.: DHEW Publication (HRA 76–51): 175–83.

Rank, S. G., and C. K. Jacobson. 1977. "Hospital nurses' compliance with medication overdose orders: A failure to replicate." *Journal of Health and Social Behavior* 18 (June): 188–93.

Reiser, S. J. 1977. "Therapeutic choice and moral doubt in a technological age." *Daedalus* 106 (Winter): 47–56.

Rizzo, J. R., R. J. House, and S. I. Lirtzman. 1970. "Role conflict and ambiguity in complex organizations." *Administrative Science Quarterly* 15 (June): 150–63.
Rosen, George. 1963. "The hospital: Historical sociology of a community institution." Pp. 1–36 in Eliot Freidson, ed., *The Hospital in Modern Society*. Glencoe, Ill.: The Free Press.
Saward, E. W. 1973. "Organization of medical care." *Scientific American* (September): 169–75.
Silver, George. 1976. *A Spy in the House of Medicine*. Germantown, Md.: Aspen Systems.
Smith, H. L. 1958. "Two lines of authority: The hospital dilemma. Pp. 468–78 in E. Gartly Jaco, ed., *Patients, Physicians and Illness: Source Book in Behavior Science and Medicine*. Glencoe, Ill.: The Free Press.
Starkweather, D. B. 1970. "Hospital size, complexity and formalization." *Health Services Research* 5 (Winter): 330–41.
Steton, D. 1977. "Hospital workers win pay increase." *New York Times*, June 29, p. B18.
Thomas, L. 1971. "The technology of medicine." *New England Journal of Medicine* 285 (December 9): 1366-68.
———. 1977. "On the science and technology of medicine." *Daedalus* 106 (Winter): 35–46.
Todd, C. D. 1971. "Hospitals' organizational structure: Trend toward the corporate form." *Hospitals* 45 (September): 55–59.
Veney, J. E., and J. Khan. 1973. "Causal paths in elaboration of organizational structure: A case of hospital services." *Health Services Research* 8 (Summer): 139–50.
Waitzkin, H. 1979. "A Marxian interpretation of the growth and development of coronary care technology." *American Journal of Public Health* 69 (December): 1260–68.

8

Unions among Health Care Occupations and Professions

Unions are associations of employees who have banded together to protect their interests. Unlike professional associations, which are created to promote the development of a field or discipline, unions focus more on the goal of extracting a contract from management that provides a certain rate of payment for work, job security in times of reduced demand for the product or the availability of a large pool of eager workers in the marketplace, and limits to what management can demand on the job. Unions strike or threaten strike as a way to gain their goals. In the past, many unions would not give up their right to strike because they felt that that was the major way of ensuring that a contract would be honored by management. Today, unions take a more practical view, acting more like business agents for workers. Recently, some unions have signed no-strike contracts in exchange for wage increases or long-term contracts.

Some unions have attempted to win broader social goals for the entire society, as in the 1930s and to some extent among new unions in the 1960s (e.g., the United Farm Workers of America), but now most are concerned with getting the highest income for their members, given the profits of employers or rates of pay received for the same kind of work in other industries.

The right to organize unions and elect bargaining agents for workers employed by firms engaged in interstate commerce was legally recognized and encouraged by the Wagner Act of 1935. In order to enforce this act, the National Labor Relations Board was set up (and later amended under the Taft-Hartley Act of 1947), its essential duty being to make sure that labor and management bargain collectively in good faith. This law gave recognition to labor as an adversary, but also as a participant in the wage-setting process, preventing management from intimidating workers who wished to form unions. Under the provisions of the law, certain industries were specifically excluded because they were nonprofit or governmental. These organizations were seen as dependent on charity or tax monies and not able to afford to bargain collectively. Among these organizations were nonprofit hospitals.

A union to represent health workers is a relatively recent phenomenon. The push among health care workers to organize unions came about through developments internal to the field itself, which made health care a large-scale service, employing vast numbers of skilled and unskilled workers at the same place. This chapter examines the conditions under which unionization came about, the occupations where they made their biggest gains, and the consequences of both. Finally, some analysis of whether or not unions can improve the quality of health care will be made.

UNIONIZATION AND THE GROWTH OF THE HOSPITAL

The increased size of workplaces is often a necessary condition for unionization. Generally, the larger the workplace, the greater the proportion of workers who belong to unions. It is no less true of hospitals than of factories. Hospital size is usually measured by bed capacity, and by 1970, 38.6 percent of the hospitals with 500 beds or more had collective bargaining contracts with unions, as compared with only 15 percent of those hospitals with 99 beds or less (Miller and Shurtell, 1969).

Nonetheless, size in and of itself does not mean very much. Small-scale workplaces, such as group medical practice, may involve frequent contact with people of different statuses, which usually means that one is exposed to different political points of view. There is less constant reinforcement from people who are similarly situated, and one may develop a perspective that may not be in accord with one's interest as part of that sector of the workplace that receives orders and carries them out.

Small work units usually mean that relatively little social distance separates management from labor. Persons in a subordinate position can direct their demands to the top relatively quickly and directly, depending on the degree of contact between boss and worker. In turn, management can also call upon past loyalties and close personal contact to induce workers to stay late or do other things for which they will not receive remuneration.

Small workshops permit workers to get to know everyone in the organization, which gives a strong sense of community and means usually that contributions are recognized. As sociologist Robert Blauner points out, a feeling of belonging can encourage a sense of participation in a shared effort:

> Membership in an industrial community involves commitment to the work role and loyalty to one or more centers of the work community. Isolation, on the other hand, means that the worker feels no sense of belonging in the work situation and is unable to identify or uninterested in identifying with the organization and its goals. [Blauner, 1964: 24]

Finally, in small work units, workers are more likely to have more control over the design, initiation, and implementation of production or service delivery tasks, enabling them to have more varied activities, understand the processes, have a greater degree of freedom, and make a greater contribution to the accomplishment of goals. In contrast, larger work units are more likely to have a refined and detailed division of labor and use more expensive technology, which often limits the variety found in the workers' daily routines and involves more middle-level management positions, making it difficult for workers to have a role in decision making.

In a more directly economic sense, large-scale work units are encouraged to introduce continuously innovations in management practices. They seek to control greater shares of their markets and to pay off investors, making it necessary to expand sales and profits in order to reduce the unit cost for each item. The same result may be achieved by using less expensive labor, an incentive for management to replace skilled labor with semiskilled or unskilled labor. The professional often works with management and gives orders to lower level personnel. Subordinates in hospitals are asked to but cannot identify with the goals of service to humanity because they are subject to the discipline of the professional in the workplace.

Unionization creates a source of identification for workers and a way for them to realize power at the workplace. In the field of health care, the trend toward unionization is a reaction to management's efforts to coordinate many complex procedures. The rules of the hospital define which positions have authority to issue orders. In this form of social organization, or bureaucracy (Weber, 1947: 328), authority is based on the position that issues an order and not the person issuing it. Consequently, workers have little *formal* opportunity to formally direct demands upward, since their right to do so is not officially recognized.

Workers in bureaucratic environments find they have little control over their own work or what can be demanded of them. In contrast, unions spell out the terms of their responsibilities and limit work demands to those agreed to in a contract. Unionization among health workers, according to Robin Badgley, a Canadian sociologist who studied a physicians' strike in that country, is a response to the constraints placed on workers by these newer forms of social organization of health services and by inflation.

> As large bureaucracies expand to encompass previously dispersed or uncoordinated institutions, two counterforces are emerging in many Western nations to challenge the established social division among workers. Reacting to the growing concentration of power in large corporations, workers increasingly are joining unions in many industries and are aggressively pressing for higher wages and increased job benefits. The trend toward unionization has been complemented by the socially corrosive effects of monetary inflation, with its invidious wage-price spread consequences for workers with various levels of training or those working in the public versus private sector of the economy. [1975: 10]

Hospitals have been particularly representative of these trends. In order to provide full patient services, a large number of new positions have been created, and more personnel have been trained and hired to perform traditional roles, as in nursing. Middle-level positions, such as laboratory technicians and dieticians, have been created in support services. Additionally, a large number of aide and clerical positions were created to free nurses and technicians from housekeeping and recordkeeping tasks. The division of labor in large hospitals has become so complicated that there may be as many as 42 pay categories for service and maintenance workers, each receiving a slightly different job title and rate of remuneration. Hospitals also have as many as 35 different grades of clerical workers, as well as 38 varieties of technical and professional jobs, each with its own job description (Ehrenreich and Ehrenreich, 1975: 44). Workers have sought to offset this growing fragmentation by identifying with a more overarching organization beyond the work units. Unions provide such an organization while also protecting the interests of workers.

Concern about representation is intensified when people make long-term commitments to their work. Nurses, who once received low wages, would drop out of the field permanently upon marrying or raising families and often not return. The increased technical demands made of nurses in hospitals has led to longer periods of education and training. In many states, only nurses who receive a bachelor's degree can become R.N.s. This upgrading has resulted in intensified demands for better pay commensurate with the new responsibilities. Nurses have joined their state associations in large numbers and have used these professional organizations in the same way as other health care workers have used unions. State nursing associations have become collective bargaining agents with associations of voluntary hospitals, municipalities, and states that employ them. Hospital management increasingly recognizes the power these organizations wield.

> By January 1974, 475 contracts had been negotiated by 33 state nurses' associations, covering approximately 65,000 registered nurses and including 38 contracts negotiated in 11 states with labor laws that protect the rights of nurses to enter into collective bargaining units. [Match, Goldstein, and Light, 1975: 31]

The recent unionization drives in health care follow a period in which several legal and cultural conditions restricted the formation of unions. In the past, the charitable nature of hospitals fused religious and philanthropic values. People who provided personal services in hospitals, such as orderlies, kitchen helpers, and housekeepers, were expected to receive low wages. In many hospitals, labor was also supplied by people who took vows of poverty as members of religious orders. In addition, physicians with admitting rights were expected to provide free services in the charity wards and outpatient clinics. An atmosphere of dedication, service, and devotion was expected to prevail. The public would have been outraged at the thought of a strike, which would endanger the lives of helpless patients. Implicit in this set of public definitions was the view that those who worked in hospitals in subordinate positions, and even those in management, were protected from the marketplace. Hospital employees were less subject to the fluctuations of the business cycle, therefore they should receive less pay than those in competitive employment. Even as recently as March 1974, according to the Department of Labor, hospital workers' average hourly earnings were $3.33, or 73 cents an hour less than the average for manufacturing workers (Davis and Foner, 1975: 19).

Another reason for this depressed wage had to do with the lack of legal protection in trying to organize unions. Because most hospital jobs were in the nonprofit or public sector of the economy, workers were legally excluded from the protection of the National Labor Relations Board. Hospital workers had little protection against harassment and intimidation by management, so union organizing efforts were few and far between. During the Kennedy Administration, an executive order made it possible for employees of federal hospitals to bargain collectively with management. On August 25, 1974, Congress passed legislation removing the exemption of voluntary or nonprofit hospitals and nursing homes from coverage under the National Labor Relations Board. Collective bargaining rights were extended to 1.5 million employees of voluntary hospitals (Davis and Foner, 1975: 19), and employers were expected to bargain in good faith with employees.

Unionization was limited among skilled and semiskilled health care workers because of their professional commitments. Many felt that joining a union would mean having to strike, an act they regarded as unprofessional because they would be arbitrarily withdrawing service from needy patients. As management became more divorced from service delivery, with specialized administrators relieving physicians of decision making in nonmedical matters, fewer middle-level workers saw strikes as aimed against patients but rather more at management. Some strikes initially demanded improved patient care as well as salaries and fringe benefits. Moreover, it became clear in the course of hospital strikes that administrators and physicians could manage to hold the hospital together on a short-term basis, dealing with emergencies without unnecessary loss of life. Some strikes removed only part of the workforce at one time, making it possible for an emergency plan to be put into effect even for months at a time.

The first major strike of hospital workers occurred in 1959 in New York City, where the union movement was strong. The newly formed Local 1199 of the National Union of Health and Hospital Care Employees sought but failed to receive recognition as a collective bargaining agent with the League of Voluntary Hospitals. This bitter battle, which lasted 46 days, did provide for wage increases. The second hospital workers' strike, in New York City in 1962, led to changes in New York State labor relations laws and to the inclusion of nonprofit hospitals under the State Labor Relations Act (Ehrenreich, 1970).

UNION POWER AND SOUL POWER

The drive for health and hospital workers to be recognized by management spearheaded by Local 1199, could not have occurred without the active support of the entire labor movement. And it came at a time when the unions were looking, in the words of the late John L. Lewis, president of the United Mine Workers, to "organize the unorganized." Taking notice of the shrinking job market for industrial work and the new growth areas in services, retail sales, clerical work, and civil-service professions, union organizers looked into department stores with large numbers of sales personnel, offices with large numbers of clerical workers, such as insurance companies, among teachers and social workers.

Hospitals were prime targets for the unions because of the large numbers employed and the subsistence wages paid to unskilled workers. Two other unions in addition to Local 1199 became active in organizing the health care field: the Service Employees International Union and the American Federation of State, County, and Municipal Employees. The leaders of Local 1199 were willing to organize the unskilled at a time when few other unions would risk such an undertaking, for traditionally those at the bottom of the occupational structure were most easily replaced and therefore most vulnerable to being fired for union activity. Nevertheless, Local 1199 succeeded. As of 1975, 20 percent or 300,000 health workers were union members.

The early success of Local 1199, was encouraged by the involvement of the Drug Workers Guild, a small union made up of pharmacists and clerks working in retail drugstores. Some members had maintained longstanding involvement in labor and left-wing politics for years, despite the repressive efforts of Senator Joseph McCarthy and FBI Director J. Edgar Hoover.

The first efforts to organize hospital workers were among the unskilled, poorly paid housekeeping staffs, porters, orderlies, nurses' aides, and kitchen helpers of the voluntary hospitals—workers who were paid a minimum wage of $40.00 per week in 1959. In contrast, by 1975 the minimum salary for a hospital worker under the contract between Local 1199 and the voluntary hospitals was up to $181.00 a week, plus an extensive benefit package (Foner and Davis, 1959: 24).

The early 1960s was a period of considerable economic expansion, and workers were in short supply. By 1964, the leadership of Local 1199 realized the importance of recruiting skilled workers whose labor could not be easily replaced by management during a strike and who had long-term commitments to health care careers. Local 1199 organized the semiskilled, skilled, and professionals working in hospitals, forming The Guild of Professional, Technical, and Clerical Workers. This distinctive organization was necessitated by the insistence of those with skills not to be in the same unit with the unskilled who could outvote them in union elections. Thus, in crucial votes such as approving a contract or calling a strike, the Guild could neutralize the actions of the other branch of Local 1199.

Success in organizing was encouraged by increased federal funding of health care through Medicare and Medicaid and special grants for research and demonstration projects. Some of these programs were part of Lyndon Johnson's Great Society program and the War Against Poverty. These new sources of income made it easier to meet the union demands of increases in wages and fringe benefits, further attracting more workers to the union's banners. Moreover, the nonmarket conditions found in health care meant that increased costs could simply be passed along to the third-party payers, either Blue Cross or the federal government. Management was willing to accede to the demands of the unions so long as funds were forthcoming. Management often blames unions for the high costs of health care because, they argue, union negotiators do not consider competitive constraints that exist in market situations. Where prices and fees are increased, consumers might reduce their demand, creating less of a need for labor and encouraging hospital closings and layoffs of workers (Match, Goldstein, and Light, 1975: 32).

Organizing health workers came at a time when the civil rights movement was at its peak. Some of the organizing drives undertaken by Local 1199 were encouraged by a coalition with the civil rights movement, led by Martin Luther King of the Southern Christian Leadership Conference. Many of the unskilled hospital workers of the big city hospitals were blacks, and these drives were for greater social equality and human dignity as much as for higher wages and other material benefits.

The chant of "union power and soul power" was heard on the picket lines at many hospitals around the country. In one strike in Charleston, South Carolina, workers stayed off their jobs for 113 days to win recognition of Local 1199 as their bargaining agent. Members of this newly formed chapter of the union found a new sense of self-worth inspired by the presence of Martin Luther King who said, "There are no menial jobs, only menial wages" (Langer, 1971: 26). The Charleston Hospital strike was won, but it

> . . . featur[ed] weeks of mass demonstrations led by the Southern Christian Leadership Conference, hundreds of arrests, a threatened closing down of the port of Charleston by the Longshoreman's union, support from unions all over the country, and the occupation of the city by the National Guard. [Ehrenreich, 1970: 6]

The open coalition of union and civil rights activity inspired hospital workers (many of them were women) to seek to improve their position in society, fighting their way in through classic trade-union tactics.

From the point of view of health care, unionization has helped to stabilize the workforce rather than creating confusion and chaos. Management has learned to live with unions, as in other industries. But what of the consequence for health care and patients? Unlike unionization in factories or offices, it has a direct impact on the user of the service, both in terms of cost and care.

UNIONS AND THE QUALITY OF HEALTH SERVICES

The record of unions in affecting the quality of health care is far from complete. Yet unions have not addressed the larger questions of who is to benefit from existing health care service, nor have they fought to participate in the major decisions in allocating resources and planning treatment procedures. In general, unions of providers have not sought to make health care more available to consumers or become more responsive to patient needs. In the larger arena of electoral politics, health care unions as well as most of the unions affiliated with the American Federation of Labor-Congress of Industrial Organizations have pushed for the establishment of a National Health Insurance Program, which would pay for all medical and hospital expenses. They have generally backed the legislation sponsored by

Senator Edward Kennedy of Massachusetts, which provides the widest coverage but would be the most expensive to operate. It also seeks to take the right to set fees out of the hands of physicians.

Nonetheless, in the long run, consumers and health workers may have common interests in finding a new way of financing health care, establishing new relations between patients and practitioners, and encouraging more consumer and worker involvement in nonmedical decision making, including the setting of fees. Accomplishing these ends requires bridging the gap between consumers and providers of health care and developing new forms of relationships between them. The editors of *Health-Pac Bulletin*, a socialist publication that is sharply critical of the American health care system, cogently states this complementarity of interests, but it does not specify the social form for promoting this recognition.

> Consumers cannot hope for decent dignified health care if they get it from oppressed, alienated, underpaid workers, from people who do not see themselves as participating in the delivery of health care but only as doing an onerous job. Just as consumers are forced to demand more money for the hospitals in order to get decent health services, they have to demand opportunities for health workers to learn about the function of their jobs, to advance to more complex and interesting and prestigious jobs, to break down the hierarchies that oppress them, and, of course, to be decently paid, decently secure, decently honored. Similarly, for the workers in the long run, better pay and longer vacations alone will not end their oppression. They need opportunities for advancement, education, and an end to the humiliating hierarchies of the present health system. And they need to be able to take pride in their "product," in the services they provide. This would only be possible if those services were something to take pride in—if they were high quality, dignified, and humane for all patients. [1979: 3]

Health workers in unions that stress the bread-and-butter issues of wages, fringe benefits, grievance procedures, and job security are often asked by organizations of physicians to join in a collective struggle for social change. Members of such organizations as the Medical Committee for Human Rights, many of whom were active as students in the civil rights and antiwar movements in the 1960s, see the physician as part of the vanguard in the struggle for a better world. Union leaders often find them to be enthusiastic supporters of worker's rights, but they also know that their own goals can be achieved within the framework of a union rather than a political organization.

Union leaders also know that collective bargaining means upholding their end of any agreement. Unions that sign long-term contracts, which include pledges not to strike during the course of the contract, become responsible for preventing workers from walking off the job. While leaders will encourage a variety of tactics short of a strike to demonstrate dissatisfaction with management (e.g., in work slowdowns), the contract makes union leaders collaborators with management in maintaining discipline on the job.

The 1970 San Francisco General Hospital strike is a good case study of how difficult it is to maintain a coalition, in this case between interns seeking a larger hospital budget, as well as salary increases, and union members seeking simply a wage increase. Since interns were vulnerable to professional pressure because they need validation of their period of training and service, a rumor to the effect that the affiliated medical school would fail to certify them led them to accepting a pay raise and call off the proposed strike. However, the interns contend that when they attempted to merge demands for improvements in patient care with the union call for pay increases, they were rebuffed by union leaders, who rejected their program for not being within the province of union interests (Bodenheimer, 1970: 19). At the same time, the interns were more concerned with their career goals than with the goals of the strike.

WHEN DOCTORS STRIKE

Professionals often do not want to join unions because of their moral commitment to serve society, making it difficult for them to withhold services from clients or patients in need. The Committee of Interns and Residents, however, have struck in New York City against the voluntary hospitals that employed them. Doctors have not been above striking to gain economic demands from national health ministries established to organize a national health care service, to gain or maintain autonomy in running their practices, or in protesting the high cost of medical malpractice insurance.

One of the most interesting cases of a strike threat by doctors was in the newly independent state of Israel in 1950–51. An association of doctors existed in Palestine before Israel achieved statehood. When the government of Israel and the general federation of labor unions, known as Histadruth, insisted that teachers, engineers, and doctors dissolve their professional association and join the general federation of labor, the doctors refused to surrender their autonomy. The medical association obtained the support of the entire profession, including those employed by the health service of Histadruth. The government gave in and never again attempted to eliminate the medical association (Ben-David, 1972: 30), although other strikes and disputes between doctors and the government over salary issues have emerged over the years. Interestingly, other professional associations, such as those for teachers and nurses, were dissolved.

Loss of economic standing seems to be just as important a basis for doctors' strikes as the threat of loss of an independent professional association. In some countries, a national Health ministry regulates and dispenses health care equally to all citizens, thus eliminating financial barriers for those who cannot pay. Such a policy could be negotiated with the ministry so that all physicians become employed by the state, either through a fixed salary or through a fee for each patient on the roster of a general practitioner or other primary care physician. This was the way the National Health Service was initiated in England.

Whatever form of payment used in a national health service, physicians are paid a fixed amount to provide care for a limited number of patients, and they cannot expand their practices (and incomes) without setting up a private practice outside of regular office hours, which are contracted with the funding agency of the government. Physicians have conducted strikes to protest a fixed salary or a capitation system, preferring fee-for-service modes of remuneration and sometimes demanding increases in salaries or per patient fees. Physicians have struck in two Canadian provinces over the transformation of the terms of payment, the most famous action taking place in Saskatchewan (Badgley and Wolfe, 1967).

Efforts to restructure health services to provide equal access to the best personnel and facilities is often a goal of socialist parties or those parties with strong labor support. An effort to create such a system, which also competed with private medicine, was attempted in Chile after the election of Dr. Salvador Allende Gossens, the first democratically elected socialist in a nonsocialist Western nation. Allende was a public health doctor who attempted to introduce a wide range of new economic and social policies in 1970. The national health service of Chile was strengthened to make medical care available for Chile's blue-collar workers and its poor, an economically depressed group at 70 percent of the population. Community participation through local health councils was also made possible, with members of local community organizations elected to serve with representatives from the Chilean medical association and various health-worker unions (Belmar and Sidel, 1975: 54).

Only 5 percent of the physicians in Chile were employed full-time by the national health service, but an additional 80 percent were employed on a part-time basis. The overall health of the country began to improve, as indicated by reductions in mortality rates and increases in life expectancy. Most significant for understanding the dynamics of the doctors' strike, the income of physicians in private practice began to decline as more people used the program. To make up for the loss of income, the Chilean medical association requested that the government permit them to charge more for services provided for private patients and at the same time institute an increase in salaries for work performed as part of the national health service. While the fees charged for private patients were not increased, those physicians who worked in the public sector were given raises, further encouraging greater physician participation in this program.

The physicians who opposed the continued erosion of their advantageous economic position joined with others in opposing government plans to bring about greater availability of services to the population. Independent truck owner-operators were natural allies to the doctors, being opposed to government plans to establish a state-owned trucking service. They called for a general strike to protest government involvement in the economy and were supported by the Chilean medical association. This strike in 1972 involved 65 percent of the country, but it did not cripple the health service. Observers of the downfall of the Allende government regard this strike as the first in a series of actions that weakened popular support for the regime. On September 11, 1973, the military dissolved the socialist government and assassinated Dr. Allende and many other high officials of his regime. Several physicians who were responsible for the establishment of the national health service were also killed and others fled for their lives (Belmar and Sidel, 1976: 60).

More recently, and less tragically, doctors have struck in California to protest high medical malpractice insurance premiums, claiming that such costs reduce their real incomes. The malpractice issue reflects upon how patients view the high cost of services and their relationships with doctors. In the context of this chapter, the doctors' strike provides further evidence for the assertion that doctors strike when their economic position is threatened.

Doctors have also struck to improve health care as well as win pay increases and create a better working environment. The Committee of Interns and Residents, which struck in New York City's voluntary hospitals in 1975, made demands of management on behalf of patients. One of the conditions of employment that encouraged this kind of unionization among physicians in hospitals was a lengthened period of training for physicians, with some residencies in specialized fields lasting several years. It is reasonable to expect that even in a training program, a lengthened period of service will encourage greater action in defending the interest of an occupational group and extensive contact among the members of that group. A long period at one hospital appointment rather than a year's required residency creates a different perspective on one's career.

In addition, the atmosphere in medicine is less hostile to unionization of physicians than in the past. The American Medical Association has not resisted this movement with the same intensity as it once did. One advocate of unionization claims that it helps deal with those institutional forces such as the insurance industry, hospitals, and government that intervene between the physician and the patient (Marcus, 1975: 37–42).

LONG-TERM TRENDS IN UNIONIZATION

Despite the growth in size of health care institutions, the likelihood of the various occupations and professions joining together to make improvements is remote. Most efforts at unionization have had to recognize the seriousness with which various health care providers take the distinctions in status, which are based on differences in skills, training, income, and prestige. Even among skilled workers willing to join unions, the more skilled were channeled into a separate unit where they could be more powerful in the local than if the standard of one member, one vote prevailed. Indeed, we are far removed from the spirit of equality among all members that existed in one branch of the American labor movement, the Industrial Workers of the World. Unionization is part of the current scene in health care, but as Krause points out

> . . . unionization, as well as the actual functioning of unions themselves, does not constitute a panacea; unions may in fact freeze existing structures in the short run. Long-term trends might drive all health workers together, and as a unified group, they might change the nature of conditions at work. But this is neither the present situation nor that of the near future. [1977: 87]

Long-term trends must be made more specific. Under what conditions and at which points will such unification take place? The team approach may be taken as such a point, despite differences in rank and salary. Teams depend on functional interdependence, producing close contact between members and a sense of solidarity. Functional interdependence is built not only on the coordination of different contributors through their specialties but a knowledge of how others do their jobs (Ehrenreich and Ehrenreich, 1975: 46). Despite this, professionals and nonprofessionals on a health care team cannot exchange jobs; nor can lower-ranked and low-paid personnel opt to move into better jobs without the appropriate education and training. The lack of internal mobility within hospitals is further reinforced when management and medicine encourage an ideology of professionalism among the skilled, letting those who carry out orders feel they are being given prestige and respect, if little decision-making responsibility.

Professionals are set apart through status distinctions from the unskilled hospital workers. In turn, housekeeping personnel, kitchen helpers, and orderlies may protect themselves from this status deprivation by being less committed to their work and becoming indifferent to their environment. Like other workers in routinized work settings, they may dissociate themselves and seek rewards outside of their jobs.

The idea of professionalism is a powerful one: When workers develop a strong sense of their importance in the service system or in productive processes, and when they perceive that their contribution goes unrecognized and unrewarded, they may begin to formulate ideas about reorganization. The health care team allows various occupational specialists to come into contact around such issues.

Similarly, patients who have continued and/or regular contact with health care facilities can learn a great deal about their own illnesses and the resources available for dealing with them. Alternatively, organizations of patients or health care consumers can hire trained people to investigate services and act as advocates for receivers of services. The importance of developing autonomy and a sense of recognition cannot be overstated. In the following chapters, the changing patterns of health services will be examined, focusing in particular on the roles of physician assistants and nurse practitioners.

REFERENCES

Badgley, R. F. 1975. "Health worker strikes: Social and economic bases of conflict." *International Journal of Health Services* 5: 9–17.

Badgley, Robin, and Wolfe, Samuel. 1967. *Doctor's Strike.* Toronto: Macmillian.

Belmar, R., and Sidel, V. W. 1975. "An international perspective on strikes and strike threates by physicians: The case of Chile." *International Journal of Health Services* 5: 53–64.

Ben-David, J. 1972. "Professionals and unions in Israel." Pp. 20–38 in Eliot Freidson and Judith Lorber, eds., *Medical Men and Their Work: A Sociological Reader.* Chicago: Aldine.

Blauner, Robert. 1964. *Alienation and Freedom: The Factory Worker and His Industry.* Chicago: University of Chicago Press.

Bodenheimer, T. 1970. "The lesson of the San Francisco hospital strike." *Health/PAC Bulletin* (July/August): 17–20.

Davis, L. J., and Foner, M. 1975. "Organization and unionization of health workers in the United States: The trade union perspective." *International Journal of Health Services* 5: 19–26.

Ehrenreich, B., and Ehrenreich, J. 1975. "Hospital workers: Class conflicts in the making." *International Journal of Health Services* 5: 43–51.

Ehrenreich, J. 1970. "Hospital unions: A long time coming." *Health/Pac Bulletin* (July/August): 3–7.

Health/PAC Bulletin (July/August 1970): 1–3. "What course for health workers?"

Krause, Elliott A. 1977. *Power and Illness: The Political Sociology of Health and Medical Care.* New York: Elsevier.

Langer, E. 1971. "Inside the hospital workers union." *New York Review of Books* (May 20): 25–33.

Marcus, S. A. 1975. "The purpose of unionization in the medical profession: The unionized profession's perspective in the United States." *International Journal of Health Services* 5: 37–42.

Match, R. K., Goldstein, A. H., and H. L. Light. 1975. "Unionization, strikes, threatened strikes and hospitals: The view from hospital management." *International Journal of Health Services* 5: 27–36.

Miller, J. D., and S. M. Shurtell. 1969. "Hospital unionization: A study of trends." *Hospitals* 43: 67–73.

Weber, Max. 1947. *Economy and Society.* Trans. Talcott Parsons. Glencoe, Ill.: The Free Press.

Part Three
CHANGING PATTERNS OF HEALTH SERVICES

9

The New Practitioners

The growth of the hospital as the major organizational form for delivering health care accounts at least in part for rising service costs. Aside from inflation and population growth during the past 20 years, increased utilization of short-term hospitals has helped to spur the rise in costs, with patient days in hospitals per 1,000 in the population increased from 1,072 in 1965 to 1,194 in 1973 (Cambridge Research Institute, 1975: 163). In 1974, hospital care accounted for 39 percent of national health expenditures (CRI, 1975: 155). Total expenses for nonfederal short-term hospitals rose from $5.6 million in 1960 to $28.5 million in 1973, a five-fold multiplication of costs. The rate of increase in the post-Medicare/Medicaid period was far higher than during the period from 1960 to 1968 (CRI, 1975: 162).

An aging population with greater access to hospital beds will take advantage of the availability of services. A health care delivery system that can count on new sources of reimbursement for services will take advantage of these financial arrangements. With federal, state, and local governments bearing 39.6 percent of the cost of all expenditures in 1974, planners have become increasingly concerned about ways to reduce the need for hospitalization. It was reasoned that if an alternative form of care could be delivered on an outpatient basis, the cost of care could be reduced. The use of new health care practitioners was brought about finally by rising costs, to which the hospital system made a major contribution. But the new practitioners provided new forms of care, and a system had to be developed for their education and training. Different work settings soon emerged, as well as a professional identity.

Planners also suggested that physicians did not have to evaluate and treat minor illness, educate and screen patients in order to prevent serious illness (e.g., hypertension), and monitor long-term, posthospitalization recovery (Sadler, Sadler, and Bliss, 1972: 10–11). Instead, under the direct supervision of physicians, nurse practitioners and physician assistants could perform some of the procedures, including physicial examinations, acquiring detailed patient histories, performing many diagnostic and therapeutic procedures, and even prescribing drugs under standing orders.

That they do not command the confidence and respect or have the aura of the medical doctor is a real problem, but it can be overcome. Competent primary care is becoming oriented to prevent emerging problems from becoming serious or permanent conditions that require inhospital care. Furthermore, by monitoring patients during recovery at home, the new practitioners prevent rehospitalization and reduce the adverse psychological consequences of separation from the family, particularly for children. Since many of the medical procedures for primary care and during recovery require careful followup examinations, the new practitioners also fit well into the general social needs for improving outpatient and home care.

EDUCATION AND TRAINING

A number of programs in universities and hospitals are now providing classroom instruction and practicums in order to educate physician assistants. According to representatives of the Bureau of Health Manpower of the Department of Health, Education and Welfare, in 1978 there were 50 training programs for physician assistants, with most aimed at primary care. As of 1980, there will be 7,400 graduate physician assistants in the United States. Early entrants to these programs tended to be young white males, often veterans of the Vietnam War.

The three-year curriculum for physician assistants involves a modified version of the first two years of medical school, with heavy emphasis on the basic sciences. Often, a general two-year junior college education is required before the study of anatomy, physiology, biochemistry, pharmacology, and related disciplines is begun. Clinic experiences are introduced during the second year and are expanded during the final year of internship in various ambulatory health services. At the end of the program, many academic-based students receive a baccalaureate degree. Plans are being proposed for a five-year program immediately following high school to train new primary care medical practitioners who

> would not be required to have a doctorate degree in medicine or the extensive knowledge of the traditional medical doctor but would have the educational background, clinical proficiency, competence and problem solving ability to make medical diagnoses, institute medical treatment and provide comprehensive preventive and primary therapeutic medical care and counseling. [Silver, 1974: 97–98]

In 1975, the American Nursing Association reported a total of 2,400 nurse practitioners in the United States, with 1,000 specialists in pediatrics. Academic programs that award Master's degrees to nurse practitioners totaled 45 in 1975. Programs that certify nurse practitioners are located in a variety of settings, sometimes in colleges and universities. But registered nurses may also become certified as nurse practitioners, both through hospital-based programs or through a tutorial program worked out with physicians in solo or group practice. The Bureau of Health Manpower estimates that the supply of these health care providers will increase to 11,400 in 1980. Nurses and nurse practitioners can also become certified as physician assistants by passing a qualifying examination.

Training programs for nurse practitioners emphasize clinical skills rather than the basic sciences curriculum for physician assistants. Clinical training also focuses heavily on primary care, and many programs provide that students carry a small case load under close supervision by physicians and graduate nurse practitioners. These programs often turn out extremely well-trained graduates, but they are criticized for being expensive and having a small number of graduates in proportion to the number of trainers. However these criticisms can be made of traditional medical education as well.

UTILIZATION

The new practitioners have different opportunities to work in various medical settings, depending on the structure of the organization (Breslau, Wolf, and Novack, 1978). Many nurse practitioners are utilized in ambulatory care settings in hospital-based clinics or neighborhood family care centers (based on the health maintenance organization model), because administrators can convert a line in their budgets for a clinic nurse with an R.N. license to a position for a nurse practitioner. In this way, nurse practitioners provide primary care and monitor home care, including the treatment of minor illnesses and the prescribing of medication under standing orders. Nurse practitioners work in special programs developed as part of outpatient programs for children and adults, often in publicly sponsored facilities such as municipal hospitals. In addition, pediatric nurse practitioners are employed in many group pediatric practices, where they conduct physical examinations and provide counseling on questions related to infant care and the management of the child in the home.

Physician assistants tend to work almost exclusively in group or solo practices, although some have been trained for special tasks such as assisting in surgery or postoperative-recovery monitoring on surgical wards (Sullivan, 1980). In private practice, physician assistants examine sutures, make house calls, perform screening functions at nursing homes, monitor patients recovering from serious illness in the care of their families, discuss laboratory tests, and make hospital rounds with M.D.s. Physician assistants have an advantage in being employed in private practices because they have some direct income-generating characteristics. Many of the procedures performed by physician assistants not only free the physician to deal with more difficult medical problems, but they are directly reimbursable to the group or solo practice from third-party insurers.

Theoretically, the cost of care should be reduced if services are rendered by a physician assistant or nurse practitioner. However, many doctors bill patients for services provided by these new health care practitioners at their customary charges. The AMA endorsed this practice in a resolution issued in December 1974 (CRI, 1975: 377). The justification is that the overall reimbursement rate from Blue Shield and other third-party payers will go down if customary fees are not charged. The fee-for-service system of payment encourages maximization of income. The same inducement is not built into group practices, which are prepaid and where the employment of physician assistants or nurse practitioners would cut costs and the financial burden to the consumer.

Despite the emphasis on classroom work, clinical skills acquired through practice often differentiate the new health care practitioners as far as competency is concerned. Nurse practitioners taken from the ranks of experienced R.N.s and trained in special hospital programs were used in one clinic as an informal resource by other nurse practitioners who were products of academic-based baccalaureate programs. At a symposium in New York City devoted to the examination of the use of all new practitioners in primary care, one nurse practitioner with supervisory responsibilities suggested that experience prior to training has distinct advantages. In a neighborhood family comprehensive care center employing nurse practitioners with both kinds of training, the nurse practitioners with no extensive background in nursing raised many questions about traditional nursing practice, answers to which were helpful in performing their assigned roles ("Proceedings," 1975: 59).

It is also likely that nurse practitioners who are trained by physicians are better prepared for primary care than those who are taught by nursing faculty in colleges. Physicians who operate nurse practitioner training programs in hospitals devote a good deal of time to imparting medical knowledge and providing close clinical instruction in both medical and psychosocial areas. Clinical experience in a supervised office practice has been found to be extremely valuable in permitting nurse practitioners to learn how to assume responsibility for patient care and to exercise independent judgment (Birenbaum, 1974: 102).

EVALUATION OF PERFORMANCE

Two major concerns about the new health care practitioners have been: (1) whether physician associates would be able to remain within the defined limits of their roles or would seek to expand them into areas beyond their training and skills, and (2) whether they would perform as well as physicians in identifying and managing illness. The physicians who began training programs wanted to prove not only that their trainees were talented but also to reassure their colleagues that the new practitioners wouldn't threaten their authority (or income).

In 1968, Henry Silver and his associates at the University of Colorado Medical School began a training program for nurses who wished to become Pediatric Nurse Practitioners (henceforth referred to as PNPs). Nurses who participated felt that their talents were more adequately utilized than they had been in the traditional nursing role. However, they were careful to note that the boundary between what they did and what physicians did was still carefully drawn: "The limits of our activities are clearly defined. We do not pretend to function beyond these boundaries" (Stearly et al., 1967: 2087).

Observant of their distinctive tasks and their limits, they were still able to take modest credit for recognizing illness and, more important, gaining the compliance of parents: ". . . a mother may come to us first with a seriously ill child and because of the sounds we hear in his chest, or the bulging eardrum we see, we advise her to see the doctor. The mother respects our advice and goes immediately" (Stearly et al., 1967: 2087).

The University of Colorado Medical School group also sought to convince physicians that the PNP was a skilled practitioner in primary care. The diagnoses of PNPs were compared with those of physicians in 278 instances (Duncan et al., 1971: 1170–76). In only two cases were the differences in judgment considered serious for the child's health status.

Physician assistants have been used in large group practices such as college medical services or in prepaid plans such as Kaiser-Permanente on the West Coast. In one study of 207 patient–physician assistant encounters, the physician assistant was able to take care of the patient without consulting the physician in 166 cases. The problem required discussion in 17 cases and referral to a physician in 24 instances (Lairson et al., 1974: 215).

The new practitioners have proven to be able performers of assigned tasks, but they are still in an ambiguous position in the organized health care delivery system. Some physicians say they will delegate more tasks to physician assistants or nurse practitioners, but they do not do so in practice. This discrepancy between what is said and what is done may vary according to the type of practice. The new practitioners are supposed to free the physician to do the more complicated and difficult work, tasks that may or may not exist in any given community-based practice. Physicians and nurses who have not been trained to work with practitioners may have difficulty ascertaining what health services they can provide.

The following section presents a case study on the making of a professional identity by nurses who became part of a PNP training program. This research identifies the social mechanism by which nurses acquire the knowledge, ability, and motivation to exercise responsibility and judgment as primary health care agents and how they manage to maintain these impressions in contact with members of the medical profession.

THE MAKING OF A PROFESSIONAL IDENTITY

Observations were made at a training program for PNPs in a general municipal hospital serving an ethnically heterogeneous working-class population of a big city. Two programs were designed to utilize the PNP in innovative special health services for children, with primary care the major responsibility.

The home care program attempts to reduce hospitalization time and its consequences for child development by using PNPs as the primary agents for children who have had serious or chronic illnesses that required hospitalization and where close monitoring and therapy can be accomplished at home. This assignment of primary responsibility is negotiated between physician and PNP, and the latter may, *de facto*, become the primary agent. This does not shift legal responsibility from the physician to the nurse practitioner. Here, clearly, the skills involved go beyond recognizing disease to include whether a child is recovering or declining and what such changes or plateaus represent developmentally, as well as what they mean for the family's management of the illness.

The PNP also is trained to work in a program providing comprehensive medical care for newborns and their siblings; thus it constitutes a general pediatric office practice, where most illnesses are managed within the unit by the nurse practitioner, although consultation with physicians is available. Although the policy of the program limits home visits, an initial postpartum home visit is made to assess the facilities available for child care, to get a medical history of the family, to answer questions on infant care, to locate potential problem areas, and to do a postpartum examination of the mother. Most of the physical examinations, diagnosis, and treatment for minor illnesses are done in the unit's offices, with the nurse practitioner acting as the primary agent.

Using the curriculum model suggested by Henry Silver and his associates (1968: 298–302), registered nurses were given four months of lectures and demonstration in pediatrics. This was followed by a twenty-month internship program for PNPs. During internship, trainees provided primary care under supervision of a pediatrician and a certified nurse practitioner, with a progressive increase occurring in their patient panel and expanded responsibility and autonomy in practice. This internship went beyond the academic training in Silver's model, where PNPs did not provide care for a panel of patients. The curriculum of the PNP training program was designed to prepare the former nurse for the major responsibility of providing primary comprehensive pediatric health care. At the end of the program, the PNP was expected to be able to:

1. Conduct a meaningful interview with the patient and/or parent
2. Obtain a full "data base" on the child and family
3. Perform a physical examination
4. Assess the health status of a patient
5. Understand the elements of normal growth and development and use them in anticipatory guidance
6. Recognize deviations from normal limits
7. Know the elements of good health care maintenance
8. Have an appreciation of major psychosocial factors and the way that they may impinge on health care delivery
9. Develop a panel of patients for whom they serve as a continuous primary source of pediatric care
10. Manage common minor illnesses of childhood
11. Begin to recognize the symptoms of more severe, acute, or chronic illnesses and participate with the physician in their evaluation and management.

These goals emphasize a more extensive role for the PNP in managing primary health care for children than are suggested by the Colorado program. (For further discussion of the pioneering efforts in Denver, see Stearly et al., 1967; Silver et al., 1968; Schiff et al., 1969; Day et al., 1970; and Duncan et al., 1971.)

In the University of Colorado Medical School program (1) PNPs were not permitted to *treat* common minor illnesses, while PNPs were participants with the physician in the screening, evaluation and management of more severe, acute, or chronic illnesses; (2) PNPs did not work in a hospital as part of an outpatient pediatric service but only in private practice with pediatricians, or in health stations in low-income areas, or later, in rural areas where no physicians were readily available, thus restricting their involvement in organized health care and limiting the nature of their contact with other professions; (3) the PNPs were not members of comprehensive health care teams, which usually include a number of medical specialties and medical social workers; and (4) PNPs were not attuned to the psychosocial dynamics of the family as it influenced the delivery of health care, although they were involved in instructing mothers of newborns concerning child-care practices.

These new tasks greatly changed the public image and the self-image of the nurse. Performing the role of the PNP called into question the prior occupational identity of the nurse in two ways: (1) as the unquestioned subordinate to the physician, and (2) as the health care agent whose day-to-day responsibilities are many, but whose medical judgments and advice are not to be taken seriously. Accordingly, some nurses as well as physicians have been threatened by this new practitioner role and have expressed concern over the efficacy of taking on expanded obligations because it creates stratification within their ranks. Indeed, officers of the nursing associations advocated that nurses concentrate on their own special tasks as the way to gain honor as an occupation (Glazer, 1966: 27).

A new professional identity cannot be assigned but has to emerge out of new responsibilities. Consequently, in its early stages, professional development is an outcome of the daily encounters between PNPs and physicians, and between PNPs and other health care professionals, resulting in symbolic identification of the task with the performer. Role definition and professional identity are forged in contact with members of a unit and in cooperation and conflict with other services.

The observations reported here were made over a twelve-month period in 1972 and 1973. Subjects expressed their personal and professional concerns to each other during the course of the working day, and the author was a participant observer in many situations: at team meetings of the two programs described above, during several home visits with PNPs to their patients and families, and when physicians in other services had encounters with PNPs. Interviews also took place casually during the working day, and respondents usually generated their own concerns rather than responding to issues that were expressly raised for their consideration, following the method of Becker and Geer (1958).

Recruitment and Training

Recruitment to this special training program brought applicants whose major motivation was to overcome the compartmentalization of tasks found in modern hospital care and to "get more into" their roles as nurses. Becoming a PNP provided an opportunity for greater patient involvement, since the strategic focus of the role is the interface between patient, family, hospital, and various medical services. All other tasks performed by the PNP are designed to be coordinated, benefiting the person's state of health and/or helping him or her make an optimal adaptation to a chronic illness or disability.

Control of the training programs and the concomitant tasks of selection and recruitment of candidates will have an important influence upon the development of the role of the PNP as an independent or quasi-independent profession. It is highly unlikely that the PNP will ever become completely independent of the discipline of medicine. Possibly some autonomy will be acquired, to the extent that the PNP achieves a "legal monopoly over performance of some strategic aspect of work and effectively prevents free competition from other occupations" (Freidson, 1970a: 123). While the PNP is unlikely to become a major source of new medical knowledge in health care, the professional autonomy of a practitioner is partly based on *controlling* "the production and particularly the application of knowledge and skill in the work it performs" (Freidson, 1970a: 123). It is possible, although not easy to convince related professionals, that PNPs can best perform the services they provide. The training program, both in the formal curriculum and the behaviors it encouraged, imparted a new way of working with medical practitioners and patients.

Selection for the training program was made by the administrative team of two physicians, a social worker, and a trained PNP. The formal curriculum was created by the members of the staff who were administratively responsible, and it was regarded as essential by both physicians and nurses. Other observers have noted the same impact of the formal training program upon nurses who became PNPs. At the 1972 meetings of the American Academy of Pediatrics, a physician who utilized a PNP in private practice said that "nurses who have left for special training acquire a special aura about them; they come back as a different person." Even after working as PNPs in the home care part of the program, prior to the formalizing of a curriculum, nurses insist on receiving the academic part of the training.

All the nurses selected for the unit were capable of handling a great deal of responsibility, such as working in a pediatric intensive care unit, supervising other nurses, or working in a hemodialysis program. The development of responsibility as a PNP was different, however. Nurses at a particular station in a hospital had more organizational supports to rely on than other nurses, house staff, and PNPs providing primary care. The new sense of self acquired by PNPs parallels that of medical students as studied by Becker and his coworkers (1961: 234). Professional responsibility extended beyond being conscientious on duty; it included direct interaction with the client, with one's peers, and with other members of the team. This rule was evident at all the team meetings attended by the author and was transmitted by the physicians and veteran PNPs during the discussion of cases. The longer the PNP's exposure to participation in team decision making, the greater the opportunity to develop responsibility because of the length of time that the program has been in existence. At team meetings in the comprehensive care program, because of its later initiation, there were numerous efforts on the part of senior staff to teach how the other members of the team might be utilized in serving one's clients.

One of the major goals of the team meetings was to formulate a plan for the management of health care for sick and well children. The PNPs in the home care program often shared the planning of care, as in the following case:

> Juan, a boy with bilateral skull fractures, was discussed. The case was presented by a PNP who met with a neurologist from a rehabilitation facility connected with the hospital. She and Dr. Pauling had asked whether transportation would be provided by the rehabilitation unit for the family. The neurologist was vague in his answers as well as to the other questions concerning follow-ups to missed appointments. The PNP thought they couldn't leave the planning to the rehabilitation unit and would try this plan only if the social worker from the Bureau of Child Welfare could remain involved. Dr. Butler asked if there was an alternative plan. The PNP wasn't sure about having just one plan ready and so suggested several, including residential placement in a rehabilitation setting.

The goals of these plans sometimes involved diagnosing and executing treatment by PNPs, which was done under physician's standing orders. In situations where the PNPs were uncertain about treatment, they consulted with the physicians. A number of other procedures, including blood tests, physical examinations, and EKGs were done by PNPs either at home or in the office.

Control over the dispensing of information to the client is a responsibility that often distinguishes the independent professional from other professions (Freidson, 1970a: 141). PNPs were increasingly able to share this task with physicians: They explained the nature of the illness and the need for procedures to the parents and the child and also interpreted the results of diagnostic tests for them.

Perhaps of utmost significance was that responsibility brought a personal reorganization of the PNPs sense of identity, from a person who does one's work upon receiving orders—direct or standing—to one who sets the pace of one's work and is self-directed; from one who works toward the goal of getting the person well to one who works toward the goal of keeping the person well; from one who sees her work as giving advice as well as providing a service, and that the advice she gives is considered necessary for solving the patient's problem; and as one whose job never ends, rather than one who can forget the job at the end of the day.

These distinctions reveal that the PNP acquired a different sense of work. When the scope of the role was extended, the direction of demands was reversed, and the demands themselves became far more reciprocal. PNPs not only made preliminary diagnoses but also sought to set up the means by which these hypotheses could be confirmed through laboratory tests or consultations with specialists. Responsibility involved making sure that a referral to a more specialized service was actually carried out by the parent and the service. Continuous concern with the well-being of the child beyond the initial illness was often demonstrated.

A PNP began a discussion on an arthritic boy whose disease had been arrested. The immediate medical problem had become inactive, but there was a feeling on her part that the family ought to be followed so that they could catch a reversal if it occurred.

While PNPs established an ongoing relationship with a family, they did not regard themselves as an endless source of service and reward to that family. If the parents of patients did not follow the advice proferred, the PNPs became more critical of ongoing family practices. In one instance, the PNP felt that she had been working well with the family but "could only go so far," if the mother did not take her advice.

However, those nurses with less experience in their new roles were less able to withdraw some support for the family when the mother would not accept assistance. The physicians in the program attempted to demonstrate that compliance was influenced by many factors:

A PNP discussed a case where a patient did not show up for an examination.

Dr. Butler: How did you feel about it?

PNP: That's what I wanted to talk about. I felt I did my part.

Dr. Butler: It could be she hates the hospital and it has nothing to do with you.

The development of a long-range perspective on one's work often involves making distinctions between what can and cannot be avoided in helping a patient. One of the tasks of the physicians in the program was to get the PNPs not to regard every noncompliant parent as a personal rejection and not to feel that they were responsible for the parent's negative behavior. In many instances, to account for a patient's anger, other factors are considered, as when a young mother seeks to compete for attention with her baby, or when a person acts contradictorily.

Dr. Butler: You want to talk about Mrs. W.?

PNP: I don't know what's going on. She gave me a brush-off. You spoke with her, Dr. Isler.

Dr. Isler: She seemed to be in and out.

PNP: This seems to be a pattern with her.

Dr. Isler: She is like the other case we discussed. We shouldn't press.

The PNPs, during the course of their training, made themselves increasingly more available to patients so as far as intervention and planning were concerned:

> PNP: Also, this job is not just eight hours a day. I think about the cases all the time. I feel I am responsible for everything. It is really a mindbending experience.

Yet PNPs also learned that immediate and constant availability to patients is not a demonstration of responsibility. Initially, staff meetings were interrupted by phone calls and messages from the secretaries, stating that a patient's mother wanted to speak to a PNP or was outside waiting to have the child examined. Staff M.D.s stressed that being well-prepared is more important than giving immediate attention, unless it is an emergency; that responsibility is not only to one's patients, but to the staff as well; that they should have some control over scheduling; and that self-mastery is an important aspect of being an independent professional. PNPs began to learn *when* to provide help. The question of *whether* to act and *how* to act were matters of acquiring judgment.

Independent Judgment

One of the central features of an independent profession is the capacity to use judgment in situations that are not clear-cut or in cases where the extension of one's service and advice may be problematic. The appearance of a client with a problem is not always a direct signal that intervention is possible. A large part of the training of an independent professional is learning when and where to attempt "solutions to the concrete problems of individuals" (Freidson, 1970b: 163).

One aspect of PNP's training is to learn how to recognize one's limitations. The medical practitioner must be able to tell when a difficult case requires a more experienced or specialized physician. The practitioner should regard this as a sign of competency, not incompetency: that is, knowing when one's judgment might endanger the patient. The physician himself is frequently faced with similar decisions in referrals to specialists. Yet there is no suspicion because the physician uses more specialized consultants.

Self-limitation, as an aspect of judgment, became part of an orientation to their work. They understood that some patients will not respond to their services. PNPs had to demonstrate that their right to accept or reject a case in the home care program was respected by the medical staff of this service and other services as well (Freidson, 1970a: 121). Sometimes, efforts were wasted if PNPs could not rely on the family to provide day-to-day home care:

> This staff meeting centered around discussion of cases not to be included in the program. In one case, the mother was inconsistent in taking the child's pulse and in giving digitalis. An aunt of the child was to be trained to do this, but when she was visiting the child on the ward with the mother, she did nothing but act as a translator. A PNP said that she "was a long way away from picking up this child" as a home care case. No one questioned her judgment in this case.

Often the home care team would accept a child on a trial basis to determine whether they could offer service:

> A child with encephalitis was discussed as a potential case for home care. The child presented no acute medical problems. The team decided to take the case on

> but would try to involve several other agencies so that the mother could get some relief from the care of the child. Homemaker services were suggested.

In this example, the PNPs found it appropriate to assess the need for their long-term involvement while providing home care. There is a major point of contact with the family, and PNPs are in the strategic position of best determining its needs.

In the area of planning, the home care team depended heavily on the PNPs' judgment. While a physician presented the details of a prospective case, PNPs made contributions and suggested procedures to use when in contact with the patient. Meetings were regarded as the appropriate forums for testing out plans.

> Billy was discussed. He is a child with abnormal head and eye movements and his head is unusually large. A PNP said that she would do a Denver Developmental Test on him the next time she made a home visit.

Sometimes contact with clients was maintained until other services were made available, as in the case of a parent suspected of child abuse. A PNP was reluctant to step out of the case because, in her judgment, responsibility could not yet be terminated. A discussion between two PNPs represents a negotiation on the limits of nonmedical involvement where no immediate health problems are found.

> PNP: We really have no medical reason to be there and we can't be interpreters for the entire city.
>
> PNP: All I can do, all I am doing, is waiting for some other agency to pick them up.
>
> PNP: This should be taken up with Rose when she gets back from vacation because it really is a social service problem.

Once the PNP agreed to take on a case, the limits of intervention were clearly outlined. Involvement could be reconsidered and reduced when the family was not responding to advice. PNPs with long-term experience were more willing to do this than the newer ones. In the illustration below, a resident, newly assigned to home care, questioned the judgment of a PNP in disengaging from a case where the mother did not take the PNP's advice. The PNP had been doing psychotherapy under a psychiatrist's supervision with this client and had made a referral to the Department of Psychiatry for the mother.

> Dr. Samler: Why was help cut off?
>
> PNP: I am not a therapist, and it was getting to the point that I could take her only so far. I felt my short-term therapy was now becoming destructive because she wouldn't seek psychiatric help since she had me to lean on.

In contrast, newer PNPs were often unsure of their level of involvement in a case and were anxious about being overly involved:

> PNP: I want to talk about Mrs. F. The baby has pustulosis. The woman told me during the information-gathering session I had with her that she had been under

psychiatric care; that she was a chronic schizophrenic since the age of 12; that she felt she had a problem of sexual identity and she couldn't satisfy her husband . . .

PNP: We ought to talk about how involved we want to get with her. She's a sick woman.

Dr. Butler: That's a good point and something we can get back to . . .

PNP: Her two-year-old is driving her up the wall.

Dr. Butler: Why?

PNP: He's very stubborn and likes to stand in front of the open refrigerator.

Dr. Butler: He sounds like a normal two year old . . . The problem with Mrs. F. is that her thought processes don't add up even if they are logical. She may not follow your advice or even resent it because she can misinterpret emotionally.

PNP (insistently): How involved are we supposed to get with these families? Maybe I'm just scared.

PNPs in the home care program constantly made determinations as to when to refer a client to another service or when to involve another service. In this sense, the programs to which referrals were made by PNPs were also being evaluated by them. Other services were sometimes found to utilize these programs because it enabled them to demonstrate more effective performance; the PNP sought to do the same. On one occasion, the home care team utilized a nursery program for a child, which also promised some therapy for the parents. Later, they reevaluated the placement because it did not deal with the parents' relationship.

Besides evaluating other services, PNPs and other members of the team wanted to reeducate the other clinical services, stressing the importance of providing comprehensive care themselves:

PNP: This sounds like a home care case, but how do we make it clear to the X Clinic that they cannot dump cases on us; that they should develop their own program which provides comprehensive care and trains parents?

Without this attitude, the home care program easily could have become a victim of its own success, assuming cases that should be the responsibility of other clinical services. Whenever it was reported that a member of another clinic service contemplated adopting some aspect of their procedures, the news was usually greeted by the PNPs with sarcastic laughter, as when a cardiologist said to one of the staff that he would make a home visit to see if a child with a heart defect could be managed at home. The home care staff did not believe that other programs would follow their lead and break the established routine of providing services only in the hospital.

Receiving Support from Other Services

However, consistent support was not received from the other services. Rather, particular individuals, scattered throughout the various services, were coopted, mainly through the personal relationships between the physicians in the unit and physicians at the hospital center. However, support was demonstrated by physicians outside the unit who worked with PNPs on special projects. Once having established a working relationship with a PNP, medical service chiefs requested the unit to train new PNPs to work in their services.

While PNPs were recruited for the program with an eye toward their prior experiences and were given training in pediatrics similar to that given in medical school, they also received informal training in how to convey their medical competency to physicians outside of the unit. Often there was covert resistance to the acquisition and usage of medical language and procedures. Yet it seems that PNPs maintained the confidence of their colleagues when they used precise medical language rather than nursing language. PNPs were corrected by unit physicians at meetings when they used the more imprecise nursing language. For example, instead of saying "has a temperature" or "temp," PNPs were expected to say "is febrile" (or has fever), the latter term being more accurate, since all people have a temperature. Rather than describing a developmental test as being "negative," they were expected to report that the results were within normal limits.

In addition, a uniform system of medical reporting was used in filling in the patients' charts. This system ultimately provided a way of profiling the patient population and enabled the unit personnel to plan services more effectively. Moreover, using a standardized system of recording allowed the innovative pediatric unit to be seen as an integral part of the medical services of the hospital. They were clues to outsiders as to the kind of professional image the unit wanted to present, as well as a way of convincing them that what they said was being understood and what they heard was accurate medical reporting. Nevertheless, at the time this case study was first reported, the PNP unit had a tenuous standing, even within the department of pediatrics.

It was evident that support from specialty clinics was limited when physicians in these clinics questioned the PNPs' right to request services on their own rather than through the physicians. PNPs had to acquire many responsibilities for specialized procedures, such as changing a catheter themselves, rather than using the urology clinic. This was done not only because they were reluctant to overload a service but also because of their willingness to take on new responsibilities when they felt able to handle them.

The avoidance of relying on other services may have had unintended consequences for the professional development of PNPs, particularly in adding new responsibilities. Indeed, too much interdependence with other services may not foster professional growth beyond narrowly defined tasks. And this program sought to encourage a sense of responsibility and independent judgment. In Chapter 10, patients' response to physician assistants and nurse practitioners will be examined.

REFERENCES

Becker, Howard, et al. 1961. *Boys in White: Student Culture in Medical School.* Chicago: University of Chicago Press.

Becker N., and B. Geer. 1958. "Problems of inference and proof in participant observation." *American Sociological Review* 23 (December): 652–60.

Birenbaum, A. 1974. "The making of a professional identity: The pediatric nurse practitioner." *Sociological Symposium* 11 (Spring): 98–118.

Breslau, N., G. Wolf, and A. H. Novack. "Correlates of physician's task delegation in primary care." *Journal of Health and Social Behavior* 19: 374–84.

[CRI] Cambridge Research Institute. 1975. *Trends Affecting the U.S. Health Care System.* Washington, D.C.: Department of Health, Education, and Welfare.

Day, L. R., R. Egli, and H. K. Silver. 1970. "Acceptance of pediatric nurse practitioners." *American Journal of Diseases in Children* 119 (March): 204–8.

Duncan, B., A. N. Smith, and H. K. Silver. 1971. "Comparison of the physical assessment of children by pediatric nurse practitioners and pediatricians." *American Journal of Public Health* 61 (June): 1170–76.

Freidson, Eliot. 1970a. *Professional Dominance: The Social Structure of Medical Care.* New York: Atherton Press.

———. 1970b. *The Profession of Medicine: A Study of the Sociology of Applied Knowledge.* New York: Dodd, Mead.

Glazer, W. 1966. "Nursing leadership and policy," in Fred Davis, Ed., *The Nursing Profession: Five Sociological Essays.* New York: John Wiley.

Lairson, P., J. Record, and J. James. 1974. "Physician assistants at Kaiser: Distinctive patterns of practice." *Inquiry* (September): 207–19.

"Proceedings of the Symposium on New Health Care Practitioners in Primary Care." 1975. Bronx, N. Y.: The Bronx Health Manpower Consortium.

Sadler, A. M., B. L. Sadler, and A. A. Bliss. 1972. *The Physician's Assistant: Today and Tomorrow.* New Haven: Yale University School of Medicine.

Schiff, D. W., C. H. Fraser, and H. L. Walters. 1969. "The pediatric nurse practitioner in the office of pediatricians in private practice." *Pediatrics* 44 (July): 62–68.

Silver, H. K., L. C. Ford, and L. R. Day. 1968. "The pediatric nurse practitioner program: Expanding the role of the nurse to private increased health care for children." *Journal of the American Medical Association* 204 (April): 298–302.

Silver, H. K. 1974. "New Health professionals for primary ambulatory care." *Hospital Practice* (April): 97–98.

Stearly, S., A. Noordenbus, and V. Crouch. 1967. "Pediatric nurse practitioner." *American Journal of Nursing* 67 (October): 2083–87.

Sullivan, R. 1980. "Help for the harried hospital doctors." *New York Times*, March 22, pp. 23, 25.

10

Patients and the New Practitioners

A major characteristic of the new practitioners is a capacity to work independently even while under the supervision of the physician.* The utilization of these new personnel in remote rural areas or in ghetto urban areas where there are few physicians makes the development of independent judgment a necessity.

A fruitful collaboration between the new practitioner and the doctor need not be based on direct supervision so long as enough time is set aside for consultation and evaluation of performance. In fact, the physical separation is made possible, if not actually encouraged, by state laws. In some states, the physician assistant and nurse practitioner can legally make house calls, prescribe medications for minor illnesses, and perform physical examinations. As a result, criteria for training have also been established in many states, perhaps before all the evidence is in on what the new practitioners can and cannot do well.

That physician assistants and nurse practitioners have some autonomy does not imply that all new health care roles will be structured with similar independence. The conditions that allow independent judgment are not available to other paramedical personnel who also work under the physician's supervision. The new role of medical assistant has been created in order to relieve doctors from routine office tasks, such as measuring blood pressures, measuring height and weight, and taking blood samples (Fowler, 1977). It may not be long before the physician's office will be similar to that

*This chapter is based on two studies of new practitioners conducted by the author. Reports of the study of PNPs were published in the *Journal of Psychiatric Nursing and Mental Health Services* (September, October, 1974). Some of the material on community mental health workers and rehabilitation workers comes from an article by M. B. Ahmed and the author, which appeared in *Intellect* 105 (October, 1977): 149–51.

of the dentist's, where the dental hygienist performs many paramedical duties.

The capacity of the new practitioners to exercise independent judgment is not only a result of their training and the environments in which they work, but is an outcome of the way their roles are defined. When they are permitted to carry their own case load and follow patients on a long-term basis, they become the experts on those particular patients. Face-to-face contact is relatively frequent between any health care practitioner and a patient when illness is being treated or monitored over a long duration. In contrast, the medical assistant or office nurse may see a patient only briefly and may not be assigned to the same patient at future visits. Also, the patient knows that the physician will be seen after the medical assistant, so he or she finds little reason to ask a question or express a concern to the medical assistant. On the other hand, the physician assistant or nurse practitioner who provides primary care may be the patient's only contact with the health care organization. Patients who do not regard them as competent may insist on seeing a physician even when it is not medically indicated, or they may seek additional opinions.

Accordingly, it is crucial to determine how patients relate to the new practitioners. No matter how well trained, medically knowledgeable, or skilled one may be, professionals who do not communicate well with patients may not be able to do their job. Of course, this holds true for physicians as well.

The sources of acceptance and rejection of the roles of the new health care practitioners are numerous. Patients may perceive some providers as ineffective, as in the case of community mental health workers and rehabilitation workers in psychiatric settings. These workers provide an interesting contrast to physician assistants and nurse practitioners, both in terms of their utilization and occupational identities. It is evident that patients not only react to their illnesses but to the health care organization and its personnel. Learning to deal with the emotional aspects of care makes care more effective, since patients will be less likely to terminate contact or fail to take medications.

PATIENT ACCEPTANCE

The general public's perception of the physician assistant is tempered by lack of experience in receiving health care from someone in this role. Where trust is established between the patient and the family physician who employs a physician assistant, approval will be forthcoming. Litman surveyed 253 rural households drawn from a probability sample in Minnesota and Iowa. He asked respondents to state hypothetically whether they would be willing to receive medical services from a former medical corpsman now trained as a physician assistant and employed and supervised by local doctors. More than 85 percent reported that they would allow a physician assistant to care for them and their families. There was a great deal of acceptance of routine care, such as taking medical histories, physical examinations, giving routine treatment for simple emergency cases, providing early childhood immunizations, or making patient referrals to specialists. Interestingly, gynecological matters such as prenatal care and routine assistance at birth were given less approval. Litman suggests this result obtained because men were the potential providers of services rather than women (1972: 345), or that the physician assistants were viewed as strange men, in contrast to the familiar family doctor, or that they may be men from less respectable backgrounds than the person with the degree from a medical college.

Gender differences can often be overcome and even reversed through acquiring high professional status, as in the case of physicians. The history of midwifery in the United States demonstrates how a standard form of health care can be terminated and later reintroduced under new sponsorship (Rich, 1976).

The rejuvenation of midwifery under the new title of nurse-midwife also demonstrates that female patients will accept a middle-level practitioner to perform essential tasks. The use of specially trained women in obstetrics is hardly a new idea, as women have shared the task of birth and delivery ever since there were stable communities on this earth. There is evidence that midwifery was an honored practice in first-century Rome ("The New Midwife," 1975). In the 1960's, the Department of Health, Education, and Welfare recognized the physician shortage in rural areas and urban ghettos and supported training programs for nurse-midwives at hospitals operated by medical colleges. Evidence from the United Kingdom, which has one of the world's lowest infant mortality rates, demonstrated and justified these programs, since nearly 96 percent of all English babies are delivered by nurse-midwives. In addition, most English births are at home rather than in hospitals.

In the United States, once a pregnant woman is declared to be medically and obstetrically within normal limits, the midwife administers periodic checkups, provides nutritional counseling, coaches the woman on managing labor, delivers the child, and provides postpartum followups. In addition, birth control information is provided if women request it and periodic gynecological screenings can be performed.

Patients are convinced that nurse-midwives are technically competent and are concerned about the mother's welfare. A director of midwife training program at a New Jersey Medical School teaching hospital said:

> We strive to inspire confidence and trust by catering to our patients' needs on a very personal level. . . . Once the physician gives the O.K.—meaning he foresees no complications in the pregnancy—we become the expectant mother's advocate. We counsel, we soothe her fears, and we help deal with problems of motherhood. If possible, we bring other members of her family into the experience to create as home-like and comfortable an atmosphere as possible. Before we know it, we're regarded as a good friend, even like a member of the family.
>
> From what she has seen and heard . . . physicians are pleased and impressed, and patients are delighted by midwife services. "When an expectant mother enters the hospital, she needs emotional support as well as professional care, and we provide both. The close relationship that develops usually lasts even beyond the delivery." ["The New Midwife," 1975]

Evidence from two sources confirms that patients approve of the care received by physician assistants and nurse practitioners: (1) consumer response studies using self-administered questionnaires, and (2) less obtrusive sources of information, such as whether patients ask to see a physician after a routine consultation with a practitioner who provides primary care or makes an outright refusal of care from a nonphysician.

Many of these studies were performed by the University of Colorado Medical School group to convince physicians to employ physician assistants and nurse practitioners. A study of acceptance of PNPs by parents at an office practice in the Denver area showed that 94 percent of parents expressed a high degree of satisfaction with their services and felt they had sufficient opportunity to maintain adequate communication with the physician. In addition, 57 percent stated that joint care was an improvement over the care received from physicians alone. Parents also were satisfied with the PNPs' home visits, her visits to the hospital after the birth of a child, and other aspects of care (Day, Egli, and Silver, 1970: 204). In a parent opinion poll conducted at a pediatric unit where nurse practitioners provided most of the care for newborns and their brothers and sisters, similar results were found. A self-administered questionnaire completed by 81 respondents at Bronx Municipal Hospital Center gave overwhelming approval to the program:

> Most of the parents felt that the PNP was very helpful in getting care after the baby was born (95%), in getting a new appointment (89%), and in explaining things so they could better follow the doctor's orders (93%). About half found help in getting birth control (59%) and having someone to talk to about problems (49%) very helpful. The PNP was very helpful least often in getting financial assistance (26%), solving housing problems (19%), and getting others in the family to see the doctor (25%). ["The Pediatric Nurse Practitioner," n.d.]

Acceptance is also reflected in the behavior of patients. Schiff, Fraser, and Walters reported less than one percent of their office practice patients preferring the pediatrician alone to joint care (1969: 65). Similar results were found when they followed and recorded patient behavior for eighteen months. Although they do not report the total number of patients followed, "less than one dozen families requested that their case be delivered the "old way." When such a request had been made, care for these patients has been given by the physician alone" (Day, Egli, and Silver, 1970: 207).

Adults who were directly examined or treated by physician assistants demonstrated similar acceptance. A study on the use of physician assistants, who were following problem-oriented protocols, or guides to examinations, in the management of patients with diabetes and hypertension, found few patient refusals. Informed consent to route patients to the physician assistants was requested of 286 patients, and six percent declined this option for care. Patients kept appointments at about the same frequency as with physicians. Only one of the 53 patients who were told they could go home without seeing the doctor asked for a consultation with a physician. Finally, patients seeing physician assistants sought out additional clinic services at other programs at about the same frequency as those being cared for by physicians (Komaroff et al., 1974: 310).

SOURCES OF ACCEPTANCE

One of the most important explanations for the acceptance of physician assistants and nurse practitioners is their accessability to patients. Silver and Duncan performed time and motion studies of the PNP, as compared with office nurses and pediatricians, in order to determine whether the new practitioner created more opportunity for contact with patients (1971: 331–36). PNPs were found to spend twice as much time with patients as office nurses, with most of the contact involved in taking histories, performing physical examinations, evaluating health problems, and counseling with parents (Silver and Duncan, 1971: 332). Other studies report a reduction in the average time spent by the physician with the patient and family in pediatric private practices that employ nurse practitioners (Schiff, Fraser, Walters, 1969).

In many private practices and hospitals, standardized protocols are used by these new health care practitioners in performing examinations or monitoring a treatment regimen. Protocols encourage a careful and systematic examination of the patient, making it incumbent upon the examiner to perform tests where indicated by answers to questions.

Patients undergoing this examination and monitoring are often reassured that a thorough procedure is being followed. In addition, comparisons have been made of physician assistant judgments using protocols for the management of diabetes and hypertension and physicians demonstrating their competent use. At Boston City Hospital, when 381 assistant visits were verified, only one serious indicator of a change in condition was ignored by the new practitioners. False indications of change in condition was found in 11 percent of the cases (Komaroff et al., 1974: 307).

An error on the side of seeing a serious change in condition when one is not really present is viewed by physicians as less damaging to the patient than overlooking a serious change in condition; the first type of error is referred to as a false-positive finding and the second as a false-negative finding. However, physicians may become increasingly concerned in the future with false-positive errors since treatment for a nonexistent illness or condition can result in failure to find the real source of symptoms, as well as possible unnecessary adverse drug reactions or surgery or psychological harm to patient and family.

Still, the study demonstrates the feasibility of using physician assistants armed with protocols to deal with these diseases of later life. Since the population is aging and diabetes and hypertension are common among the elderly, monitoring of conditions by the new practitioners may become an important part of standard medical care. However, as Celentano (1978) points out, the high quality of care provided may be an artifact of the extreme selectivity of the trainers, an outcome that might disappear when new health care practitioners are educated in large numbers.

From the patient's perspective, the clearly observable use of the protocol may represent the presence of planning and technique, instilling confidence in the health care organization. An important determinant of patient satisfaction may reside in the advance knowledge of what to expect and how services will be delivered. More research on the impressions made on patients, on their expectations, and on the services received may account for the high level of acceptance of the new practitioners.

Some observers have suggested that the communications skills of the new practitioners result from their similarity to the patients they serve. For example, mothers may tend to trust and confide in the female PNP rather than the male pediatrician. Are new health care practitioners accepted by patients because of similarities of social characteristics? Do patients also expect demonstrations of skill? Perhaps persons from the same social class and ethnic group background encourage communication between patients and practitioners (Cambridge Research Institute, 1975: 380). Being a peer may encourage conversation, but patients may often leave an encounter feeling that nothing has been done. Spanish-speaking patients may feel more comfortable receiving help from someone who speaks their language, but this may not be a replacement for a well-trained practitioner who can both perform a thorough examination and ask the right questions (Bernstein, Bernstein, and Dana, 1974).

SOURCES OF PATIENT SELECTION

Patients are able to sort out those who can help them from those who cannot, but the problem of getting to see those who can help remains. For many poor people, second-class care is the only care available. On the other hand, those who can afford to pay for physicians have been willing to receive care from nurse practitioners and physician assistants because they have been convinced that they have genuine skills. A similar movement to substitute new practitioners in the field of social psychiatry was attempted, with the development of the roles of community mental health worker and rehabilitation worker. The procedures differed, as did the results.

The idea of using nonprofessionals in human services as paid employees began to take root in delinquency prevention programs in the early 1960s. Using the informal leaders of the neighborhoods, these programs upgraded traditional community voluntary positions to the status of full-time paid employment. A few years later, community mental health centers were established, which also made use of nonprofessionals to provide services as paid employees. Starting as a social movement that was backed by the federal mandate of the Community Mental Health Act of 1963, many people expected that these centers and their programs would help develop communities through achievement of shared aspirations (Bellak, 1974: 3).

Concern for community development was based on the belief in the social psychiatry field that an important means of preventing mental illness lay in building mutual supports through membership in informal social networks. Gradually, planners at community mental health centers have developed more specific goals, becoming more concerned with the problems of ongoing care and treatment associated with psychiatric patients, both in and out of hospitals, and the provision of individual group, and family therapy to people under less severe stress who do not require hospitalization. In addition, new programs provide services in areas traditionally the concern of other institutions or agencies of social control, such as the family, hospitals, the courts, and the police (Dinitz and Beran, 1971). Consequently, such problems as alcoholism, addiction, juvenile delinquency, difficulties of children in schools, and difficulties during the process of aging have come to be defined as appropriate targets for community mental health center programs and services.

Given this shift in goals, a redefinition has been required in the tasks of the nonprofessional staff. Now generally referred to as *paraprofessionals*, these workers are being assigned specific tasks within service teams. Paraprofessionals are now subject to new work situations where contact with clients and supervision by professionals takes place on a regular basis; and standardized methods have been instituted for performance appraisal. Under the title of rehabilitation worker, some paraprofessionals work closely with patients for long periods in the hospital, day hospital, and various rehabilitation services and programs. Community mental health workers are assigned to specific tasks, such as doing short-term therapy, crisis intervention, or working in the community with adolescents. Community mental health workers are supervised by a professional, usually a psychiatric social worker or a certified psychologist.

Paraprofessionals are an integral part of service delivery in community mental health. The 1973 Community Mental Health Center profile of the United States indicates that the median hours of total staff time was 23 percent for paraprofessionals (National Institute of Mental Health, 1975: 11). An earlier study found that half of the community mental health centers in the New York City area listed at least 16 percent of their personnel as paraprofessionals (Gottesfeld et al., 1970). Interestingly, 24 percent of the directors surveyed reported that the paraprofessionals performed essentially the same tasks as professionals. However, Gottesfeld and his associates have raised appropriate questions concerning the quality and quantity of training received by paraprofessionals who performed tasks that overlap with professionals. Other writers have indicated that paraprofessionals themselves are interested in more training, particularly when they are first employed (Kaplan and Roman, 1973: 114).

Several other studies have raised questions about the current practices in the field of community mental health and their impact on service delivery. According to Cowne, "effective training" and "career ladder incentives" are necessary to prevent high turnover among paraprofessionals (1969). He also advocates the inclusion of paraprofessionals in professional associations, further training, and certification according to national standards, all to achieve the goals of keeping up interest in professional issues and knowledge.

One argument in favor of employing paraprofessionals in community mental health centers is that clients will be better able to relate to them. Advocates of these new-practitioner roles argue that clients would perceive their services as more helpful and effective than those performed by professionals from outside the community. In other words, they suggest that an empathic person with little in the way of technique can do more to help people with psychiatric histories or those facing personal stress than the well-trained but distant professional.

Nevertheless, the research has not borne out the expectations. A study conducted in Texas among 102 Mexican-American clients found that while the subjects thought the paraprofessionals were indeed similar to them in social and cultural backgrounds, they also thought professionals were more helpful. Andrade and Burstein (1973: 397) concluded that "the much-emphasized view of the advantages of using indigenous, nonprofessional aides in CMHCs is ill-founded empirically." This finding does not rule out the possibility that better trained paraprofessionals or professionals of the same social class backgrounds as clients would be perceived as more helpful than professionals from different backgrounds.

The strong trust of both professionals and laymen in people trained in an established health care institution to provide help may also affect perceptions of who can perform what services. A patient may feel better simply knowing that help is on the way, as when an asthmatic person in the midst of an attack finds it easier to breathe knowing the doctor is about to arrive. Community mental health centers have attempted to introduce new ideas about understanding and treating mental illness while "trying to maintain the traditional conceptualizations of mental illness which carry implicit the idea that nonprofessionals cannot heal" (Minuchin, 1969: 722). The emphasis in the utilization of the paraprofessional in community mental health was originally on prevention, not treatment. The shift of goals in the field to more precisely defined functions of patient care has left community mental health and rehabilitation workers without a distinctive role. Many of the tasks they perform overlap greatly with better trained social workers and psychologists.

Professionals who work in community mental health centers have more clearly defined roles than paraprofessionals, making it easier for patients to understand what they do and how they can help. Training helps to define roles clearly, as can be seen in the case of nurse practitioners or physician assistants. Community mental health workers or rehabilitation workers cannot project a convincing image of skill to the patient unless they have a set of techniques to demonstrate.

The ancillary personnel in community mental health can be strongly committed to the goals of the agency in providing psychotherapeutic services to all, regardless of ability to pay. In a study of 39 workers employed at one well-known center, 46 percent of the paraprofessionals were defined as having primarily a *psychotherapeutic* orientation to their work, 39 percent were considered to have an *interpersonal* orientation, and 15 percent saw their goal as providing *support* services. The psychotherapeutically-oriented respondents referred to their responsibilities as developing a treatment plan for patients, motivating patients, and helping them to cope with reality or doing insight therapy. The interpersonally-oriented described their responsibilities as based on being able to get along with patients, understanding their situation, or caring about the person's well-being. A support service orientation was characterized by seeking social assistance from welfare agencies or providing recreational and activity therapy.

While respondents did not always express their psychotherapeutic orientation in the technical language used by professionals, the examples they used in describing their work indicated that they understood these implications of their role.

> I get satisfaction by just getting one of my patients to do something that he hasn't done in a long time. I have one patient, in particular, who won't leave his house. And I spoke to him for a while—I started seeing him the end of July—and he's going out to the bank by himself, which is really great. I started first to get him to go out for little walks . . . because he was so afraid to go outside and be hurt by someone. . . . But now he's really doing well.

Alternatively, respondents who were interpersonally oriented indicated that they were not as involved in active efforts to motivate patients. While no less enthusiastic about their work, they did see empathy and rapport with clients as the basic responsibility of the role: "If you can care for them and understand them, then you can deal with them."

Given the basic responsibilities of paraprofessionals, what skills did they see as necessary for their work? Interestingly, only 18 percent of the respondents mentioned such skills as an ability to develop a treatment plan for clients, motivating patients, or doing diagnoses. In contrast, 82 percent described their skills as interpersonal and empathic: "A certain flexibility in one's thinking, dealing with patients, dealing with their family, dealing with other staff in getting the job done; a need to be able to work on a team, to reach team decisions at times."

Respondents who spoke about their psychotherapeutic skills were aware of the importance of interpersonal skills, but they also expressed the view that the interpersonal skills were a means of accomplishing their goals of affecting the patient's life.

> Well I guess therapy would be the most important skill . . . the ability to do therapy one to one . . . the ability to communicate with a patient and get through to them. That's a skill you've got to really—sometimes it's really kind of hard with patients—to communicate with some of them. [Birenbaum and Ahmed, 1978: 122–34]

DEALING WITH PATIENT REACTIONS TO HEALTH CARE

Every health care practitioner must deal with the problem of maintaining the confidence of the patients and families in their knowledge and ability. New practitioners are more likely to be conscious of this problem than more established professional disciplines because their contacts with patients may be punctuated by comments or questions concerning the status of the practitioner. Physician assistants and nurse practitioners are often mistakenly addressed as "doctor." While these new practitioners may be flattered by such titles—and such misidentifications are often cited by them as evidence of their acceptance by patients—confusion can occur when the real doctor is present.

A second source of concern is also evident when a new practitioner is working with patients and their families. The response to nurse practitioners and physician assistants can interfere with the care delivered or the compliance with a treatment regimen. The attitudes and behaviors of patients toward the practitioner can be based on a variety of prior experiences and current expectations of or about the organized system of health care in general. Nevertheless, these factors must be dealt with, and the practitioner must be able to put the patient at ease. Being attuned to the context of health care delivery is an important way in which new practitioners learn to exercise judgment in dealing with patients and their families.

The following case study was derived from observations made at the same training program for PNPs discussed in Chapter 9. Observations made for more than a year at team meetings where treatment plans were discussed suggested that the psychosocial environment of the child was a central area of concern for PNPs. Concern with the parents' attitudes toward the PNP, the child, or toward each other became important sources of information for planning primary care. The anecdotal material presented here from field notes collected at team meetings and at home visits demonstrates the sensitivity of PNPs to patient reactions to health care organizations and their agents.

The population served by the PNPs is often said to receive second-class care because of its economic position in the United States. Many critics and observers of how the poor receive health care have made this comment (Strauss, 1973). It is not unusual for the poor to resent receiving care from any source. Precisely because patients at municipal general hospitals can command so little in the way of services, it is more difficult to convince them that the care is adequate.

Resentment grows when people feel that they are using a service because they cannot afford anything else. Poor families who have had incompetent medical aid or had it provided by callous people, are likely to generalize from these experiences and, in so doing, condemn the entire hospital. Thus pediatric services may receive criticism based on incidents that had nothing to do with personnel. Similarly, the families of the children seen at the two programs may demonstrate great reluctance to receive care at a hospital where they watched suffering and death. PNPs often had to deal with the problem of accounting for what happened when medical help failed to cure or arrest a condition treated at the hospital. Manifestly, the PNP was there to provide health care and medical aid to the child, but in reality, she helped a family overcome the loss of confidence many people express toward the system available to them. Sometimes the family confronted the PNP with past traumatic experiences, as when the mother had experienced poor treatment, or the father had lived in a convalescent hospital for several years as a child.

A second reaction to health care personnel was related to lifestyle differences between the poor and those who provided health services. Some parents whose children were cared for by PNPs were unprepared for parenthood because the child's birth resulted from an unwanted pregnancy, which interfered with other plans, especially in the case of adolescent parents who had expected to work or finish their education. Young mothers on occasion were found to make invidious comparisons with the PNPs, who were often little older than themselves. PNPs attempted to help these mothers develop individual goals, find ways to return to school, or even to find employment. Under these conditions, it was not unusual for parents to be extremely provocative to PNPs, and questions were often raised at team meetings about the best way to deal with such provocations. In addition, and not unexpectedly, PNPs had to deal with their own anger toward women who could be abusive to those providing services.

Beyond these general reactions to practitioners and the institutions they represented, PNPs had four other functions to perform that enhanced patient and family compliance with treatment regimens. First, PNPs played a major role in preparing children and their parents for hospitalization, for medical procedures of a surgical or diagnostic nature, preparing them to leave the hospital, and how to manage the illness at home; they also explained diagnostic results and prepared parents for positive findings of illness or disease. In so doing, PNPs attempted to help the family avoid the disruptive effects of anxiety on family functioning and relationships.

Second, in a similar way, PNPs tried to get parents to express their anxieties about potential psychiatric problems in children and to learn how to deal with them. Moreover, they were able to help parents see how such behavioral manifestations were likely to be induced or exacerbated by lengthy hospitalization, chronic disease, or strained parental relationships.

Third, PNPs worked with parents who either had a past history of psychiatric care or who were in immediate need of such care on a short- or long-term basis. This preventive work was usually done through close consultation with psychiatrists and psychiatric social workers.

Finally, PNPs had to recognize the signs of child abuse or neglect and the need for referring families to legally mandated agencies, compared to working directly with the parents.

Psychological Preparation for Medical Procedures

PNPs participated in the task of explaining new procedures to be utilized in treatment or care of a child. This involved telling a family about the need for surgery and its chances for success, as well as preparing the child. Similarly, PNPs often presented the results of such procedures in conjunction with physicians. Explanations were often made by PNPs when a child left the hospital under supervision in order to let the child know that ending a stay in a ward is not equal to being completely well. Care often involved occasional returns to the hospital for a child to undergo new tests. In the case of a child who was hospitalized for extensive reconstruction of his stomach and who went home on tube feeding in order to allow the surgery to completely heal, returning to the hospital could be misinterpreted by the child to mean a lengthy stay. In a home visit, a PNP prepared the child for his short-term visit for an esophagram:

PNP: I have something to tell you, Fred. You can come to the hospital to play, not to stay. The doctors are going to take an X-ray. Do you know what X-rays are?

Fred: X-rays?

PNP: It's a picture. You have to drink something to make the picture work.

Fred: By my mouth?

PNP: Yes, Fred. Do you remember how to drink things by your mouth? Do you know what day you are going to the hospital?

Fred: Tomorrow?

PNP: No. Tuesday. You'll be able to come upstairs and see the play lady. What happens to you when you get pictures taken in the hospital?

Fred: I have to drink chocolate.

PNP: Do you drink a big or a little glass?

Fred: A big glass.

PNP: . . . Were you scared the last time you went for a picture? Did you take a special toy with you? Would you like to take one on Tuesday?

Fred: Yes, a car.

PNP: It shouldn't hurt at all. I am going to come see you when you come in for your X-ray on Tuesday. Now, I am going to talk to Mommy for a while.

Parental Anxieties about Their Children

Parents often want a complete report of how injured a child might be as a result of a birth defect, and they demand this information from PNPs even before a complete assessment can be made. The question arose concerning how much to tell when the physician's suspicion of organic impairment, particularly neurological damage, was not fully confirmed. In these instances, the PNP shared the reporting of medical information about children to the families, a task that physicians usually reserved for themselves in more traditional settings.

In the unit described here, medical status information is given under the physician's guidance and authority. Nurses may give clues and hints to families about the condition of patients in hospitals, and physicians do not always discourage this. The PNP must also answer questions and deal with reactions to receiving bad news.

Parents often suspected that their children had developmental problems, hinting to PNPs that problems existed aside from those requiring hospitalization and home care. Sometimes they became anxious about behavior that was typical for a particular stage of development and regarded it as aberrant, requiring special intervention. At other times, they felt that PNPs and other health care deliverers were not telling parents the complete diagnosis and that the child suffered from an emotional disorder. Fred, the child discussed above, was regarded by his mother as possibly in need of psychiatric help because he received thorazine, a medicine given to "crazy people." In addition, the child had a head tic. The PNP tried to allay the mother's anxiety:

> PNP: This is a whole area I would like to talk to you about some more. Particularly, the tensions in these relationships.
>
> Mrs. F: Yes, I get up in the morning tense. This happened with my husband the other day. Fred is no problem anymore.
>
> PNP: I would like to talk privately to you about this, when Fred isn't present.
>
> Mrs. F: I get so impatient with Fred sometimes. When I'm trying to teach him.
>
> PNP: Sometimes it is good to talk about these tensions with a third party who is not too close to all this.

Finally, the social consequences of disability were often a concern of the PNPs. Team meetings were devoted to discussions of the problems that emerge when a chronically ill child is in the family and the kinds of changes in relationships between family members that occur as a result. Team members considered such problems as happening to any family in which a child is chronically ill and/or had severe developmental lags.

Parents Who Need Psychiatric Consultation or Therapy

PNPs occasionally found that mothers of their patients had psychiatric histories or were undergoing current emotional stress, including postpartum depression. One woman reported several psychiatric hospitalizations in a nearby state facility and long-term involvement with outpatient care, dating back to a diagnosis as a chronic schizophrenic at the age of twelve. This parent also mentioned a variety of interpersonal problems related to her condition.

The PNPs attempted to be supportive of this woman and of mothers in general who expressed anxiety about their capacity to cope with their children. They attempted to help by setting limited goals for them to accomplish, usually after consulting with psychiatrists and other mental health personnel familiar with the person's problems. In acute situations, PNPs helped arrange for child care, so mothers would not feel unable to fulfill parental obligations. Children who were admitted to day-care programs were able to interact with other children outside of the home and, even more important, with other adults.

In order to promote the entry of the parent into a therapeutic relationship and to provide short-term therapy, under psychiatric supervision, the PNPs sought to recognize that they could take parents only to the point of getting more specialized help. Occasionally, the PNP played the role of the confidante for a child who was having a difficult time with parents or a foster home. Often PNPs had to control their urge to intervene in cases when there was little they could do. Team meetings provided psychiatric, pediatric, and social work advice for the PNP and helped determine whether it was useful to intervene when those efforts might be regarded negatively by the parent.

PNPs also worked with parents who were addicted to alcohol and illegal drugs to assist them to voluntarily join addiction services programs, to get them to recognize the potential health dangers to the child and future children; and to get them to act more responsibly toward their children. Yet this was not easily accomplished, for the PNPs themselves often expressed doubts about the possibilities of success. They did not feel that addict parents trusted and they were wary of people who were subject to arrest; nor did they want the responsibility for reporting addicted children or parents to health agencies or the law.

Child Abuse and Neglect

Because of the frequent contact between a PNP and a child, the latter became increasingly aware of cases of child abuse and neglect. A PNP might notice that a child had suspicious bruises; that the children were never dressed; that they were frequently out of school with upper respiratory infections; that there was little or no food in the house; that other children in the family were never immunized; and that a child's medication was not being administered. Such observations were discussed in team meetings, and the staff weighed the advantages and disadvantages of reporting the family to the preventive service unit of the children's division of the Department of Social Services.

Where the PNP thought she had a therapeutic relationship with the family, there was some reluctance to report marginal incidents of child abuse and/or neglect because of the fear that her work with the family would be more difficult if the parent found out. PNPs were more likely to attempt to provide education for the parents in child development and forms of discipline that did not depend on the use of corporal punishment.

In addition, homemaker services were often suggested to help a disorganized parent develop a more acceptable routine and provide some opportunity for that parent, usually a mother without another adult to help, to find some time away from the children. Attempts to report incidents of questionable child abuse and/or neglect occurred only when alternative solutions failed to change parental behavior and there was genuine fear for the child's health and safety.

In reporting on the four ways in which PNPs responded to patients and their families, a number of paramedical tasks were identified, which if performed can induce compliance. The functions of PNPs can be arranged on a continuum: from those that overlap with other nonmedical practitioners of short-term counseling and those who assess the need for more specialized intervention, to those that make it possible for important medical procedures to be performed. The practice of PNPs as primary health care deliverers not only enables parents and their children to receive better care, but it can provide a model for other practitioners, including medical personnel.

In order to make this potential a reality, the new practitioners must encourage patients to regard them as independent professionals. This may be more necessary in a hospital setting, even at an outpatient clinic, than in a private group or solo practice. Patients may impute limited skills to nurse practitioners or physician assistants by virtue of their position in the hospital's organizational hierarchy.

While physicians and patients have generally accepted the new practitioners, a number of interesting forms of competition have emerged between the various occupations.

REFERENCES

Andrade, S. J., and A. G. Burstein. 1973. "Social congruence and empathy in paraprofessional and professional mental health workers." *Community Mental Health Journal* 9 (Winter): 388–97.

Bellak, Leopold. 1974. *A Concise Handbook of Community Psychiatry and Community Mental Health.* New York: Grune and Stratton.

Bernstein, Lewis, Rosalyn S. Bernstein, and Richard H. Dana. 1974. *Interviewing: A Guide for Health Professionals,* 2d ed. New York: Appleton-Century-Crofts.

Birenbaum, A., and M. B. Ahmed. 1978. "Recruitment, training and utilization of community mental health workers." *Sociological Symposium* 23 (Summer): 122–34.

[CRI] Cambridge Research Institute. 1975. *Trends Affecting U.S. Health Care System.* Washington, D.C.: Department of Health, Education, and Welfare.

Celentano, D. D. 1978. "Critical issues concerning new health practitioners—Quality of care." *Sociological Symposium* 23 (Summer): 61–77.

Cowne, L. J. 1969. "Approaches to the mental health manpower problem: A review of the literature." *Mental Hygiene* 53 (April): 176–87.

Day, L. R., R. Egli, and H. K. Silver. 1970. "Acceptance of pediatric nurse practitioners: Parents' opinion of combined care by a pediatrician and a pediatric nurse practitioner in a private practice." *American Journal of Diseases of Children* 119 (March): 204–8.

Dinitz, S., and N. Beran. 1971. "Community mental health as a boundaryless and boundary-busting system." *Journal of Health and Social Behavior* 12 (June): 99–108.

Fowler, E. H. 1977. "Careers: Medical assistants—a new field." *New York Times,* July 6: D11.

Gottesfeld, H., R. Chongik, and G. Parker. 1970. "A study of the role of paraprofessionals in community mental health." *Community Mental Health Journal* 6: 285–91.

Intellect 103, 1975: 417–18. "The new midwife—Sophisticated and caring."

Kaplan, Seymour R., and Melvin Roman. 1973. *The Organization and Delivery of Mental Health Services in the Ghetto: The Lincoln Hospital Experience.* New York: Praeger Special Studies.

Komaroff, A. L., et al. 1974. "Protocols for physician assistants: Management of diabetes and hypertension." *New England Journal of Medicine* 290: 307–12.

Litman, T. J. 1972. "Public perceptions of the physician assistant: A survey of the attitudes and opinions of rural Iowa and Minnesota residents." *American Journal of Public Health* 62: 343–46.

Minuchin, S. 1969. "The paraprofessional and the use of confrontation in the mental health field." *American Journal of Orthopsychiatry* 39 (October): 722–29.

National Institute of Mental Health. 1975. *1973 Profile for Federally Funded Community Mental Health Centers.* Rockville, Md.: Survey and Reports Branch, Division of Biometry, National Institute of Mental Health.

no date "The pediatric nurse practitioner program: A parent opinion poll."

Rich, Adrianne. 1976. *Of Woman Born: Motherhood as Experience and Institution.* New York: W. W. Norton.
Schiff, D. W., C. H. Fraser, and H. L. Walters. 1969. "The pediatric nurse practitioner in the office of pediatricians in private practice." *Pediatrics* 44 (July): 62–68.
Silver, H. K., and B. Duncan. 1971. "Time-motion study of pediatric nurse practitioners: Comparison with 'regular' office nurses and pediatricians." *Journal of Pediatrics* 79 (August): 331–36.
Strauss, Anselm L. 1973. *Where Medicine Fails*, 2d ed. New Brunswick, N. J.: Transaction Books.

11

Cooperation and Conflict among New and Old Health Care Practitioners

The major thrust since World War II has been the realization that health care is not the exclusive province of medicine. In many places where services were unavailable, alternative systems had to be created. For instance, in the Haight-Ashbury district of San Francisco in the 1960s, an indigenous health care system emerged when the established institutions avoided dealing with the problems of adolescents and young adults involved with drugs and casual living (Smith, Luce, and Dernberg, 1973). Traditional practitioners from rural areas who advocate various folk remedies used by farmers and local naturalists did not disappear with the growth of modern medicine. In fact, healing itself is sometimes seen as a gift, rather than a learned technique, and it does not always involve medication from botanic or artificial sources. Spiritualists or faith healers have often been sought by people in need of care. In fact, spiritualism and folk pharmacies are combined in Puerto Rican communities (Borrello and Mathias, 1977).

Some health practitioners compete directly with the field of medicine, claiming to have a theory of disease and an appropriate therapy. In employing the impression-management techniques of professionals, chiropractors are often viewed by laymen as identical to physicians. Medicine has always regarded the chiropractic theory of "subluxation," or the misalignments of vertebrae as the principal causes of disease, as questionable scientifically. Contemporary chiropractic has modified this singular theory of disease to encompass the germ theory and knowledge about the body's immune system (*Consumer Reports*, 1975: 542).

Chiropractic has come a long way in gaining acceptance by state and federal regulatory agencies, mainly because of fervent public support from satisfied patients. Despite their distinctly marginal status before the 1970s (Wardwell, 1952), chiropractors are now licensed in every state, are eligible to render services under Medicare and Medicaid, and have their own evaluational agency for colleges that train chiropractors. Since 1974, the United States Commissioner of Education recognizes the Council on Chiropractic Education as the official agency to accredit chiropractic colleges.

Chiropractic followed the path toward respectability taken by osteopathy a few years earlier. Osteopaths are now trained in schools where the curriculum resembles that of medical colleges. Both osteopathy and chiropractic have modified their claims of competency, becoming more specialized and limited in their focus. Chiropractors and osteopaths are now legally permitted to treat many illnesses, can prescribe medication, and take X-rays. In other words, outside of performing surgery, most of the tools and techniques of medical doctors are at their disposal. In addition, chiropractors and osteopaths have their own boards in each state to issue and regulate licensing (*Consumer Reports*, 1975: 610). No physicians or any other health care practitioners serve on these licensing boards.

Other independent nonphysician specialists in health care are more limited in scope, generally treating one area of the body (Krause, 1977: 45). Dentists and podiatrists also control their own licensing boards and are permitted to treat and prescribe for a limited range of diseases. The podiatrist is not legally allowed to treat diabetes with insulin, although care of the feet of a diabetic in order to prevent the serious complications of ingrown toenails is permitted. However, dentists are less circumscribed; for example, they might be called on to treat the effects on the teeth and gums of a serious calcium deficiency that is being handled by a physician who specializes in nutrition. Dentists and podiatrists are legally permitted to use all the techniques and tools of the field of medicine, including surgery, so long as they apply these techniques only to the parts of the body of their specialization.

Many health care practitioners—laboratory technicians, nurses, X-ray technologists, physician assistants—can use the techniques and tools of medicine only under direct medical supervision or standing orders. To diagnose or treat would be considered practicing medicine without a license. However, in the 1940s X-ray was used by some shoe stores to help fit customers, a practice discontinued because of evidence that frequent exposure to radiation is dangerous. In short, the legal responsibility to define disease remains firmly in the control of the medical profession.

A key difference between paramedical personnel, such as nurses, X-ray technicians, and physician assistants, and independent nonphysician specialists is that the occupational licensing board is primarily made up of physicians in the fields serviced by the paramedical personnel. The same control over the paradental field is exercised by dentists, who sit on licensing boards for dental hygienists, technicians and assistants. Pathologists, a recently formed group of specialists within medicine, control the licensing boards of their laboratory technicians. In essence, the paramedical practitioners possess an official inability, recognized by the state, to diagnose, prescribe, treat, and perform surgery, except under standing orders (Krause, 1977: 47).

Today, some medical specialties have been concerned about the threat to their livelihood posed by both other physicians and health care practitioners. While surgery can legally be performed by any licensed physician, the boards that certify surgeons have attempted to prevent nonsurgically trained and certified physicians from doing these procedures. The American College of Surgeons claims that nonsurgeon physicians are inadequately trained, do not have proper equipment, and are not able to make the correct decisions about whether surgery is necessary. This group has also attempted to prevent graduates of medical colleges from becoming residents in surgery because they claim there are sufficient numbers of surgeons available. The United States may indeed have more surgeons than it needs.

> While 24 percent of our doctors are surgeons, U.S. prepaid group practices find it necessary to have only 20 percent of their physicians be surgeons, and in Britain only 8 percent of physicians are surgeons. There is a suspicion that the abundance of surgeons in our health system is a major reason that the U.S. population as a whole undergoes twice as much surgery as the British population or as members of U.S. prepaid group practices. [Cambridge Research Institute, 1975: 362]

Physician assistants are now being trained and used to replace interns and residents in teaching hospitals that have cut back on the training of surgeons (Sullivan, 1980). Yet M.D.s often become indignant when federal legislation is suggested to encourage medical schools to train their students for primary care. In 1976, President Ford signed into law a $2.1 billion health manpower bill that linked federal support for medical colleges with residency training programs to allocate more training positions to primary medicine, including general and family practice and pediatrics. This bill gives medical colleges four years to comply voluntarily before the federal government will step in and impose a quota. Schools that fail to meet such a quota would lose a subsidy of $2,000 per year per student, called capitation funds. This was a compromise to a bill voted favorably by Congress in 1974 limiting the choice of new doctors in selecting their practice locations, but which was never signed into law (Hicks, 1976: 20).

Physicians still jealously guard their exclusive rights to diagnose and treat disease. Opthamologists have opposed a bill in New York State that would have legally permitted optometrists to use drugs in order to diagnose eye diseases. One physician opposed this procedure:

> The optometric society, in an attempt to enhance the optometrists' allure as an "eye doctor," has long sought entrance into the practice of medicine without undertaking medical training. To such an optometric mind the instillation of drops into the conjunctival sac is the only artifice missing from the shop.
>
> Optometrists currently are not adequately or properly trained in the diagnosis of eye disease. Those in practice have had very limited exposure (if any exposure) to qualified training in the recognition of disease processes. Legislative action will not suddenly endow them with knowledge and experience. There is no known eye drop that gives a diagnosis.

> If the proposed legislation becomes law, then one must ask about the mechanics of the use of drugs by optometrists. Optometrists could acquire the drugs they are longing to use only by prescribing them. Ultimately, they would administer the medication (this without training in pharmacology or any knowledge of the systemic effects of such drugs). In addition, therapeutic trials would certainly become part of a diagnostic procedure. Would not this then be treatment? Is this not the practice of medicine as it relates to disorders of the eye? [Taffet, 1976: 27]

Three instances of conflict between various health care practitioners, and the causes and consequences of these disputes, will be examined. While each case involves different health care occupations, they all raise similar questions about how decisions are made relative to the formation and recruitment of new occupations, and how various public and private organizations contribute to cooperation and conflict.

The division of labor in health care is deeply affected by societywide structures of law, financial arrangements, and corporate control. The validity of this proposition will be demonstrated in examining the occupational rivalry between physician assistants and nurse practitioners, the movement to revitalize pharmacy, and the incipient conflict between paraprofessionals and professionals in community mental health. Finally, we will discuss the idea of how the division of labor in health care fits into the social divisions in American society.

OCCUPATIONAL RIVALRY AMONG HEALTH CARE PRACTITIONERS

Rivalries within the burgeoning field of practitioners, such as physician assistants and nurse practitioners, focus on jurisdictions of competency, training, and licensing. In many settings, the two groups perform almost identical tasks, each seeking to prove its superiority in delivering primary care.

At an earlier point, physician assistants received specialized technical training and were not utilized in primary care. This pattern appears to be changing as group medical practices have adopted their services for primary health care. Nurse practitioners are also performing similar roles, particularly in publicly financed programs for the medically indigent. Despite the differences in target population, the similarity in function has produced competition (mainly between organizations representing both occupational categories) over who can do what tasks better. Moreover, people performing different tasks and at different levels of competency are referred to by the same title (Vogt and Ducanis, 1977: 38–44).

This competition is confounded by several factors. First, most nurse practitioners were women, whereas physician assistants were predominantly men. While some physician assistants now are women, the initial maleness of the group has engendered high prestige. Second, physician assistants tend to work closely with the socially more highly ranked physicians, in private group practice rather than as employees in publicly owned hospitals, and they tend to serve a population drawn from the middle class rather than the poor. The impact of such features on the development of these occupations should provide some clues to sociologists as to how occupations do or do not receive prestige from the general public. In the nineteenth century, physicians and apothecaries evolved differently as a result of serving different social classes.

However, nurse practitioners have an almost exclusive monopoly on the pediatric field, by virtue of their gender and early affiliation with children in the field of nursing. There is still some reluctance among the general population to permit male nurses to have intimate contact with women and children. The nurse practitioner has an advantage in this area of health care.

Another form of competition is emerging between nurse practitioners and the nursing leadership found in supervisory positions in hospitals, associations of nurses, and schools of nursing. Here, the traditional spokeswomen for the field may prevent nurse practitioners from developing their own leadership and from organizing separately. The physician assistants do not have to work in an environment where an established leadership already exists.

A further form of conflict has resulted from the apparent downplaying of the older paramedical professions of nursing and pharmacy, as a result of efforts to create new health care practitioners. Both nursing and pharmacy have upgraded their education and training through four- and five-year baccalaureate programs, respectively. In the future, all registered nurses will have to have a college diploma and academic training as well as practical experience.

THE REVITALIZATION OF PHARMACY

The field of pharmacy in particular has recently experienced both an expansion in the utilization of pharmacists in hospitals and nursing homes and, at the same time, a threat to its survival as a profession. David Mechanic considers pharmacy to be in the midst of a crisis of purpose.

> Increasingly . . . with manufactured drug combinations the technical role of the pharmacist has eroded and, despite his training, the typical American pharmacist appears to be more of a businessman than a professional, and he provides the consumer a limited technical service. [Mechanic, 1970: 536]

Also, the number of small retail pharmacies in the United States has declined, with the larger discount drug stores replacing several pharmacist-owned stores in any given area.

> Aggressive chain operators are dispensing prescriptions at lower cost to the patient. They are charging roughly $3 to $3.25 a prescription, whereas a typical independent pharmacy averaged $3.60 per prescription in 1966. These lower charges are possible due to dispensing procedures and increased promotion of the prescription department. [Knapp and Knapp, 1968: 749]

In 1975, there were 19,820 "small independent" retail pharmacies in the United States, and it is estimated that by 1980 there will be only 6,620

(Anderson, 1975: 36). This projected two-thirds loss will limit still further the economic opportunities of licensed pharmacists.

The opportunities for hospital pharmacists may also be limited. Hospitals with a large volume of prescriptions could introduce automated dispensing. Along with automation, new pharmacy assistant and technician roles are being created to service these machines. Pharmacy technicians, trained in six-month programs at community colleges, are utilized now in hospitals to free the pharmacists from simple and routine tasks, allowing them to do more clinically oriented work.

Pharmacy has traditionally had a less professional status than other health care fields because the pharmacist in the United States could be a self-employed businessman, selling products as well as using his expertise. He was often the town grocer, and for many years ran a soda fountain or luncheonette as part of his drugstore. Norman Denzin, a sociologist, designates this phenomenon as one of incomplete professionalization (1968). The economic position of the pharmacist is further threatened by the end of compounding, the computerization of dosages, and the creation of technical and assistant roles. It comes as no surprise, then, that pharmacists feel a loss of control over their field and their place in health care.

Anthony F. C. Wallace, an anthropologist interested in religious movements among dispossessed peoples, created the concept of "revitalization movement," denoting "any conscious, organized effort by members of a society to construct a more satisfying culture" (Wallace, 1966: 30). This is based on the assumption that new beliefs and practices

> . . . always originate in situations of social and cultural stress and are, in fact, an effort on the part of the stress-laden to construct systems of dogma, myth, and ritual which are internally coherent as well as true descriptions of a world system and which thus will serve as guides to efficient action. [Wallace, 1966: 30]

Applied to the field of pharmacy, the idea of a "revitalization movement" helps us understand what is happening in health care generally, and in pharmacy specifically.

Pharmacy is attempting to change the status it receives from other health care practitioners, particularly the medical profession, and gain control over the dispensing of drugs in hospitals and nursing homes. Central to this effort is a reorganization of the education of pharmacists so that they will receive recognition for their knowledge. Currently, undergraduate education in pharmacy is similar to a premedical curriculum. In addition, undergraduate pharmacy students take a large number of courses in pharmacology, their specific area of expertise.

The model followed by pharmacy for revitalization of the field is similar to that undergone by medicine after the publication of the Flexner Report early in the twentieth century. The Study Commission on Pharmacy, established by the American Association of Colleges of Pharmacy in 1973, and headed by John Millis, a noted scholar and philosopher, was to thoroughly examine the current practices and education of pharmacists. After a two-year period of investigation, involving review of written material and testimony from eighty consultants from the field of pharmacy, the results were published in 1975. Colleges of pharmacy have already made extensive curriculum revisions on the basis of the Millis Report's recommendations, including the introduction of social science courses.

A major thrust of the revitalization of pharmacy has been to expand the clinical role of the pharmacist, including increased contact between patients and pharmacists and greater responsibility in informing other health care professionals about the potential dangers of administering combinations of medications at the same time. For the advocates, this shift is justified by the awesome consequences of mistakes. Like medicine, pharmacy is regarded as a sacred trust. For the reformer, no prescription is routine.

> The trouble is that *every* prescription, *every* situation, *every* question from a physician, nurse, or patient, is potentially crucial. The pharmacist's response, his action, his answer can do the utmost good or cause the utmost harm or even death as a result. A major question for pharmacy and for pharmaceutical educators is how to orient the individual practitioner to view his practice in such a light. [italics in original] [Knapp and Knapp, 1968: 755]

A great deal of evidence suggests that medications are not always administered correctly, particularly by elderly people with chronic illnesses.

> Two studies of elderly patients receiving care in clinic settings revealed that 59 percent of the patients had made one or more errors in taking prescribed medications and roughly one quarter had made errors that could be classified as potentially serious. [Smith, 1977: 223]

Yet other practitioners perceive the pharmacist as having little patient involvement and was encouraged to become more involved. In one survey, other professionals saw review of drug utilization in hospitals as the pharmacists' major clinical activity (Lambert et al., 1977: 253).

Recent research appears to justify the expanded clinical role of pharmacists. A controlled study of compliance among hypertensive patients showed a significant improvement in the number of patients who complied with prescribed therapy and in the number whose blood pressures were kept within the normal range when clinical services were provided by a pharmacist (McKenney et al., 1973: 1104). Deviation from prescribed drug regimens among discharged hospital patients was found among a control group receiving no consultation prior to going home, while two study groups showed 90 percent compliance (Cole and Emmanuel, 1971: 960). However, one study of efforts to teach a group of patients about their medications and to label their drug containers did not significantly decrease the number of errors made at home (Malahy, 1966: 292).

The revitalization movement is the rational result of witnessing a decline in pharmacy as a profession. Pharmacists have seen responsibilities delegated to nurse practitioners and physician assistants by physicians, including prescribing under standing orders. Pharmacy is making a greater effort to define its roles more clearly, to receive recognition, and to exclude those who are untrained and unlicensed. Pharmacists also advocate charging a separate fee for their services, quite apart from the price of the drug that they dispense. In a hospital setting, this movement would take the form of separate billing as consultant and educator. This quest for a new identity is also found in the colleges of pharmacy, where courses on Pharmacy and Society are introduced and where students are taught that pharmacy is a profession and not a business. Interestingly, a recent study of 53 pharmacists in the Midwest showed that both a strong professional and business orientation coexisted, with community-based pharmacists having stronger service orientations than their hospital-based colleagues (Kronus, 1975: 179).

Perhaps one of the most important reinforcing tendencies to the revitalization movement in pharmacy today exists outside of the field itself. Pharmacy traditionally attracted people who were upwardly mobile but had some early vocational contact with pharmacists in their families or neighborhoods. Whether pharmacy was a profession or a business was not an issue to people who would have an opportunity to buy into a community store. Now by virtue of the limited opportunities in the sciences and the difficulties of getting into medical school, many people are entering the field who might have gone on for advanced degrees during an era of more vocational opportunity. Many pharmacy students and recent graduates are experiencing the shock of finding out that while they may start with good salaries in a community practice or a hospital, they soon reach the top of their earning power. Furthermore, the prestige of pharmacy is low in a hospital, and it is not particularly high in affluent communities, where doctors and lawyers earn more and are held in higher esteem. The pharmacist in the working-class community is admired because he is independent, while in the upper-middle-class community, he may be looked down upon because he has to tend the store. The ambitious and talented person who becomes a hospital pharmacist may learn that his control over his work setting is limited compared to the physician.

Revitalization is supported by other factors in health care in general and the education of pharmacists in particular. The expansion of pharmacy is dependent on the continued use of drugs in treatment, making for growth in the area of hospital and nursing home pharmacy. There is far more interaction between pharmacists in larger departments, and they are less isolated than in the past. Recent graduates maintain continuous contact with schools of pharmacy because of the use of preceptorship programs to give on-the-job training to future pharmacists. Recent graduates are used to train students in the last two years of pharmacy college. Linkages are maintained with the idealistic pharmacy educators, who advocate increased professionalization through performance of clinical roles in health care. A greater sense of obligation to the field is engendered by this type of intense contact, producing a sense of a shared fate, and one which the pharmacists themselves control.

An important source of social solidarity among hospital pharmacists arises from the exchange of stories (some perhaps exaggerated or apocryphal) about how nurses or doctors were ignorant about medications and about to make a disastrous error until the pharmacist was consulted. Some hospital pharmacists have mounted campaigns to become cosigners of all prescriptions and to gain the right to substitute generic-named drugs for brand names, without the need of permission by the doctor (a practice opposed by some retail pharmacists, who would make less profit from generic-name drugs).

PARAPROFESSIONALS AND PROFESSIONALS IN COMMUNITY MENTAL HEALTH CENTERS

The role of paraprofessionals in community mental health centers has undergone some interesting changes as a result of their direct competition with social workers and psychologists for staff lines. Many rehabilitation workers and community mental health workers were hired during the 1960s, when federal funds were available. Since then, they have received steplike salary increases, often as part of union contracts, making their remuneration similar to that of social workers and psychologists starting out in the field as therapists. Despite their early arrival in the field, paraprofessionals are subject to increased questioning of their role as part of the community mental health care team by both professionals who provide services and administrators who are accountable to funding agencies for productivity.

The most direct constraint has been imposed by funding agencies, which are demanding greater accountability of the daily activities of service-giving employees. To maintain eligibility for contracts, fee reimbursement, and grants of public funds, agencies must introduce new management practices for careful recording of client contacts and use of staff time. In order to demonstrate the delivery of effective services in a measurable way, the limits of the day-to-day activities of clinicians, both professionals and paraprofessionals, are being narrowed. The definition of the paraprofessional role is becoming more specific and rationalized.

Yet the role was conceived of and initially implemented as a fairly diffuse one. The community mental health worker reinforced the work of the therapist. Siegal sees the paraprofessional as adding a new dimension to therapy by performing those special efforts for patients "that may mean the difference between success and failure" (1974: 320). Lynch and Gardner conceive of the central functions of this component as an expression of "the treater's empathy and utilization of certain treatment techniques that we have endeavored to abstract from the psychiatrist's role and to construct therefrom a new role that can be performed by a paraprofessional" (1970: 1477).

These therapeutic tasks are often carried out in an innovative and untraditional way. Paraprofessionals who fill this role not only have direct contact with patients, but they must work as part of a service delivery team. Contact with professionals, such as psychiatrists, social workers, psychologists, and nurses, involves establishing formal and informal relationships to determine daily responsibilities for patient care and treatment.

Community mental health teams must make decisions about a patient's progress through various phases of a rehabilitation program, the continued use of medication, and action to be taken against disruptive patients. The question of the scope of the contribution to be made by paraprofessionals in planning the course of a client's treatment and activity program can generate problems for the team. Paraprofessionals who have considerable day-to-day contact with clients may feel that they should have major input in such decision making, and they may regard professionals as not being close enough to the clients to make wise decisions in a particular case, despite their greater formal knowledge and training. The uncertainty of the paraprofessional's role in decision making strains the relationships among team members and thus reduces its effectiveness.

These direct relationships are also affected by the increased competition between professionals and paraprofessionals in a tight labor market. Some professionals, particularly social workers, feel that paraprofessionals are rivals for the same budget lines at service agencies. As a result, professionals must improve the skills of paraprofessionals with whom they are in direct competition. In turn, those who supervise and train paraprofessionals are skeptical of their contribution, given their limited training, to community mental health.

The structure of this professional-paraprofessional relationship is as likely to produce conflict as cooperation. One way to locate the sources of conflict is to examine and compare the mutual perspectives of both. The author conducted such a study at a community mental health center in which a total of 39 paraprofessionals and 38 professionals were interviewed.

Professionals were more likely than paraprofessionals to want to limit the role of the latter to coordinative or "backup services," with 67 percent of the first group mentioning service activities, compared to 53 percent of the second group. Sixty-one percent of the professionals said they would use interpersonal or personal criteria to evaluate paraprofessionals, looking for such characteristics as the ability to make contact and get along with others; capacity for growth and change; willingness to recognize limitations in abilities and knowledge and to use available supervision and expertise when needed. In contrast, 41 percent of the paraprofessionals evaluated their own performance according to organizational or administrative conformity, mentioning such traits as ability to follow the rules, punctuality, and submitting reports on time. A significant number (38 percent) stressed psychotherapeutic criteria, including clinical judgment and evidence of improvement in patients; these criteria were mentioned by only 29 percent of the professionals.

Professionals, particularly social workers, pointed to the lack of uniformity in the paraprofessional group, both in terms of training and performance. Professionals said that paraprofessionals did not present a clear image as a well-defined occupational grouping, representing certain levels of competency and training. In so doing, professionals also noted that paraprofessionals had no organizations to represent them and no journals and academic forums where issues pertinent to their work could be discussed. Paraprofessionals explained this failure to organize as the direct result of a lack of financial resources to encourage these kinds of developments. Although paraprofessionals are often verbally encouraged to attend national conferences of community mental health center personnel, they are rarely selected to attend such meetings at the center's expense. When travel funds are in short supply, the tendency is even stronger to send professionals deemed most capable of representing the center or benefiting from contact with others in the field.

Professionals do not view paraprofessionals as coworkers capable of exercizing independent judgment. Frequently, professionals characterized their relationship with paraprofessionals as similar to their role as supervisors of students in field placement. What appears even more significant is that a greater proportion of professionals than paraprofessionals pointed out problems of uncertainty related to authority. Sixty-five percent of the professionals mentioned areas of uncertainty in authority concerning procedures undertaken by paraprofessionals in treating patients and failures to recognize organizational and role-related boundaries in the community mental health center. In contrast, only 32 percent of the paraprofessionals mentioned any areas of uncertainty or ambiguity about their authority, with most specifying similar organizational and role-related problems. Both groups agreed that professionals had far more input in shaping new programs, while paraprofessionals were seen by both groups as having significant involvement in development of treatment plans for individual patients.

Despite the lack of agreement on the present limits of paraprofessionals, there was strong agreement on what they *should* be doing. Both groups advocated the utilization of paraprofessionals primarily as providers of necessary support services. Professionals took the cautious position that the paraprofessionals needed more training. Such a perspective enhanced the professionals' authority. Professionals spoke at length about the enormous variation in attributes of different paraprofessionals and the personal nature of their relationship wtih those they regarded as particularly competent. The idiosyncratic nature of the relationship was evinced in frequent statements made by professionals that competent paraprofessionals shaped their jobs in negotiation with supervisors. Professionals felt that paraprofessionals needed more education in order to effectively treat patients. Few professionals recommended on-the-job training for currently employed paraprofessionals, even though only 10 percent of the latter were ever subject to a training program before being employed at the community center. When training was advocated by professionals, the program outlined was so rigorous that the interviewer often suggested that paraprofessionals who successfully completed such a course of training would be professionals. The response to this was usually a statement that the work currently performed by many paraprofessionals required such training.

THE DIVISION OF LABOR, THE DIVISION OF SOCIETY

The sources of conflict among various health care practitioners are many; some challenge the professional dominance of medicine, while others exist within the currently changing division of labor among paramedical personnel, including pharmacists, nurse practitioners, physician assistants, community mental health workers, social workers, and rehabilitation workers. Some of these conflicts result from the differences in recruitment into these different occupations, organizational and technical change, and new financial arrangements rather than from questions related to technical and clinical assignments.

The study of the changing division of labor in society reveals a struggle between those with and those without power as well as those who seek to gain more honor. While many people in the United States believe there is open and free competition between individuals to gain access to educational opportunities, the acquisition of property, and job advancement, group mobility through virtual monopoly on certain occupations makes individual mobility difficult.

Individual competition between various health care practitioners does not take place because medicine controls decision making. Only physicians command and order the changes in the division of labor. Elliott Krause, a sociologist engaged in the study of occupations, emphasizes the unique position of physicians in the division of labor in health care by focusing on their legal monopoly in the field. "Physicians, it should be noted, are the only group that can both own and use such technology for profit in the community, such as doctors who privately own a kidney dialysis machine" (1971: 55).

Ownership, however, may be far less important than possession of the legal right to use certain techniques. Since equipment and hospital beds are expensive, individual ownership has been replaced by collective, corporate ownership. Yet many corporations are nonprofit and provide services, living off patient fees, third-party payments, or government grants. Consumers pay for these services regardless of the form of remuneration, whether they make direct payment, purchase group health insurance, or pay taxes. The health care industry, both in the profit-making corporations that manufacture and sell drugs and the profit and nonprofit companies that sell insurance, depend on these voluntary and government organizations. Physicians depend on their fees. Michael Harrington, a well-known critic of American capitalism, refers to such a situation as "socialism for the rich" (1972: 334).

This system of service combining private enterprise and public funding is monopolized by physicians. Some doctors have a greater stake in seeing this system reformed, while others see the need to maintain it. Robert Alford, a political sociologist, has summarized the current situation and the possibilities of change from within, led by medical planners whom he labels "corporate rationalizers."

> . . . medicine seems to be a classic case of the socialization of production but the private appropriation of the "surplus" by a vested interest group—the doctors—who maintain control through their professional associations of the supply of physicians, the distribution of services, the cost of services, and the rules governing hospitals. The gradual decline of solo practice has created the social

conditions for the challenge of this professional monopoly by the corporate rationalizers. [Alford, 1973: 142]

Any discussion of conflict within the health care field, between physicians and direct competitors, between the new practitioners and old, or among other providers of care, is illuminated within the larger framework of society. These struggles can be brought out in the open through protest or mediated through collective bargaining between unions and management.

Elliott Krause notes the importance of structured accumulated disadvantage: "the social class distinctions of the wider society are reproduced in the way different social groups—by sex, race and social class—are tracked into the division of labor in health work" (1977: 42).

Thus there is a never-ending cycle of conflict and accommodation among various health care practitioners. It is highlighted in the issues of unionization; and it becomes even more complex in community and consumer participation in decision making. The development of new practitioners has been jointly encouraged by the need to reduce the cost of health care and by efforts to avoid the depersonalization of people subject to long-term hospitalization.

REFERENCES

Alford, R. 1972. "The political economy of health care: Dynamics without change." *Politics and Society* (Winter): 1–38.

Anderson, John, et al. 1975. *Remington's Pharmaceutical Sciences.* Easton, Pa.: Mack Publishing Co.

Borrello, M. A., and E. Mathias. 1977. "Botanicas: Puerto Rican folk pharmacies." *Natural History* 86 (August/September): 64–73.

[CRI] Cambridge Research Institute. 1975. *Trends Affecting U.S. Health Care System.* Washington, D.C.: Department of Health, Education, and Welfare.

Cole, P., and Emmanuel, S. 1971. "Drug consultation: Its significance to the discharged hospital patient and its relevance as a role for the pharmacist." *American Journal of Hospital Pharmacy* 23 (December): 954–60.

Consumer Reports 40 (September 1975): 542–48. "Chiropractors: Healers or quacks? Part 1: The 80-year war with science."

Consumer Reports 40 (October 1975): 606–10. "Chiropractors: Healers or quacks? Part 2: How chiropractors can help—or harm."

Denzin, N. 1968. "Incomplete professionalization: The case of pharmacy." *Social Forces* 46 (March): 375–81.

Harrington, Michael. 1972. *Socialism.* New York: Bantam Books.

Hicks, N. 1976. "Ford signs medical training bill to send doctors to areas of need." *New York Times,* October 14, p. 20.

Knapp, D. A., and Knapp, D. E. 1968. "An appraisal of the contemporary practice of pharmacy." *American Journal of Pharmaceutical Education* 32: 747–58.

Krause, Elliott. 1977. *Power and Illness: The Political Sociology of Health and Medical Care.* New York: Elsevier.

Kronus, C. 1975. "Occupational values, role orientations, and work settings: The case of pharmacy." *Sociological Quarterly* 16 (Spring): 171–83.

Lambert, R. L., et al. 1977. "The pharmacist's clinical role as seen by other health workers." *American Journal of Public Health* 67 (March): 252–53.

Lynch, M., and Gardner, E. A. 1970. "Some issues raised in the training of paraprofessional personnel as clinical therapists." *American Journal of Psychiatry* 126 (April): 1473–79.

Malahy, B. 1966. "The effect of instruction and labeling on the number of medical errors made by patients at home." *American Journal of Hospital Pharmacy* 23 (June): 283–92.

McKenney, J. M., et al. 1973. "The effect of clinical pharmacy services on patients with essential hypertension." *Circulation* 48 (November): 1104–11.

Mechanic, David. 1970. "Social issues in the study of the pharmaceutical field." *American Journal of Pharmaceutical Education* 34: 536–43.

Millis, John. 1975. *Pharmacists for the Future: The Report of the Study Commission on Pharmacy*. Ann Arbor, Mich.: Health Administration Press.

Siegal, R. L. 1974. "Do we really need paraprofessional mental health workers?" *Hospital and Community Psychiatry* 25 (May): 320.

Smith, D. B. 1977. "A cooperative pharmacy project: An autopsy on a community health intervention." *Journal of Community Health* 2 (Spring): 222–31.

Smith, D. E., J. Luce, and E. Dernberg. 1973. "The health of Haight-Ashbury." Pp. 25–50 in Anselm L. Strauss, ed., *Where Medicine Fails*. New York: Transactions Books.

Sullivan, R. 1980. "Help for the harried hospital doctors." *New York Times*, March 22, pp. 23, 25.

Taffet, S. 1976. "Forum: For better eye care." *Mamaroneck Daily Times*, (New York) February 16, p. 27.

Vogt, M. J., and A. J. Ducanis. 1977. "Conflict and cooperation in the allied health professions." *Journal of Allied Health* 6 (Winter): 38–44.

Wallace, Anthony F. C. 1966. *Religion: An Anthropologic View*. New York: Random House.

Wardwell, W. 1952. "A marginal professional role: The chiropractor." *Social Forces* 30 (March): 339–48.

12

New Concepts and New Practices

The emergence of the hospital as the centralized unit of health care production resulted from an intersection of changes in the patterns of work, family life and medical techniques.* The hospital became the major organization of health care and physicians learned to rely on it even when diagnostic tests and simple surgical procedures could be performed for outpatients or when illnesses could be managed in the home. Further, disabled people who could live in the community with assistance were often kept in long-term care.

The justification for attempting to maintain people in need of health care in the community, rather than in long-term hospitalization, came from the consequences of World War II. Many returning veterans, whose lives were saved by battlefield surgery, refused to remain hidden from public view in chronic disease hospitals as charity cases. In addition, the greater availability of prosethetic devices for amputees, coupled with low-cost automobiles and fuel, made it possible for thousands of wheelchair-bound people, or those who used crutches, to become highly mobile.

Another important source of the thrust toward home and community care came from the child development specialists writing on the effects on children of long-term separation from the family. The English were particularly concerned about the consequences of separation because of their program to evacuate thousands of children from the cities during World War II during the Nazi air war against urban and industrial targets. Children left their families to live in small towns, and some went into institutional settings. Spitz, a psychiatrist, first noted that children separated from their parents

*Part of this chapter first appeared in *USA Today* 107 (July 1978) as "Home Care: An Alternative to the High Cost of Hospitalization," pp. 52–54.

showed signs of depression, which he called "hospitalism" (1945, 1946). Bowlby and others (1956) began a series of studies of the effects of maternal deprivation on children.

Not long after the appearance of Spitz's work, Montefiore Hospital in the Bronx began a home care program which extended the wartime findings to adults confined for long periods in hospitals. In 1946, some hospitalized patients at Montefiore were given the opportunity to return to their homes, provided the family was willing to accept the responsibility for care. No diagnosis was excluded from consideration, and even the terminally ill could be cared for at home. When the family was unwilling to perform even minor medical procedures for a member, however, the person remained in the hospital (Silver, 1976: 76). The hospital provided extensive support services, such as training in the use of equipment, emergency care, and short-term readmission to give families some respite.

The growth of home care services came about primarily because of the concern over the high cost of hospital care to the consumer and third-party payers. Home care costs only about 25 percent of hospital care, because the custodial tasks and even many of the nursing tasks are carried out by the family. Hospital charges include housekeeping costs and amortization of the expenses of financing and building of the hospital itself.

The diminishing use of hospital care could serve to reduce the total health care bill in the United States considerably. As of 1975, more than 39 percent of the $118.5 billion dollars spent on health care went for hospital care (Department of Health, Education, and Welfare, 1976: 26). It is reasonable to expect that extending home care administered through outpatient services will help reduce costs substantially. George Silver, one of the originators of the home care program at Montefiore Hospital, points out how this can happen:

> Another cost sharing element provided is that those who are engaged professionally in home visiting are spending only a part of the time on any patient and can therefore see many more patients during the day than they would if they were taking care of one patient all day in an institution. [1976: 158]

By eliminating the need for hospitalization for minor surgical procedures, which can be performed on an outpatient basis, further reductions of time spent in hospitals can be effected. Convalescence at home can follow operations for hernia repair and varicose veins. In particular, children subject to surgery find the experience traumatic, since it involves separation from parents and handling from many strangers. One-day units for hernia repairs or tonsillectomies permit parents to be present during preoperative procedures and recovery. Unless there are complications, children who arrive at the hospital at 7 A.M. can go home by 6 P.M. Generally, little nursing care is required after these surgical procedures, and ordinary parental attention promotes recovery quickly.

A further incentive to home care comes from the recent technological advances that have reduced the size of many machines. Now portable diagnostic devices such as electrocardiograph machines and some treatment devices such as hemodialysis units can be taken to or installed in a patient's home. Some physicians have argued that home-based dialysis units are less costly than those in hospital clinics and equally successful. Patients with end-stage kidney disease can be dialyzed at home, after they and their families have received rigorous training to learn to operate the machine and avoid infection.

In a Seattle-based program started in 1966 at the Northwest Kidney Center, 23 patients learned to perform their own dialysis, and 21 were alive after 2,500 home treatments had been performed. The only complication of uremia, the consequence of renal failure, was anemia. The team claimed that they had created a practical way of treating end-stage kidney disease and questioned the need to continue kidney transplant programs using live donors (Fox and Swazey, 1974: 225). The success of this project did slow the introduction of the less certain kidney transplant operations in this area.

Some think that the hospital environment may be inappropriate for people with chronic diseases, although acute care, it is argued, cannot be provided at home. Research indicates, that on the contrary, even acute illnesses of a very serious nature can be managed at home. Hospitalization for acute myocardial infarction is standard medical practice, and many hospitals have established intensive care units exclusively for cardiac cases. Mather and his colleagues found no evidence that patients recovered more quickly from heart attacks in hospitals compared with home care. He randomly assigned 343 men from four English communities with episodes of acute myocardial infarction either to home care under the supervision of a family physician, or hospitalization, with early treatment in an intensive care unit. The results showed a similar rate for both. Men with no history of high blood pressure, however, did somewhat better at home than in the hospital (Mather, Pearson, and Read, 1971). While no method is available to foretell whether given patients will do better in which treatment environment, clearly the home can be a suitable place for care, even when families are not selected according to any strict criteria. Additional English studies report similar results (Hill et al., 1978; Colling et al., 1976; Dellipiani et al., 1977). Further research is needed in other countries to determine whether these results are independent of the English family and health care delivery system.

The development of organized home care depends on the willingness of the health care system to reach out into the community. Home programs are critically important in helping to keep the elderly out of old-age and nursing homes and chronically ill and disabled children out of hospital-like institutions. The availability of home care can be a decisive factor in reducing the need for institutions that provide custodial service but do not encourage personal growth and development.

The effectiveness of home care varies with the availability and willingness of families to extend themselves when the patient requires more than occasional help. In some types of serious chronic illness, such as end-stage kidney disease, the family's competent use of the machinery can be a lifesaving activity. The sense of responsibility for the life of a family member can be awesome for some people, producing tensions in the relationship.

The beneficiary of such complex medical activities may also resent the person providing these procedures, since there are no ways of demonstrating reciprocity. Merely saying thanks may leave the recipient feeling that something remains undone (Fox and Swazey, 1974: 9).

The involvement of the professional is useful in dealing with the social dynamics of such an unusual relationship, putting it into the perspective of the larger framework of what members owe to society rather than what they owe to each other (Titmuss, 1971: 226). Home care for seriously ill individuals is dependent on informal social supports that can be mobilized into an organized system.

HOME CARE AND THE ELDERLY

The national health care needs in the United States reflect the context of changing demographic patterns. As is true in such other highly industrialized countries as Sweden, England, and Denmark, lengthened life expectancy combined with a reduced birthrate are profoundly altering lifestyles and health costs. Along with longer lives come increased health problems associated with the diseases of later life, such as heart ailments, high blood pressure and other impairments of the arteriovascular system, diabetes, and cancer.

Poor health is a major concern of the elderly, with 21 percent claiming it as a very serious problem for themselves and another 29 percent as a somewhat serious problem (Louis Harris, 1975: 29). Moreover, reduced physical mobility is often a consequence of poor health, reducing the capacity of persons to maintain contact with others, particularly relatives and peers. Shanas reported that in five industrialized countries

> . . . from 4 to 5 older people in every 100 are institutionalized. From 8 to 15, depending on the country are either bedfast or housebound and living in their own homes. An additional 6 to 16 in every 100 are able to go outdoors with difficulty. [1971: 39]

The health status of the elderly is also related to their sense of social involvement or isolation. When elderly living alone were compared in an international study, those in poor or fair health said they were often lonely (Shanas et al., 1968: 60). Home care activities do not reduce the isolation for the elderly in poor health, but it can increase their chances of remaining outside of extended care facilities, environments that generally do not promote a sense of well-being (Mendelson, 1975).

A controlled study comparing elderly discharged hospital patients who received home aide services with those who did not found that the experimental group had fewer days of institutionalization in long-term facilities such as nursing homes. The group receiving home aide services was also more content, but there were no differences in the mortality or survival rate of each group (Nielson, 1970). A nine-year study conducted by Philadelphia Blue Cross demonstrated that home care clearly reduced the need for hospitalization (Trager, 1972: 22).

Without the availability of medical programs, the elderly often have no alternative but to become patients in nursing homes. Those who live alone and have some difficulty in managing daily activities may also find that home care in a more limited form can help them remain in the community. For instance, some can cook and clean for themselves but cannot do marketing; others can do marketing but cannot take a bath without assistance.

The elderly living alone are possible candidates for nursing homes so long as some necessary daily activity remains undone, even though most elderly manage quite well alone. In the United States, many elderly people prefer to maintain a separate residence from their children, and many of the widowed live alone without any feeling of isolation or loneliness (Chevan and Korson, 1972). These preferences are idealized ways of aging with dignity, but they are influenced by reality. Moving in with children is the last resort for many when there is little money and health is poor, making self-care impossible (Troll, 1971: 266). Yet many of the elderly feel a loss of self-worth when they cannot maintain their own households. Home care allows the elderly to maintain their dignity because it avoids dependence on their children.

Thus the needs of the elderly for home care range from concentrated, intensive short-term services, involving a complicated treatment regime and a highly skilled medical and nursing staff, to some simple homemaker services. There are also a variety of intermediate services during a period of convalescence in which recovery is subject to regular medical monitoring (Trager, 1972: 6).

The range of services required does not reveal the frequency with which each service is called upon by the elderly. The most often needed services are not strictly medical, but are those related to personal hygiene and homemaking. These tasks can be performed efficiently by trained aides, even though supportive or therapeutic intervention may also be required (Trager, 1972: 28).

Intermediate services can be provided by nurse practitioners or physician assistants, who, besides providing direct medical services, also assess progress through ongoing observations. As with any form of medical treatment, followup is important. Despite recognition of the preventive quality of homemaker services, mainly in keeping people out of hospitals and nursing homes, Medicare insurance for the elderly does not reimburse patients for the cost of a homemaker. It does pay for short-term, acute home care, with an upper limit established on the amount of service it will support. Moreover, it is difficult to receive reimbursement for home service, even for acute care, unless a patient had previously been hospitalized for an acute condition. As a result, physicians have not often recommended home care for Medicare patients, and during 1969–71, only one percent of Medicare insurance expenditures were allocated to home care (Trager, 1972: 14).

By 1971, 2,256 participating home health agencies were receiving Medicare reimbursements for services rendered. Only 263 programs were hospital-based, making coordination of services difficult in many instances because the same administrative authority did not supervise service delivery. In general, the participating hospitals were large and could afford to implement this program because it placed no strain on their bookkeeping and billing services. In 1973, all state agencies administering social security funds from the federal government were required by law to provide homemaker services to clients in need of assistance.

Homemaker services are provided for the elderly to assist in daily activities such as cooking and cleaning or help with personal hygiene, dressing, or transportation. Some group homes are designated "domiciliary care homes," where personal services are not provided. Others are called "personal care homes," where assistance is available to those who cannot fully take care of themselves. In either category, a paid staff conducts the custodial tasks of cooking, cleaning, and household maintenance. While these facilities are useful substitutes for nursing homes, only about 91,000 people were living in them as of 1971, as compared with more than one million in nursing homes and personal care homes with nursing care (Cambridge Research Institute, 1975: 281).

Alternatives to nursing homes have been created in England through the development of the geriatric day center, a facility that provides daily medical treatment and recreation and opportunity for socializing, as found in senior citizens' centers. Only two percent of the elderly live in nursing homes in Great Britain, as compared with five percent in the United States. Those who attend geriatric day centers live at home, making the costs for the program only 25 percent of the cost of institutional care. Day care centers help to prevent deterioration of the elderly who are in poor health (Cambridge Research Institute, 1975: 284).

COMMUNITY CARE FOR THE MENTALLY ILL AND RETARDED

The philosophy of care for the emotionally disturbed or mentally retarded has gone through various changes. Not long ago the conventional wisdom in the medical profession was that people with psychiatric histories and the mentally retarded could not manage to take care of themselves in the community and required asylum in long-term facilities, usually large institutions located in isolated settings.

In the 1950s, the idea was put forth that the social environment had a substantial impact upon the behavior of normal people and those with psychiatric histories as well. A new concept in psychiatric care developed, leading to the creation of a therapeutic community. It was reasoned that if psychiatric patients were treated with respect, they would begin to take control over their own lives (Jones, 1953). In addition, the development of major tranquilizing drugs such as thorazine made it possible to limit some of the acute psychotic behavior of psychiatric patients, leading psychiatrists to conclude that they could also be managed in the community.

Psychiatrists began to become more aware of the treatment environment, and a number of organizational studies of residential services for psychiatric patients were conducted by sociologists and anthropologists (Stanton and Schwartz, 1954; Belknap, 1956; Caudill, 1958). Perhaps for the first time, state hospitals and other asylums were conceptualized as social environments, where patients and staff interacted and attempted to influence each other. Some questions were raised in these studies about the structure of institutions and whether or not such social environments reinforced the incapacities of people who were patients, making it impossible for them to take care of themselves. Not long after, Erving Goffman's (1961) brilliant essays on how the "self" is structured in "total institutions" suggested that much of a person's typically aberrant behavior was situational and institutionally induced. Moreover, Goffman argued that patients' behavior must be seen within the restrictive context of the psychiatric hospital. It became evident that institutional living constituted a kind of cruel although not very unusual punishment for many people who were rarely dangerous to themselves or others.

Institutions for those who are regarded as incapable of taking care of themselves, whether psychiatric hospitals or state schools for the mentally retarded, have come to be considered as social environments radically differing from those in the outside world. These asylums were set apart from the mainstream of life, often in the country (to effect segregation, symbolized by surrounding fences and high walls). Isolation was one source of understimulation for patients in state schools or state hospitals. In addition, much of their day was spent in enforced idleness. The restrictiveness of the scheduling and social distance between staff and inmates appeared to make for what George W. Brown refers to as "clinical handicap" (1973). In his comparative study of several residential psychiatric institutions, lack of activity, particularly lack of opportunity for self-initiated activity, was shown to be a major impediment to recovery during hospitalization of chronic schizophrenics (Wing and Brown, 1970).

Later studies demonstrated great variability in institutional care and opportunities for personal development. King, Raynes, and Tizard (1971) identified important differences in child management practices in residential institutions for handicapped children. (However, no attempt was made to examine the effects of these practices on the child's behavior, self-regard, or social skills.)

Some evidence suggests that institutional care induces patients to conform to regulations in asylums but makes them maladaptive for community living. Consequently, the staffs of state schools and psychiatric hospitals are reluctant to plan for the return of their patients to the community. In a study of the impact of four years of institutional care on mentally retarded children and adults at a state school, for example, a significant decrease in the measured I.Q. of mentally retarded children occurred, but the change in test scores for adolescents and adults was not as striking (Sternlicht and Siegal, 1968). Most interestingly, the changes in verbal intelligence were far greater than the changes in performance, ability, or visual-motor coordination. Perhaps the social situation of the state school patient was undemanding in the area of verbal skills. Dentler and Mackler (1961), in a field study of the socialization of retarded children to cottage living, showed that patients were successfully trained by staff for institutional living through the use of rewards and punishments.

One of the important variables in explaining why residential institutions for the mentally retarded and psychiatric patients are understimulating and impersonal is the size of the facility. Since American institutions are generally large, it is difficult to specify the effect of size on behavior of residents and staff because there are no ways to compare institutions of varying size. Jack Tizard points out that more than 67 percent of the state institutions for the mentally retarded listed in the *1962 Directory of the American Association on Mental Deficiency* have more than 500 beds (1970: 301). However, he adds that it is too soon to generalize that the big institution is a bad institution (Tizard, 1970: 308–9). In his previous work on residential care for children in England, there was no correlation between size of institutions, size of child-care units, staff-child ratios, and type of care.

Large size creates conditions for the formation of primary groups among attendants that may subvert rehabilitation goals. The social organization of the residence is often considered central to understanding child-care practices. Tizard found that when the person in charge of the unit spent a great deal of time in direct contact with the children and delegated administrative and domestic responsibilities to others, child-oriented rather than institution-oriented practices prevailed. Supervisors who spent time in direct contact with residents functioned as models for attendants.

Ongoing social interaction between staff and children varied a great deal, depending on the orientation of the directors of the residential facility. Where institution-oriented management practices prevailed, the staff "spoke to them less often, played with them less, and physically handled them much less frequently than did their counterparts in the hostels" (Tizard, 1970: 309).

Other students of institutional life have pointed out how important the role of employees and staff is to an understanding of the social situation of patients. Scheff found attendants in state psychiatric hospitals exercising informal means of social control upon each other as a way of preventing new programs from being successfully introduced into the life of the ward (1961). Similar observations have been made at state schools for the mentally retarded (Morris, 1969). Dorothy Smith has also noted how organizational goals can be subverted by front-line staff (1965). Attendants are often cynical about the motives of administrators for introducing new programs (Bogdan et al., 1974).

Community care for psychiatric patients was encouraged by the recognition of the difficulties in establishing innovative programs in environments that were hostile to rehabilitation. During the 1960s, an alternative to the massive, isolated, impersonal psychiatric hospital was developed in the form of a halfway house; this small community-based, informally run facility was first intended to be a "transitional environment following hospitalization and before resumption of normal independent living" (Landy and Greenblatt, 1965: 2–3). The purposes of these programs were later expanded to include: (1) reducing the length of hospitalization and its negative effects for psychiatric patients; (2) providing a way to reintegrate people who have been hospitalized into the community; (3) offering an alternative program to hospitalization; and (4) developing a permanent living arrangement for people who no longer need to be hospitalized but either cannot return to their families or who need a residential program while living in the community (Glasscote et al., 1970: 22–23). While the goals of halfway houses have expanded, a recent survey showed that 77 percent of the referrals still come from state hospitals rather than from the community (Glasscote et al., 1971: 21).

In a case study of a halfway house for women in Boston, a positive relationship was found between the establishment of "mutually satisfying relationships with other women in the house and having an adequate adaptation to community living" (Landy and Greenblatt, 1965: 107). It is not clear, however, which variable is independent, or whether both success in establishing interpersonal relationships and community adaptation are the results of other social factors, such as the length of hospitalization, etiology, therapy, or nature of the condition.

The concept of the halfway house is not always carried out in a comprehensive way when former psychiatric patients are placed in a community. Neighborhoods with high concentrations of single-room occupancy hotels or former resort hotels can be overwhelmed by large numbers of former mental patients, many of whom attend no programs or are unemployed (Schumach, 1974). Aftercare services for those psychiatric patients who were formerly hospitalized have not been effective in preventing rehospitalization, even when they do remove idle people from the streets (Birenbaum and Seiffer, 1977).

Small residential facilities for the mentally retarded are somewhat more effective in reducing idleness and getting their residents involved in more independent living (Birenbaum and Seiffer, 1976). Current efforts in California to return mentally retarded adults to the community have involved extensive use of board-and-care facilities (Bjannes and Butler, 1974). These residential programs are run for profit and house 30 to 40 persons or more. Lacking supportive services and individualized goals to increase the independence of the residents, the board-and-care facilities are located in the community but do not utilize it for programs in vocational rehabilitation or recreation. Nor do they instruct residents in how to use the community transportation system.

Edgerton has observed that the economic arrangements that reimburse proprietors in these facilities provide few incentives to train residents for independent living. Caretakers operate at a profit when their beds are filled to capacity. Consequently, there is great reluctance to permit a resident to strike out on his own unless a replacement is immediately available (1975). However, other investigators have compared the activities of residents at board-and-care facilities with group homes and family care and found that the former encouraged more independent behavior (Bjannes and Butler, 1974). Furthermore, board-and-care facilities seem to realize more closely the goals of developing social skills by making possible a more varied round of life than other domiciliary arrangements in the community. Extensive exposure to the community was found by Bjannes and Butler to be an important aspect of reintegrating former state-school patients (1974).

A longitudinal study conducted by the author and Samuel Seiffer examined what happened to a total of 63 men and women who left three large and isolated state schools for the mentally retarded and went to live at a community residence (1976). 63 persons were resettled in 1973, as of April 1977, 42 were still living at the facility. Among the 21 who left, 5 had gone to live with their families, 1 moved into the community, 3 were participating in an apartment-living program, 1 was in a nursing home because of physical problems, 1 had voluntarily returned to a state school, 9 were transferred back to the original state school because of unacceptable behavior, and 1 was struck by a car and killed.

The purpose of the study was to see whether changes in self-image, interpersonal relationships, work experience, use of leisure time, personal decision-making, and social competency would occur. Interviews were conducted on three occasions with the 48 respondents who remained for at least 16 months at the facility. A fourth interview took place with 42 respondents 40 to 44 months after resettlement, and the results were compared with those found in the third interview to determine whether any further changes had occurred in their reactions to community living, relations with peers and staff, and involvement in the wider community.

From these studies it appeared that residents not only approved of the new way of living but also wanted to acquire even more independence. The new experiences of community living and learning to work in vocational rehabilitation programs at sheltered workshops permitted more conventional activities and greater involvement in adult activities than in their past situations. However, while residents became more self-reliant and developed more personalized social relationships with their peers, they still remained dependent on the staff for many services they could probably learn to perform for themselves. Most evident was the general lack of skills in the area of travel to distant locations. Other than travel to workshops, they could not determine the logistics for scheduled events: when they took place, when to leave, and how to get there. The fourth wave of interviews was designed to see whether these patterns had changed.

The most recent study of the facility found new restrictions imposed on self-determining behavior of residents, limiting their right to choose what time to go to bed and wake up in the morning. Many residents continued to express desire to live more independently; their goals in almost half the cases were to find apartments of their own or to move in with their families. Moreover, certain self-management skills had been acquired and maintained, including careful management of money and ability to describe how to make breakfast. Finally, the period of personal exploration and the acquisition of new experiences that initially accompanied resettlement had given way to a prosaic routine of sleep, work, and at-home recreation of a passive nature; weekends were often reserved for visiting the family or receiving visits. This lifestyle is not too different from that of those who are not mentally retarded but are marginally employed or mostly unemployed (Birenbaum and Re, 1979).

The most dramatic changes in behavior of mentally retarded persons were made in a small experimental unit, Brooklands, a residential program for children who had previously been in a large institution. Organized in such a way that the daily routines of life were guided by concerns for maintaining a normal home life, the children at Brooklands were observed to be "able to play socially and constructively, at a level approaching that of their mental age" (Tizard, 1964: 79). The children also made gains in verbal abilities and lost many of the behaviors traditionally associated with mental retardation (for example, rocking). A matched control group who remained in the traditional hospital continued to exhibit these behaviors and made few gains in verbal abilities.

In a similar comparison of severely retarded children living in a small locally-based residential care unit and in a hospital unit, Kushlick reported change in 9 out of 13 behavior areas (1975: 334). Children improved in their ability to feed and dress themselves, and in their exercise of appropriate general behavior. Children who could not walk made the most progress, in a comparison between those who lived in locally-based units and their counterparts who remained in hospital care (Kushlick, 1975: 335).

One of the concepts guiding the development of community care networks is the idea of *normalization*. Using Scandinavian and English social welfare policies as a model, some planners have attempted to apply normalization to the establishment of services in the United States and Canada (Wolfensberger, 1972). Their aim is to create programs that are coordinated but not centralized, "making available to the mentally retarded patterns and conditions of everyday life which are as close as possible to the norms and patterns of the mainstream of society" (Nirje, 1969: 181). Implicit in this concept is a sociological generalization, namely, that social surroundings will deeply influence opportunities to lead conventional lives. In addition, the social environment is subject to judgment by others, not only as to who lives there, but as to how they are to be treated and what can be expected from them. Those who live in institutions are often regarded as not having potential for growth and development. Normalization involves an approach that takes growth and development into account as needs of the mentally retarded, and an understanding that mentally retarded people change during their life cycle, not because their impairment is substantially altered, but because of the unimpaired self that remains. Indeed, the principle of normalization insists that the retarded person be defined as having a life cycle and personal career independent of his or her socially defined status as inmate, patient, and resident (Nirje, 1969: 181–83).

The planners of services for the mentally retarded are now concerned with the ways in which programs that, among other things, separate mentally retarded persons from society interfere with the conventional rhythms of daily life and with the establishment of ordinary social relationships and rewarding experiences. Therefore, they pattern services to enhance community involvement beyond focusing simply on the level of impairment of the population served.

PEDIATRIC HOME CARE SERVICES

Perhaps a good illustration of normalization is found in the efforts to humanize health care for all children. These efforts provide dramatic and convincing evidence of the importance of home care services as a way of promoting normal life for sick children, whether they are recovering from acute illness, major or minor surgical procedures, or learning to live with chronic illness of a partial or profoundly disabling kind. Home care programs for children with specific diseases have been particularly effective in reducing the number of days in which children do not attend school and are rehospitalized for complications following treatment. These efforts to deliver services at home not only make health care more humane but help to avoid later dependencies on public funds for the care of people never able to acquire skills needed to be economically and socially independent. Moreover, avoidance of hospitalization or rehospitalization reduces the risk of acquiring crossinfections, which are prevalent in hospitals.

Reducing hospitalization for children can begin at birth. Low-risk mothers and infants are sometimes sent home as few as twelve hours after delivery (Yanover, et al., 1976). In most of the current pediatric home care programs, early discharge from the hospital is accompanied by both parent training in care of the infant and home visits by a nurse practitioner to monitor the mother's and the child's health.

While a few days in the hospital for mother and child may be of little consequence to their health and the child's psychological development, long-term hospitalization does inhibit the development of parent-child interaction. Observers of the social consequences of disability and chronic illness have noted how different the socialization experiences of children growing up in hospitals are when compared with those raised at home (Richardson, 1969). The former learn rather early to fend for themselves, since there is no protecting adult around, but they also have diffiulty getting emotionally close to adults (Davis, 1963). Although they are often kept in hospitals because of the fear that medical complications will arise at home, children with major diseases show a great deal of success in managing illness at home. A two-year study of the medical, economic, and social aspects of the treatment of hemophiliacs demonstrated advantages in home care when compared to hospitalized cases. The great majority of bleeding incidents encountered in the home care group did not require hospitalization, nor were other complications noted. While more bleedings were reported—and they were revealed more quickly by the home care group than the hospitalized group—the consequences were more limited, and school attendance for the experimental group was better than for the control group (Strawczynski et al., 1973).

The management at home of children with special medical appliances has also been implemented in standard pediatric home care practices. Tracheotomies can be managed at home when parents are trained in the proper maintenance techniques, where homes are evaluated, where support services are provided, equipment distributed, and emergency and followup care available (Stool and Tucker, 1973).

Effective home care is not simply delegation of responsibility of nursing tasks to the family; rather, it involves active intervention by professions. Chronic and recurrent respiratory diseases are sometimes managed at home without supportive medical services. In a review of 402 patients selected for home care during a two-and-one-half-year period, more than 60 percent suffered from chronic or recurrent respiratory diseases. These children had mist tents at home and facilities for intermittent inhalation therapy. Mothers were trained to administer various physiotherapies. In the same patient panel were 28 cases of cystic fibrosis, a well-defined diagnostic group. In 12 of these cases, the various equipment and techniques were available to patients in their home without medical support services. This subsample was followed for a year without medical support services and then for a year with support services. The results were striking, and the researchers found that "the total number of hospital days for the group without "home care" was 369, as compared with 70 hospital days after the home care services were commenced" (Finkel and Pitt, 1968: 163).

A ten-year followup of a home care program in London suggests that nursing care at home is a central component of a pediatric program. Out of 2,923 patients, nursing intervention took place in more than 85 percent of the cases. As in other studies, a substantial proportion of the total number of cases seen involved respiratory diseases (Bergman, Shrand, and Oppe, 1965). Most of the referrals (67 percent) for home care came from the family physician, indicating that hospitalization is being prevented in many cases. In all of these studies, parental satisfaction with the program has been extremely good.

The organization of health care around the hospital has made dying an even more harrowing experience for the terminally ill and their families. Parents of children ill with a fatal disease are particularly dissatisfied by hospital management of death, since they cannot do anything for their children, and if the child is separated from them when death occurs, as is often the case, it is particularly traumatic. While the death of a child is always distressing, parents of children who died of cancer were able to experience a great deal of accomplishment and comfort through caring for their children at home. A three-year Minnesota study of home management of terminal illness revealed, at its midpoint, many possible economic psychological and social benefits. Parents expressed great feelings of completion of their obligations and satisfaction in knowing that the child died among loved ones in familiar surroundings. Control of pain was accomplished equally well at home as in the hospital (*Medical News*, 1977).

SUPPORT NETWORKS

While all of the new concepts and practices use the new health care practitioners to deliver services, their success largely depends on the availability of informal social support networks. The family is clearly the first line of support, but in numerous instances where people are living alone, as is the case with many of the elderly, the availability of neighbors and friends to help with daily activities can make the difference in determining whether a chronically ill elderly person can remain in the community and avoid transfer to a nursing home. While two-thirds of the elderly respondents in a representative sample of the 400,000 noninstitutionalized elderly living in

New York City say they have neighbors who help them when they are ill (and they in turn provide similar assistance), they define these sources of mutual aid as based on occasional emergency needs, rather than being available on a regular basis (Cantor, 1975: 7–8).

As home-service health agencies become increasingly aware of the limited amount of informal support services, they may be able to encourage and assist the formation of social networks among various households. Some of these networks might be developed among the elderly or among parents of children who live close to each other. This method can be particularly effective among parents of children who are physically disabled but mobile, making it possible for one parent to care for two or more children on a short-term basis. If local health aides are used to gather information, such health affinity groups could be initiated.

REFERENCES

Belknap, Ivan. 1958. *Human Problems of a State Mental Hospital.* New York: McGraw-Hill.

Bergman, A. B., H. Shrand, and T. E. Oppé. 1965. "A pediatric home care program in London: Ten years' experience." *Pediatrics* 36 (September): 314–21.

Birenbaum, A., and M. Re. 1979. "Resettling mentally retarded adults in the community: Almost four years later." *American Journal on Mental Deficiency* 83 (January): 323–29.

Birenbaum, Arnold, and Samuel Seiffer. 1976. *Resetting Mentally Retarded Adults in a Managed Community.* New York: Praeger.

———. 1977. "The effectiveness of aftercare referrals for previously hospitalized schizophrenics." Paper presented at the Annual meeting of The Society for the Study of Social Problems, September 5, Chicago.

Bjannes, A. T., and E. W. Butler. 1974. "Environmental variation in community care facilities for mentally retarded persons." *American Journal of Mental Deficiency* 78: 429–39.

Bogdan, R., et al. 1974. "Let them eat programs: Attendants' perspective and programming on wards in state schools." *Journal of Health and Social Behavior* 15 (June): 142–51.

Bowlby, J., et al. 1956. "The effects of mother-child separation: A followup study." *British Journal of Medical Psychology* 29: 211–47.

Brown, G. W. 1973. "The mental hospital as an institution." *Social Science and Medicine* 7 (July): 407–24.

Cambridge Research Institute. 1975. *Trends Affecting U.S. Health Care System.* Washington, D.C.: Department of Health, Education, and Welfare.

Cantor, M. H. 1975. "The formal and informal social support system of older New Yorkers." Paper presented at the 10th International Conference on Gerontology, June 25, Jerusalem, Israel.

Caudill, William A. 1958. *The Psychiatric Hospital as a Small Society.* Cambridge: Harvard University Press.

Chevan, A., and J. H. Korson. 1972. "The widowed who live alone." *Social Forces* 51: 45–53.

Colling, A., A. W. Dellipiani, and R. J. Donaldson. 1976. "Teeside coronary survey: An epidemiological study of acute attacks of myocardial infarction." *British Medical Journal* 2: 1169–72.

Davis, Fred. 1963. *Passage Through Crisis: Polio Victims and Their Families.* Indianopolis: Bobbs-Merrill.

Dellipiani, A. W., W. A. Colling, and R. J. Donaldson, et al. 1977. "Teeside coronary survey: Fatality and comparative severity of patients treated at home in the hospital ward, and in the coronary care unit after myocardial infarction." *British Heart Journal* 39: 1172–78.

Dentler, R. A., and B. Mackler. 1961. "The socialization of retarded children in an institution." *Journal of Health and Human Behavior* 2 (Summer): 243–52.

Edgerton, R. 1975. "Issues on the quality of life of retarded adults." Pp. 127–40 in Michael J.

Begab and Stephen A. Richardson, eds., *Mental Retardation and Society: A Social Science Perspective*. Baltimore: University Parks Press.

Finkel, K. C., and S. E. Pitt. 1968. "Pediatric home care program: Review of two and a half years' experience at the Children's Hospital of Winnipeg." *Canadian Medical Association Journal* 98 (January 20): 157–64.

Fox, Renée C., and Judith P. Swazey. 1974. *The Courage to Fail: A Social View of Organ Transplants and Dialysis*. Chicago: The University of Chicago Press.

Glasscote, Raymond M., Jon E. Gudeman, and J. Richard Elpers. 1970. *Halfway Houses for the Mentally Ill*. Springfield, Ill.: Charles Thomas.

Goffman, Erving. 1961. *Asylums: Essays on the Social Situation of Mental Patients and Other Inmates*. New York: Anchor Books.

Harris, Louis, and Associates. 1975. *Myth and Reality of Aging*. Washington, D.C.: National Council on Aging.

Hill, J. C., J. R. Hampton, and J. R. A. Mitchell. 1978. "A randomized trial of home-versus-hospital management for patients with suspected myocardial infarction." *Lancet* 1: 837–41.

Jones, Maxwell. 1953. *The Therapeutic Community*. New York: Basic Books.

King, Roy D., Norma V. Raynes, and Jack Tizard. 1971. *Patterns of Residential Care: Sociological Studies in Institutions for Handicapped Children*. London: Routledge and Kegan Paul.

Kushlick, A. 1975. "Epidemiology and evaluation of services for the mentally handicapped." Pp. 325–44 in Michael J. Begab and Stephen A. Richardson, eds., *Mental Retardation and Society: A Social Science Perspective*. Baltimore: University Parks Press.

Landy, David, and Milton Greenblatt. 1965. *Halfway House: A Sociocultural and Clinical Study*. Washington, D.C.: Department of Health, Education, and Welfare.

Mather, H. G., N. G. Pearson, and K. L. Read. 1971. "Acute myocardial infarction: Home and hospital treatment." *British Medical Journal* 3: 334–38.

Medical News 1977, 24 (June 13): 2591–93. "Taking the dying child home: What effect on patient, family?"

Mendelson, Mary Adelaide. 1973. *Tender Loving Greed*. New York: Vintage Books.

Morris, Pauline. 1969. *Put Away: A Sociological Study of Institutions for the Mentally Retarded*. New York: Atherton Press.

Nielson, Margaret. 1970. *Home Aide Service and the Aged: A Controlled Study. Part I. Design and Findings*. Cleveland: Benjamin Rose Institute.

Nirje, B. 1969. "The normalization principle and its human management implications." Pp. 179–96 in Robert B. Kugel and Wolf Wolfensberger, eds., *Changing Patterns of Residential Services for the Mentally Retarded*. Washington, D.C.: Department of Health, Education, and Welfare.

Richardson, S. A. 1969. "The effect of physical disability on the socialization of a child." Pp. 1047–64 in David A. Goslin, ed., *Handbook of Socialization: Theory and Research*. Chicago: Rand McNally.

Scheff, T. J. 1961. "Control over policy by attendants in a mental hospital." *Journal of Health and Human Behavior* 2 (Summer): 93–105.

Schumach, M. 1974. "Halfway houses for former mental patients create serious problems for city's residential communities." *New York Times*, January 21, p. 31.

Silver, George. 1976. *A Spy in the House of Medicine*. Germantown, Maryland: Aspen publications.

Shanas, E. 1971. "Measuring the home health needs of the aged in five countries." *Journal of Gerontology* 26: 37–40.

Shanas, Ethel, et al. 1968. *Old People in Three Industrial Societies*. New York: Atherton Press.

Smith, D. E. 1965. "Front-line organization of the state mental hospital." *Administrative Science Quarterly* 10 (December): 381–99.

Spitz, R. A. 1945. "Hospitalism: An inquiry into the genesis of psychiatric conditions in early childhood." Pp. 53–74 in O. Fenichel et al., eds., *Psychoanalytic Studies of the Child*. New York: International Universities Press.

———. 1946. "Hospitalism: A follow-up report." Pp. 113–17 in O. Fenichel et al., eds., *Psychoanalytic Studies of the Child*. New York: International Universities Press.

Stanton, Alfred H., and Morris S. Schwartz. 1954. *The Mental Hospital*. New York: Basic Books.

Sternlicht, M., and L. Siegal. 1968. "Institutional residence and intellectual functioning." *Journal of Mental Deficiency Research* 21: 119–27.
Stool, S., and J. Tucker. 1973. "Tracheotomy in infants and children." *Current Problems in Pediatrics* 3 (March): 20–33.
Strawczynski, H., et al. 1973. "Delivery of care to hemophilic children: Home care versus hospitalization." *Pediatrics* 51 (June): 986–99.
Thompson, Edward P. 1963. *The Making of the English Working Class.* New York: Vintage.
Titmuss, Richard. 1971. *The Gift Relationship: From Human Blood to Social Policy.* New York: Pantheon Books.
Tizard, Jack. 1964. *Community Services for the Mentally Handicapped.* London: Oxford University Press.
———. 1970. "The impact of social institutions in the causation, alleviation and prevention of mental retardation." Pp. 281–340 in H. Carl Haywood, ed., *Social-Cultural Aspects of Mental Retardation.* New York: Appleton-Century-Crofts.
Trager, Brahna. 1972. *Home Health Services in the United States. A Report to the Special Committee on Aging.* Washington, D.C.: U.S. Government Printing Office.
Troll, L. E. 1971. "The family of later life: A decade review." *Journal of Marriage and the Family* 33 (May): 263–90.
U.S. Department of Health, Education, and Welfare. 1976. *Forward Plan for Health: 1978–82.* Washington, D.C.: U.S. Government Printing Office.
Wing, John K., and George W. Brown. 1970. *Institutionalism and Schizophrenia.* Cambridge: Cambridge University Press.
Wolfensberger, Wolf. 1972. *The Principle of Normalization in Human Services.* Toronto: National Institute on Mental Retardation.
Yanover, M. J. 1976. "Perinatal care of low-risk mothers and infants: Early discharge with home care." *The New England Journal of Medicine* 294: 702–5.

Part Four
EMERGING SOCIAL ISSUES

13

The Women's Health Movement

Women today are often actively engaged in work roles once thought to be the traditional domain of men. The family is undergoing sharp and nonreversible transitions, involving greater equality of the marital partners and fewer children. Consequently, parental obligations for women are not full-time roles, and child rearing is now of more limited duration. Women in the United States may marry and remain childless, channeling their energies into other activities without feeling empty or incomplete.

Once women began to attend college in large numbers (and they now outnumber men in the ranks of college students), it seemed unlikely that traditional roles could be performed without a complaint or alteration. Writers of the contemporary novel, such as Mary McCarthy, pointed out the disparity between the life of the mind, found in elite coeducational and women's colleges, and the limited world of the suburban matron, organized around childbearing and homemaking. Betty Friedan, the godmother of contemporary feminism, named the amorphous sense of isolation and unfulfillment the "Problem That Has No Name," and many of her readers recognized this condition in themselves. The concern with the role of women in society has spawned ideological manifestos that question all institutions and the distribution of power within them.

The issue of the role of women in society is not new. Women of the middle and upper classes in the nineteenth century were considered to be not only weaker in strength than men, but to have a weaker constitution. They lived a protected and sheltered life, partly justified by viewing them as sickly and in need of care. Their sickness was seen to be the result of the strain of their biological destiny to be the bearers of children. This perspective was shared among members of the medical profession, and even those who introduced new ideas, such as Freud, found women to have different diseases from men. Freud completely revolutionized the study of psychopathology with his clinical work on hysteria, a disease closely identified in his thinking with females who resisted their place in society (Ehrenreich and English, 1973a).

At a time when infant and maternal mortality rates were still quite high, men were concerned about any impediment to having male heirs to carry on the family business or daughters who could be married off to families with good names, thereby lending prestige to the family. In an age of personal capitalism, where wealth was directly controlled by property owners, women and their offspring were economic advantages.

These ideas could not completely rule out the existence of an enormous population who lived in abject poverty. Women of the working class were hardly placed on a pedestal. The perspective of women as weaker and sicklier was not directly called into question by the capacity of female factory workers or domestics to engage in hard work during menstruation or pregnancy. They were seen by some observers not as sickly, but as a source of sickness, and a potential source of mentally incompetent children who would become a burden to society.

Some feminists of the late nineteenth century were concerned about the conditions of the laboring poor, particularly the lives of women and children, and they sought to introduce social reforms that would make improvements in housing and shorten working hours. In a sense, they extended the protection of their privileged status to poor women, advocating legislation protecting poor women and children from the stresses of factory work.

OLD MYTHS, NEW MYTHS

Beliefs in the natural inferiority of some human beings, buttressed with what historians have designated as "Social Darwinism" (Hofstader, 1955), do not die easily. But the women's health movement has been particularly effective in dispelling some of these myths. The women's movement has been sharply critical of medical practices, particularly those that seem to be more for the convenience of physicians than for promoting the health and safety of the patient. Today, however, patients are better educated and therefore more likely to expect rational explanations for treatment procedures. Patients are also less likely to accept the physician's authority as a social superior, as in the past, because they are aware that certain technical procedures are not based on the extraordinary talent of the doctor but on the availability of diagnostic equipment. The clinical role of the doctor, while still extremely important, is somewhat narrower in scope than in the past.

Some doctors still see themselves as a source of moral authority and expect their patients to listen to them respectfully. Women may find male physicians, particularly pediatricians and gynecologists, expressing traditional attitudes that reinforce the place of women as mothers and homemakers (Gross, 1977: 15). Women not only find moralistic statements offensive, but they sometimes suspect that the technical skills and knowledge are equally antiquated.

It would be a myth to suggest that all doctors hold this patronizing attitude. Gross found that a sizable minority of Chicago gynecologists surveyed were *not* holders of traditional attitudes, or at least were diplomatic enough not to express them in a self-administered mailed questionnaire

(1977). At the same time, women's health groups are alarmed at efforts by the American College of Obstetricians and Gynecologists to claim that it speaks for women's health care. Critics such as the National Women's Health Network view this claim as an effort to gain domination if pending national health insurance legislation is passed. Thus the exclusive services of this specialty will be reimbursable in the insurance program, creating a disincentive for women to use other providers, including nurse-midwives. This organization is predominantly male, and critics feel its members have a trained incapacity to do primary care since they specialize in surgery. The National Women's Health Network argues that primary care is too important to be left in the hands of obstetricians and gynecologists (Women and Health, 1977: 16).

Women's health groups have been active advocates of informed consent for patients, and they have been sharply critical of physicians who perform procedures without explaining the consequences to patients. They insist that explanations not only be offered, but that they be made in clear, nontechnical language. Members of the movement have encouraged gynecologists to allow patients, for example, to choose among treatments for breast cancer, if there is no evidence that one is more effective. They have also been concerned about the failure of physicians to inform poor young black women who were sterilized through surgical techniques. Through these types of involvements, the women's health movement has been a driving force for creating protections of patients' rights.

The movement generally views health care as a right and not a privilege, and it has been concerned with questions of equal access to services of rich and poor alike. Since almost 40 percent of health care is publicly subsidized, legislation affecting the procedures to which poor women are legally entitled will have a deep impact on their ability to control their own lives. Originally under Medicaid, eligible women could have abortions performed at public expense, cutting down the number of medically unsafe abortions performed by incompetent practitioners or without adequate safeguards. Opponents of all legal abortion led the fight to restrict, at least, this practice of Medicaid subsidized procedures, through the successful passage of the Hyde Amendment to the Labor-HEW Appropriations bill, H.R. 7555. The bill was passed by both houses of Congress in late 1977 and was bitterly opposed by an organization established by the women's health movement, the National Abortion Rights Action League. In the summer of 1980 the Supreme Court upheld the constitutionality of the Hyde Amendment.

Abortions are viewed by many people as the least desirable form of birth control, a last resort to prevent an unwanted pregnancy. Recent advances in surgical procedures have made it a relatively safe operation, no more risky than having a baby. Many health planners in the United States have advocated making access to abortions easily available to all, regardless of ability to pay. Most advanced industrial societies, including France, Germany, and Italy, have made safe legal abortions a right of all women, thus eliminating some of the public health costs of poorly performed illegal abortions, and perhaps as well, the long-term welfare costs of unwanted births.

The opponents of abortion have argued passionately that every fetus has a "right to life." This position is not included within a general principle that all living creatures should be safe from harm or an overall position of pacifism; there is no suggestion that capital punishment should be abolished; there is little reluctance to take a human life on the battlefield or another extreme situation. What seems to be at issue among the opponents of abortion are the quests for self-determination among women, which threaten the traditional organization of the family and other institutions.

BIOLOGICAL AND SOCIAL ASPECTS OF MOTHERHOOD

Mothers ordinarily find themselves in frequent contact with physicians. Parents of handicapped children, and mothers in particular, may have extensive contact with health care establishments in their efforts to find rehabilitation or even educational services. In some instances, mothers often become experts on the quality of care they receive from diagnostic clinics, physical therapists, and psychiatric social workers. Mothering can become a full-time social role for women whose children are disabled. New patterns of coresponsibility, however, could change these tendencies in the future.

Many of the voluntary agencies devoted to serving the handicapped started as programs for children excluded from public schools because public philosophy and limited resources suggested that the disabled could not be integrated into the mainstream of American society (Katz, 1961). In some instances, the women who began these organizations "embraced" a stigma by virtue of their affiliation with their children, and in others, they sought to achieve a more normal life for their offspring and themselves.

People who bear a courtesy stigma—those regarded by others as having a spoiled identity because they share a web of affiliation with the stigmatized (Goffman, 1963: 30)—are in an ambiguous situation in society. They are "normal" yet "different." Their normality is obvious in their performance of conventional social roles; their differentness is occasionally manifested by their association with the stigmatized during encounters with normals.

The mother of a handicapped child bears a courtesy stigma, but mothers of mentally retarded children face a special dilemma, since the more they become active on behalf of their children, the more visible—and therefore stigmatized—they become. The person who adapts to a courtesy stigma seeks a careful balance between the world of the stigmatized and the world of the normal, being involved in organizations for the handicapped but not neglecting other activities (Birenbaum, 1969). Those with courtesy stigmas assiduously avoid overinvolvement in the world of the stigmatized, thereby minimizing the extent to which normals will regard them as deviant, even in the presence of the stigmatized (Birenbaum, 1970).

Mothers of mentally retarded children provide an outstanding example of persons with courtesy stigmas who seek to maintain a normal-appearing life. Their actions and attitudes bring others in their communities to regard the retardate's family as conventional members of that community. In so doing, they have helped to create a climate of greater tolerance of nonconformity for all the disabled in society.

THE IDEA OF SELF-HELP

The desire to live a normal life on the part of mothers of disabled children helped them overcome any hesitations in starting organizations that provide services unavailable elsewhere. This movement has been called "self-help," because it follows in the American tradition of voluntarism, of eschewing charity. The women's movement stresses self-help for a different purpose: as a step toward becoming independent. Part of becoming independent involves learning to select the expert health care one needs rather than take what is available. But to be selective requires developing alternative forms of care.

The family physician of years gone by played a curiously ambivalent role with regard to women in a male-dominated society, particularly since he was the guardian and promoter of the middle-class lifestyle. Women who were barren or who gave birth to disabled children were often blamed by others, particularly the husband's family (Birenbaum, 1971). The family doctor could point to the biological bases for such outcomes, thus supporting the woman. However, there may also have been some sound sociological reason for him to believe in the life-sustaining features of family living. Durkheim's classical social interpretation of suicide ([1897] 1951) clearly demonstrated that married life was a way of preventing self-destruction. Other studies also made the point, for whatever reasons, that married people live longer than single people. One may argue that these beliefs and knowledge were self-serving, and that there are life-sustaining functional equivalents to marriage. However, fifty years ago, these alternatives were considered backward rather than progressive.

In the 1970s, women began to seek even greater control over their own bodies than was permitted by established medicine. Armed with the knowledge that medical expertise was fallible, some feminists, under the encouragement of a few sympathetic gynecologists, began to teach vaginal self-examination done by using a plastic speculum and a mirror. The special aura of the medical surroundings were missing; so was the examining table, the drape, the white-clad physician and aides.

> An old church basement, a long table, a woman, a speculum—and pow! In about five minutes you've just about destroyed the mystique of the doctor. I saw it happen this week when Carol, a woman from the Los Angeles Self-Help Clinic, slipped off her dungarees and underpants, borrowed somebody's coat and stretched it out on a long table, placed herself on top and with her legs bent at the knees, inserted a speculum into herself. Once the speculum was in place, her cervix was completely visible and each of the fifty women present took a flashlight and looked inside. [Frankfort, 1973: vii]

While this unceremonious but nevertheless strong ritual defiance of the medical establishment had a deep impact, some advocates of self-care are less than enthusiastic about other procedures. Ellen Frankfort, a journalist, observed self-care advocates demonstrate menstrual extraction, a procedure she readily admits can have some harmful side effects (Frankfort, 1973: xiii).

Self-help advocates feel that the medical expert controls and withholds information from patients. In its extreme form, self-help denies the use of expert knowledge. The ideological nature of any self-help concept deserves special caution, since modern living requires access to expert advice. At its best, self-help encourages self-awareness, representing the right to know—the free access to knowledge and the free use thereof—rather than liberation from knowledge and expertise.

In another way, self-help is a critical probe of the health care system because patient education has been seriously neglected. The patient-practitioner relationship is dependent on mutual aid and an exchange of information. A patient can best decide when to undergo a particular procedure when all the appropriate questions have been asked, not after the procedure has been performed. Therefore self-help can educate physicians, making them aware of issues that were previously taken for granted. And as one sympathetic physician points out, these questions are medically heretical.

> They imply that health professionals have no intrinsic expertise about the moral, social and political wisdom of a given health care system. They imply that given the facts and an honest explanation of them, the American public can decide, as well as the Establishment, what a reasonable national health care system should be. They imply that patients could actively decide about their medical treatment, as they decide whether to accept the advice of counsel. It is of course true, or ought to be, that doctors know more about the medical aspects of patients' problems. That is why patients consult doctors in the first place, rather than consulting plumbers or mathematicians. But given the facts and an honest explanation of what the problem is, patient should *be able* to decide and *should* decide for themselves, for example, whether the risks involved in a particular procedure are acceptable. But this is heresy. [italics in the original] [Costanza, 1973: xxi]

WOMEN AND HEALTH CARE

The women's health care movement can be seen as a microcosm of the larger feminist movement taking place in many countries. The concern over health care is part of the struggle to secure equal protection under law, be evaluated on their merit, and be accorded respect. In this sense, feminism is a legal, economic, and social struggle, similar to other movements for greater equality.

The feminist critique of the position of women in society has become a powerful tool for challenging current health care institutions, and it goes far beyond some of the simple truths about the role of consumers in participating in their own care. Feminists recognize that the special needs of women are either overlooked or are provided by men in an unsympathetic way. One may also argue that male patients are treated no better than female patients—but they are examined less often and given fewer opportunities to recognize their own depersonalization. Furthermore, simply because all are treated equally poorly is not evidence that women are making inappropriate claims and unwise suggestions for change. Traditionally, feminists have always sought to make life more human and caring, and at times they have sacrificed their own ambitions in the process.

Women who seek to humanize society do not always wish to do so at the expense of their own freedom for self-realization. In order to accomplish both goals, feminists are committed to gain control over their biogenic reproductive capacities. And by virtue of their function as producers of children, they have presented these demands to those who currently have technical information and can strongly influence legislative action. Historically, this demand for control over the reproductive functions by women has been met with strong opposition from various interest groups, influential people who seek to speak in behalf of the entire society or for posterity (Ziem, 1975: 168). Those who control major institutions in society, such as government, business, and medicine, often try to universalize their special interests.

Women have often been looked upon as subordinate to their biological function. Such views have been put forth to mask the interest of others to control women as property or a resource to be used to ensure the destiny of a family fortune. In contrast, the views held by founders of the current women's health movement sharply contest the rights of others to restrict the self-determination of women in questions related to reproductive functions. Helen Marieskind, one of the leading spokeswomen of the movement, succinctly puts forth this position.

> Irrespective of their socioeconomic class or their relationship to the corporate structure, women in the Women's Health Movement have concluded that their reproductive potential is a central cause of their oppression. Women recognize that the means to control their reproductive potential is determined not only by the government but by the preponderance of males in the top ranks of the health care industry. Medical knowledge and therefore "scientific" definitions of women are known to be made by men and legislation concerning women's health needs is created by men. [Marieskind, 1975a: 218]

What are the goals of this movement? The movement is not merely aimed at preventing pregnancies, a conclusion that some critics of feminism may come to prematurely, but is equally active in combatting sterilization among poor young women who are threatened by professional health care personnel or misled into believing that sterilization is reversible. Deliberate procedures for providing an opportunity for informed consent have been fought for by women who feel that the full consequences of sterilization are not explained to unwed mothers.

The women's health movement has complex educational and political facets in its efforts to redefine the place of women in society. First, free access to information and its free use is a primary goal where the subject of reproduction is concerned. Therefore, the movement seeks to change attitudes in society that restrict this information, both before and after conception. Also, it endeavors to change the perceptions held about women: that women should not be perceived in terms of their childbearing and child-rearing functions, and alternatively, that men should learn to share emotional participation in the former and direct responsibility in the latter.

Second, the movement seeks to gain the resources necessary to run their own clinics. It is not sufficient that men change their attitudes toward women, or that women develop new ways of looking at themselves, but that new institutions be created where women can shape the way things are done in the delivery of services. Some feminists assert that women have lost control over their bodies when medicine gained an almost legal monopoly over the delivery of babies (Ehrenreich and English, 1973b).

Finally, feminists are concerned about changing existing health care organizations so that not only information but safe devices are distributed as part of gynecological services or through nonmedical auspices, as they were in the early days of the birth control movement before its leaders were accepted by the medical profession (Gordon, 1975: 274; Marieskind, 1975a: 220).

Women's health advocates are concerned with redefining the boundaries between general knowledge and expert knowledge. Spokeswomen feel that some aspects of gynecology could be made available to every woman. The movement has sponsored self-examination groups in which women learn how to check their breasts and cervix, using safe, standardized techniques employed by gynecologists and nurse-midwives. This kind of program helps to break down the often self-imposed attitudes of viewing the body as open only to medical inspection, and women give and receive mutual support. This kind of monitoring becomes similar to other procedures performed by patients at home, as in the case of diabetics checking on the sugar in their urine. And there is no reason that the concept of self-examination cannot be extended still further.

In seeking to change existing institutions, the women's health movement has taken its ideas to the medical profession and other health care workers; as such, it is not a strictly separatist phenomenon. For example, the movement has been involved in negotiating for space in the San Francisco General Hospital, making it possible for clinics run for and by women to be part of a major organization providing health care. In addition, they have sought to act as patient advocates where issues related to reproduction are involved (Marieskind, 1975a: 220–22).

The movement comes up against some deeply ingrained attitudes about the place of women in society. The strong cultural emphasis upon the role of women as childbearers encourages women to see themselves as incomplete if they do not reproduce. In a number of tragic instances, this attitude has led to the use of a powerful drug to keep women from having spontaneous abortions (miscarriages) when they had a history of failing to carry a fetus to term. Physicians endorsed a drug whose full impact on future generations went untested. Administration of the estrogen DES resulted in a high incidence of vaginal cancer among female offspring of users of the drug. The drug was approved for human application without fully examining the potential side effects (Weiss, 1975).

The consequences of the women's health movement could generate a greater concern for patient participation in the health care they receive, the education of providers, and even the selection and recruitment of providers. The development of women's clinics adds a great deal to consumer influence. Most important, it focuses on preventive and primary care, areas in which patients can participate most actively, as opposed to therapeutic intervention, where patients can have less involvement. Moreover, it creates an environment in which patients can receive support from others in the situation. A description of a women's clinic, although perhaps idealized, offers a rendering of this atmosphere.

> A typical women's clinic offers routine gynecological care—Pap tests, breast examinations, treatment and education to prevent minor vaginal infections—contraceptive services, abortion care, and maintains a referral service for more complex needs. A few clinics offer basic primary care. Self-help groups are part of a clinic's outreach program and may be organized around such topics as breast cancer, hysterectomy, menopause, childbirth or for young women—puberty.
>
> In breast cancer groups, for example, women learn the alternative operative procedures available to them, the importance of breast self-examination is stressed, and much needed support is offered to the woman who is a breast cancer patient.
>
> Clinics are generally staffed by lay women health workers who function to provide all the routine services, and a physician who performs the medical responsibilities defined by law. Many clinics seek to include nurse-practitioners on their staff and to encourage their clients to utilize midwives, recognizing the superior infant and maternal mortality records enjoyed by countries in which midwifery is widely accepted. [Marieskind, 1975b: 118]

The future will probably bring increasing involvement of consumer groups of various kinds in the planning, implementation, and operation of health care services. Any health insurance program for the United States that is cost-conscious will probably attempt to eliminate duplication of facilities, increase preventive services, and extend health education to all Americans so that early detection of disease is possible. Since many of these measures depend upon community cooperation if not direct involvement, organizations with prior experience, some legitimation in the community, and techniques for mobilizing people to become active in their own behalf will be more likely than strictly professionally dominated organizations to be approved to establish community health centers. Consequently, the idealized views of the women's health movement might have practical advantages in a contest as to who represents the community. In addition, it will be ready to become operational in a relatively short startup period. Whether there is one form of health insurance or another, the effort to control costs will be strenuously made by funding agencies; and those who can mount an effective program for fewer dollars will be looked on favorably.

REFERENCES

Birenbaum, A. 1969. "Helping mothers of mentally retarded children use specialized facilities." *The Family Coordinator* 18 (October): 379–84.

———. 1970. "On managing a courtesy stigma." *Journal of Health and Social Behavior* 11: 196–206.

———. 1971. "The recognition and acceptance of stigma." *Sociological Symposium* 7 (Fall): 15–22.

Costanza, M. 1973. "Introduction," in Ellen Frankfort, *Vaginal Politics.* New York: Bantam Books.

Durkheim, Emile. 1951. *Suicide: A Study in Sociology.* Trans., John A. Spaulding and George Simpson. Glencoe, Ill.: The Free Press.

Ehrenreich, Barbara, and Deidre English. 1973a. *Complaints and Disorders: The Sexual Politics of Sickness.* Old Westbury, N.Y.: The Feminist Press.

———. 1973b. *Witches, Midwives and Nurses: A History of Women Healers.* Old Westbury, N.Y.: The Feminist Press.

Frankfort, Ellen. 1973. *Vaginal Politics.* New York: Bantam Books.

Goffman, Erving. 1963. *Stigma: Notes on the Management of Spoiled Identity.* Englewood Cliffs, N.J.: Bobbs-Merrill.

Gordon, L. 1975. "The politics of birth control, 1920–1940: The Impact of the Professionals." *International Journal of Health Services* 5: 253–75.

Gross, H. E. 1977. "Women's changing roles: The gynecologists' view." *Women and Health: Issues in Women's Health Care* 2: 9–15, 18.

Hofstader, Richard. 1955. *Social Darwinism in American Thought.* Boston: Beacon Press.

Katz, Alfred H. 1961. *Parents of the Handicapped.* Springfield, Ill.: Charles C. Thomas.

Marieskind, H. I. 1975a. "The women's health movement." *International Journal of Health Services* 5: 217–23.

———. 1975b. "The women's health movement: Political, social and working roles for women in health care delivery." Proceedings of the International Conference on women in health. Washington, D.C.: DHEW Publication (HRA 76–51): 117–21.

Weiss, K. 1975. "Vaginal cancer: An iatrogenic disease." *International Journal of Health Services* 5: 235–51.

Women and Health: Issues in Women's Health Care 2, (1977): 16. "Exchange."

Ziem, G. 1975. "Introduction to the theme: Women and health." *International Journal of Health Services* 5: 167–71.

14

National Health Insurance or Service?

Control of the means of delivery of health care in the United States is generally in the hands of providers, even when the equipment, space, and support services are owned by nonprofit community organizations. Community efforts in the tradition of self-help groups were often considered the best ways to acquire health services. Nevertheless, concern for health care was one of the goals of political parties seeking to limit the inequalities in industrialized and urbanized societies, resulting in social legislation to protect those who may not be able to pay for medical and hospital services. By the early twentieth century, national health insurance was established in almost all the industrialized countries of Europe (Glaser, 1972).

Under a national health insurance program, funds are collected in advance from employers and employees. Payment is made for services rendered, similar to the way private insurance programs or Medicare and Medicaid work in the United States. In other countries, national health insurance provides protection first for those who are in the labor force, and it is defined as an earned benefit of workers rather than a program for people unable to pay. Therefore, national health insurance never has acquired the reputation of being for those who needed charity or public assistance.

National health *insurance programs* should be distinguished from national health *services*, as in England, where physicians are directly employed by the government and are paid either on a *per capita* basis or in a straight salary arrangement. Physicians paid on a capitation basis must provide equipment, rent office space, and pay other expenses out of their income, whereas the government provides these to salaried physicians. These different financial arrangements encourage or discourage doctors from maintaining modern equipment in their offices, according to whether they have to pay for it themselves. A similar result can be predicted concerning whether little-used equipment will be ordered when the costs are not going to affect income (Mechanic, 1968: 331).

In national health services, the physicians depend on remuneration from the government, but technical decisions involving medical knowledge remain in the control of the profession of medicine. Even in countries where a highly centralized authority structure existed, and where political interference might be anticipated in the sphere of medical decision making, as in the case of Nazi Germany or the Stalinist period in the Soviet Union, there was little evidence of dictating to the medical expert on health matters (Freidson, 1970: 39–44).

In many countries where national health services exist, medical associations remain extremely influential and often become the bargaining agents for doctors in matters related to working conditions, number of patients per physicians, rates of pay, and so forth. Other decisions related to where hospitals or clinics will be established, where expensive equipment will be located, or whether a particular medical service will be closed are made by administrators—who themselves are not physicians—who plan services and allocate resources on a national or regional basis (Glaser, 1972).

The push for national health insurance programs came mainly from socialist political parties in Europe and the United States seeking to make services available to all who worked, regardless of their ability to pay. Sometimes other political parties adopted similar programs in order to ensure a stable labor force and reduce the voting appeal of the socialist parties. Therefore, social legislation was not limited to countries where socialist parties acquired power. Germany, in the late nineteenth century under the conservative chancellorship of Bismarck, was one of the first countries to introduce state-sponsored worker's compensation for injury, unemployment insurance, and old-age pensions. Prior to this some unions in nineteenth-century Europe initiated their own "sick funds" to provide financial aid for members. A few of these programs directly employed physicians (Glaser, 1972).

In the United States, some employers as well as unions have created their own programs, contracting with health care providers on a large scale, particularly in industries with high rates of injury or disease, and where local private resources were inadequate. The United Mine Workers Union established its own clinics and hospitals, directly employing physicians and other health care providers in order to make sure that help would be available in isolated rural mining areas. This program is still in existence.

PREPAID HEALTH SERVICES

One of America's major industrial magnates, Edgar Kaiser, will probably earn a place in American social history for his contribution to health consumers. In fact, Kaiser himself suggested that he was most proud of starting the Kaiser-Permanente Health Care Partnership (Keene, 1971).

This project came from the modest need to provide modern health care in locations where such services were minimal. The urban development and agribusinesses of southern California were dependent on getting water from remote mountain areas, far distant from the coastal locations where cities were being built. Teams of construction workers were employed in the 1930s to build reservoirs, pumping stations, and lay pipe for the aqueducts that carry water to the coastal areas. Sidney Garfield, a young physician, had tried to establish a private practice in towns near this construction. He found plenty of demand for his services among the construction crews but no way to receive adequate compensation. Garfield developed a scheme whereby each worker would contribute a small amount every week on a contract basis, paying in advance for any medical care he provided. In exchange for these payments, he agreed to provide all medical care, no matter how often required. Garfield even built a small mobile field hospital that could be moved on skids to follow the crews as the project advanced (Cutting, 1971: 17–18).

In 1937, some five years after Garfield started this program, Edgar Kaiser was building the Grand Coulee Dam in Washington. This massive undertaking was financed out of public monies and employed large numbers of construction workers. Kaiser asked Garfield to create a program of health care for the workers and their families. This program was jointly paid for by employee and employer contributions, and it was considered a great success.

Kaiser Industries did not specialize only in dam construction. During World War II, it build cargo and troop ship carriers, popularly known as "liberty ships." In 1942, this massive effort employed 90,000 workers in the San Francisco Bay area. Garfield was called upon again to create a new program. After the war, the shipyards were closed and workers were dispersed. Garfield was left with a substantial group medical practice and a few thousand patients still employed by Kaiser Industries. Rather than reduce the size of the practice, he sought to keep it going by soliciting subscribers throughout the community, depending mainly on referrals (Cutting, 1971: 19).

This recruitment drive was successful enough to keep the Kaiser-Permanente program going. Still known by the name of the original employer (and the site of one of his cement factories), it had 970,000 members in several states in 1970. Consumers view the program as a way of getting good care at a reasonable price. Membership increased significantly during the late 1960s, when health care costs increased at a much higher rate than in the preceding decades. In areas where programs are long established, members comprise 17 percent of the general population. Recently, Kaiser-Permanente has moved east of the Mississippi, and groups have been established in Ohio (Weissman and Anderson, 1971: 35).

Most of today's members or subscribers voluntarily join through health plans offered by large employers. Groups of 100 or more account for 87 percent of the membership; public employees make up 40 percent of the total membership (Weissman and Anderson, 1971: 35). Almost all members are covered fully or partially through payments made by employers. Employers sometimes offer other health care plans as well, such as Blue Cross and Blue Shield. The difference is that the former provides without cost almost all routine office visits as well as treatment and hospital care, making it a more economical way of getting care for families with young children who need frequent visits to the doctor. Controlled comparisons show that the cost of prepaid group-practice health care is less than the cost of Blue Cross and Blue Shield insurance contracted for through commercial insurance companies, where an average-size family is involved (Klaw, 1975: 166). In 1970, 44 percent of the subscribers at Kaiser-Permanente were families of three or more members (Weissman and Anderson, 1971: 36).

Similar prepaid health services are provided by group or individual subscription in New York State through the Health Insurance Program, popularly known as HIP. Some observers claim that the quality of care provided by physicians employed by HIP groups is not up to the standards set by Kaiser-Permanente. Employment by HIP does not prevent a physician from having a private practice, while Kaiser-Permanente doctors are limited by their contracts to practice only in the group practices to which they are assigned (Klaw, 1975: 174–75).

The success of the Kaiser-Permanente groups has been the inspiration for federal legislation to create a favorable atmosphere for other prepaid programs. The model of care provided by Kaiser-Permanente has been given legislative sanction and modest funding by the passing of a 1973 law to promote the creation of Health Maintenance Organizations. The formation of HMOs is supported by planning grants for medical groups and loans to cover losses during the early period when subscribers are being acquired. Companies with 25 or more employees are required under this legislation to offer group-practice services if they have group health insurance as a fully or partially paid fringe benefit, provided an approved HMO is available in the community where the corporation is located.

A number of legal problems have arisen, however, some having to do with the right of a union to bargain collectively over the fringe benefits available to members, and others having to do with the costs involved in meeting federal guidelines for planning grants and loans.

COMMUNITY REPRESENTATION

Organizations, such as hospitals, that provide a substantial amount of health care to patients, usually involve some nonmedical personnel in decison-making positions, for example, service on a board of trustees. Membership on these boards does not reflect a cross section of the community but consists primarily of people of influence, those who control scarce resources, or, sometimes, special skills in management. Many hospitals were founded by religious organizations, enlightened citizens who sought to relieve the suffering of the working poor, or wealthy people who wanted to do good works and/or gain respect and recognition. The same people were also members of the boards of trustees of nonprofit hospitals, running them as proprietary enterprises despite their nonprofit character. It was rare that an ordinary patient or an unknown in the community became a member of these boards.

As the techniques of medicine became more complex, increasing hospital-based practice, physicians gained control over the decison-making bodies. Then, as hospitals themselves became highly complex, both internally through their variety of services and externally because of the dependence on third-party payers such as Blue Cross and the need to meet standards for reimbursement, grants, and certification, administrators and lawyers became more important as decision makers. In fact, lawyers became distinct assets and often were asked to serve on boards of trustees. A recent survey reported that 15 percent of the members of hospital boards in Boston were lawyers (Cambridge Research Institute, 1976: 340).

In general, hospital boards are made up mostly of wealthy businessmen and lawyers, with very few women or working-class members, even though these are the groups that comprise most patients and who make up the labor in health care. Except for hospitals established by unions, labor leaders are rarely found on these boards. Navarro estimates that wealthy property owners and managers of corporations make up 3 to 5 percent of the membership of boards of voluntary hospitals, even though they comprise only 1.3 percent of the labor force (1975: 182). Even more striking are his estimates that 80 percent of the members of the boards of voluntary hospitals are upper-middle class in occupational and educational background (e.g., lawyers, doctors, engineers), with males outnumbering females six to one (Navarro, 1975: 182). Even consumer-oriented health services such as Kaiser-Permanente have no representatives from the broad patient population on the board of directors of the hospitals or the group medical practices they operate. Consumer input, however, has led to a broadening of benefits, such as the inclusion of services where behavioral problems produce medical disorders, as in alcoholism-related diseases (Weissman and Anderson, 1971: 43).

Many federally funded programs now require community representation on governing boards. Some of the health care projects funded under the Economic Opportunity Act of 1964 expressly mandated that programs be "developed, conducted and administered with the maximum feasible participation of the residents and members of the groups served." The general principle of local involvement in decision making has been extended to other programs that receive federal funds, such as community mental health centers. However, few governing boards have a full-time staff to collect information independently from what is given to them by professionals and administrators in health care organizations, nor are they trained to ask the most significant questions of personnel to find out this information. Finally, authority to hire and fire is usually in the hands of the director of the program rather than the community advisory board. Therefore, despite formal inclusion in health care organizations as representatives of the community, there is little evidence that consumers wield significant authority.

A more direct form of authority in the hands of consumers is exemplified by the self-help organizations founded by parents of handicapped or disabled children who could not find needed services in the community. Organizations such as the Association for Retarded Citizens and United Cerebral

Palsy have remained consumer-controlled organizations despite the employment of professionals and administrators to run their programs. These organizations have often been able to achieve goals directly tied to the various needs of the disabled. As the disabled children got older, the parents worked for the establishment of services for adolescents and adults, providing an unusual momentum for organizational change. Consequently, parents of younger children who joined the organization at a later point sometimes found themselves in conflict with the founding parents (Birenbaum, 1968).

The case of parents of disabled children providing a deep and determined interest in health care (as well as other services) indicates that recurrent contact with provider organizations may be the basis for establishing community representation or even including representatives from different providers in the division of labor. Consumers whose interest in health care is short-term and sporadic may not find it very interesting or attractive to become involved as representatives, even when opportunities to do so are available. Similarly, providers who have no long-term commitment to their work may also find no advantage to having greater control over their own work.

CONSUMER PARTICIPATION: AN INTERNATIONAL PERSPECTIVE

The brief history of the women's health movement presented in Chapter 13 suggests that one way consumers can participate in health care delivery is through the acquisition of knowledge about matters related to disease and its prevention. In fact, there are a number of books written by physicians on the subject of how to increase the lay person's knowledge, such as Dr. Keith W. Sehnert's, *How to Be Your Own Doctor (Sometimes)* (1975). Consumers can also become involved in the selection and recruitment of health care personnel, particularly those who become doctors. To make the health care delivery system more responsive to the needs of consumers, it may be necessary to attract people to medicine who are willing to take on these tasks.

One of the most important problems in health care today is the lack of primary care physicians. Even if physician assistants and nurse practitioners provide most of the direct services in primary care in the future, a substantial number of physicians are still required to supervise, train, and work with such personnel. The number of doctors in the United States per 100,000 in the population is on the increase, but more and more are becoming specialists. Those in general practice have declined from 28 percent of all doctors in 1963 to 17 percent in 1973 (Cambridge Research Institute, 1976: 359).

The growth in specialties has been encouraged in part by the selection of students for admission to medical school who are academically proficient, particularly in biology, chemistry, and physics. The selection committees of medical schools appear to choose those who are most technically competent, ensuring the presence of those who will most benefit from a medical education but not necessarily those who will best serve the needs of society. The technically competent may be overtrained for the delivery of primary care. Moreover, the selection of students with the highest grades may exclude those who are capable of mastering the technical side of medicine but bring additional aptitudes to the role of the doctor.

Beyond ensuring a minimal level of technical competency, are there not other criteria to judge those who want to pursue medical careers that will be helpful in meeting the health needs of the entire population? Simply choosing those with the highest grades ignores the nature of the relationship between the patient and the health care provider and how important that relationship is in healing. Two professors of community health, who are also physicians, emphatically underscore the importance of this combination:

> The technically *and* socially competent physician, given an adequate minimum of scientific and intellectual ability, may be the one who can best respond to the needs of patients. [Geiger and Sidel, 1976: 23]

Some countries have already attempted to involve consumers in the selection of candidates for further training in health care, using social as well as technical criteria for evaluating those who will enter educational institutions. Socialist or communist governments have generally taken medicine, including the operation of medical colleges, out of private hands. These governments have been particularly concerned about preventing the concentration of medical services in the cities and the consequent lack of services in rural regions. Furthermore, while achievement is rewarded, and those with more education and technical skills are more highly paid than those with less education and skills, efforts have been made to reduce the economic and cultural advantages for subsequent generations.

These governments have been particularly concerned with the problem of preventing the sons and daughters of highly educated professionals, managers, technicians, and party officials from gaining an accumulated advantage over those of other families where learning and technical competency might not be as enthusiastically encouraged. Therefore, they have broadened the criteria of selection for admission to medical school (as well as other professions) and have used groups on the local level to help select indigenous talent. One way this is done is through the process of peer selection for middle-level health care practitioners. "Barefoot" or peasant doctors in rural Chinese communes or "worker" doctors in factories or other work places are chosen by their peers and paid out of funds directly derived from the constituency served. They are trained to work with medical doctors as well as provide primary care services (Sidel, 1973: 161).

Recruitment was done somewhat differently in Cuba after Fidel Castro came to power. After 1959, when all health activities were placed under the authority of the Ministry of Public Health, more than 3,000 Cuban doctors, or half of all the physicians in the country, left because of their objection to nationalization of health care, or because of objections to the new regime in Cuba. At this point it was necessary to recruit and train more doctors, and the health ministry began to admit and subsidize students previously excluded from consideration. Larger numbers of working class, black, and women medical students were now admitted to medical schools (Guttmacher and Danielson, 1976: 8).

While both Cuba and China operate within the framework of centralized planning of production and services, serious efforts were also made in both countries to decentralize the location of technically competent health care so that rural areas would receive a fair share of services. In Cuba, physicians are required to give national service for three years after becoming licensed and are generally sent to practice primary medical care in remote areas (Breo, 1977: 12). China used volunteer physicians who were willing to serve in health brigades in rural areas. As part of their duties, physicians trained middle-level personnel from among the local residents of rural areas, concentrating on preventive public health medicine, such as learning how to make water safe for drinking. Peasants were also trained to diagnose and treat a few diseases commonly found in the area, using some 40 drugs (Horn, 1969: 136). "Barefoot" doctors who demonstrated skill and motivation were sent to medical schools upon the recommendation of the physician.

The examples provided by the experiences of China and Cuba are meant to suggest what could be done to make health care more responsible and responsive to users of the system. Even in the United States, few physicians are willing to set up practices in remote areas or even in low-income neighborhoods in large cities. (The National Health Service Corps has recently been established to make up for these deficiencies.) Correcting these imbalances may also be possible through positive incentives, such as the financing of students who attend medical colleges in exchange for national service in neglected areas. Alternatively, federally sponsored national health insurance will certainly make practices in remote areas and urban inner areas more attractive because the purchasing power of the population will be able to compete with that of more desired communities. Nevertheless, while each society seeks to learn from the innovations, experiences, successes, or failures of others, there is a limit to the extent that mechanisms instituted in newly industrializing collectivized nations can be utilized in our competitively individualistic, advanced industrialized country.

CHANGE AND STABILITY

Health care services in the United States are moving in the direction of greater organization, mainly in the form of larger units providing services, a greater division of labor, increased dependence on technology, and reliance for financing on third-party payers and publicly funded programs such as Medicaid. This growth in bureaucratization has not meant the end of private-practice medicine, as some physicians have feared, but rather has increased the prosperity of doctors (Sidel and Sidel, 1978: 42). Moreover, prosperity has been maintained through the use of public financing, nonprofit insurance programs, and voluntary hospitals (Alford, 1975).

This form of capitalization has meant that physicians, as those who have used their investment in acquiring knowledge and skill, have had to risk little in realizing profits from the work of others or the investments by taxpayers and contributors to the building of hospitals. In addition, patient fees have also led to the development of complex facilities. Since the advent of Medicaid and Medicare, attending physicians who have admitting rights at hospitals no longer provide free clinical services to the medically indigent. The teaching duties of attending physicians are also minimized, since interns and residents are more likely to seek knowledge from full-time hospital physicians or those on the faculties of medical schools where such affiliations exist (Miller, 1970).

Finally, the encounter between physician and patient rarely involves a joint search for the answer to the patient's medical problem or even joint responsibility for treatment. Insofar as physicians do not enrich the patients' knowledge or ability to control their own lives, patients remain dependent on the physician's monopoly of services. In addition, since the physician's intervention is usually based on a model of the patient as an object needing repair rather than a partner seeking to improve health and combat disease, the patient may resent being physically manipulated and not consulted.

The outcome of all these developments is contradictory; there is collective ownership of health care services and facilities (i.e., voluntary and public ownership), meaning that they are no longer considered to be private property, but authoritative control remains in the hands of the medical profession and hospital administrators.

Such arrangements have not made it possible for all the health care needs of the nation to be met (Rogers, 1977: 81–103). Patients still lack information, and as a result, there are strong movements for consumer control. Moreover, many providers of care now share these criticisms of health care delivery in the United States (Wildavsky, 1977: 105–23). It is ironic that as more services are provided, there is a greater sense of dissatisfaction, part of which can be explained by the image that most Americans have of health care as a necessity, if not a right. As a result of the increasing cost to consumers despite third-party involvement, many Americans feel insecure. Americans who are not eligible for publicly funded programs such as Medicaid and Medicare and who are unable to pay enormously high medical and hospital bills are particularly concerned about the specter of higher costs.

The experiences reported from other countries indicate that health care need not be an unsolved social problem. Observers of systems in various societies similar to the United States in per capita income, wealth, and age structure report that England, Sweden, and other European countries spend less per person on health care and may get more for their money (Sidel and Sidel, 1978: 75). There is simple security: ordinary citizens do not have to worry about losing their savings or selling their homes to pay costly bills. While their taxes are higher, they get something back for their money, and state planning agencies can exercise some control on the performance of unnecessary services. In addition, objective indicators report overall that health care is doing a more than adequate job. Sweden and England have lower rates of infant mortality and lower death rates for comparable age and sex categories compared with the United States (Sidel and Sidel, 1978: 14–19).

NATIONAL HEALTH INSURANCE OR A NATIONAL HEALTH SERVICE

While most consumers need not be impressed by the objective indicators of overall health, few would argue against them. Moreover, public opinion in the United States has moved in the direction of approving a national health insurance program that would cover the entire population. Several laws have been introduced in Congress to bring about a national health insurance program. There are limits to the utility of such programs in dealing with the major problems built into a fee-for-service and third-party payment financial structure. National health insurance provides protection from disaster and guards against a loss of savings, but it also freezes the division of labor according to current arrangements. In addition, if efforts are made to keep costs down, it will be through attempts to increase productivity, a burden that will fall most heavily on health care providers paid by the hour rather than by the procedure; and increasing the productivity of labor may reduce the quality of care.

The advocates of national health insurance have been found in organizations that represent people who are most at risk. Labor unions represent a vast number of workers who are employed in organizations that have grown in size as a result of capital growth. These corporate entities and other bureaucracies are fertile grounds for organizing because of the more impersonal nature of relationships and lack of opportunity to move into ownership or management positions.

The union movement, successful as it has been in organizing most large industrial organizations, has not aimed at the elimination of private ownership of productive organizations; nor has it helped members to become entrepreneurs themselves (Brooks, 1964). Unions basically are defensive organizations, and material benefits won at the negotiating table or through strikes have not substantially increased the wealth of the majority of union members (or even nonunion members in the same industries). Quite often, dreams of wordly success are deferred to the next generation, a process that has been ongoing in the American working class for more than a hundred years (Chinoy, 1955).

Health care is an expenditure in the family budget that becomes totally unpredictable if a member has a serious or prolonged illness and convalescence. People with limited assets want protection against unanticipated health care problems, just as they might want protection against the destruction of their homes from fire or storm damage. As a result, unions have fought for hospitalization insurance and later for medical insurance for employees. These benefits are seen as a necessary way of protecting people of moderate means against financial disaster. At the same time, third-party payment has been responsible for the stability and extraordinary growth of hospitals in the United States, since it guaranteed a predictable income.

Private insurance plans such as Blue Cross have provided some protection. However, many private insurance plans do not cover all medical bills, or they require the subscriber to pay the first-dollar costs, or deductibles, for all medical care received through office visits. In addition, private insurance plans have upper limits to their benefits, such as a maximum number of days of hospitalization, forcing the patient to pay substantial amounts once these benefits are exhausted.

Some private insurance plans also encourage hospitalization, because medical fees are reimbursable only when a patient is seriously ill and requires admission to a hospital. The consequences of such plans for the relationship between provider and consumer should be evident. Patients often delay going to physicians when faced with serious symptoms as a way of avoiding first-dollar costs on deductible policies. Alternatively, patients are sometimes hospitalized unnecessarily as a way of accommodating those patients whose medical bills are paid only when hospital care is given (Klaw, 1975: 134–48). Some of the proposed legislation in Congress, such as the labor-backed Health Security Bill, have encouraged the elimination of the deductibles because it discriminates against those of moderate means.

A second problem with existing health benefits provided by employers through group health insurance contracts is related to the economic impact of a fixed deductible on the subscriber. Employer contributions to these plans are based on a fixed per capita basis, and the fees paid for each employee are not adjusted to the income of the subscriber but are the same for everyone. The same formula also applies to payroll deductions for employees who are required to make contributions to these plans. Consequently, lower-paid employees are getting less for their money than better-paid employees because they are in control of fewer dollars to start. A percentage-based payroll tax according to the income of the employee would be a fairer way of paying for a national program, a feature of only some of the pending health insurance legislation.

Any planning of a national health insurance scheme will have to face a third problem; *how much* to allow as charges for services, and *who* will be involved in setting fees now and in the future. In order to prevent a national health insurance plan from enriching doctors, hospitals, and drug supply companies, some way of limiting fees paid for service and supplies would have to be developed. Without such a ceiling there would be no way to limit costs, and Americans would be paying even more on a per capita basis than in the past.

Fixing rates of reimbursement on a national scale, even when local customs and cost of living variations are noted, will take fee setting out of the hands of physicians (Klaw, 1975: 221). No doubt this step will be strongly resisted by the AMA and the American Hospital Association. Even having a fixed-fee schedule set by administrators can be a problem unless the services provided are monitored carefully. The fixed-fee system of Medicaid has encouraged the development of overtreatment of patients in order to maintain expected income levels. And no mechanism was established to guarantee the quality of care provided under these conditions.

The problem of keeping costs down cannot be solved without a different social form for the delivery of health care, requiring incentives for keeping people out of hospital beds, for the performance of preventive procedures and educational work, and for maintaining and improving skills. Paying the doctor for procedures performed may permit patients to know concretely what they are getting, but it also encourages impression management along the same lines. Doctors perform unnecessary work, some of it resulting in avoidable death when they are concerned about maintaining their share of the patient market rather than treating patients' needs. The assignment of patients according to other criteria, such as responsibility for a fixed panel of patients, may eliminate these unnecessary procedures.

Finally, there is the inevitable problem of administration. Who will run this system of national health insurance so that money goes to doctors and hospitals for services rendered? The private insurance plans represent a vast private bureaucracy in which the costs of administration are higher than publicly run programs, such as those in Canada. It would make some sense to use the private insurance programs' organizational skill and technical facilities to handle the billing and payment, rather than make a large investment of public funds to start from the beginning. However, using an existing resource is not the same thing as turning the entire task over to private hands. Perhaps the government could gradually take over the operation of Blue Cross and Blue Shield, non-profit corporations. In this way, there would be no long-term dependence on private insurance programs, and some public accountability could be established. Finally, the plan for gradual takeover would limit any schemes within these private bureaucracies to expand at public expense.

THE RIGHT TO HEALTH CARE

The goal of adequate health care at reasonable cost in America will not be achieved through national health insurance, because the same influences in decision making will ensure that all interest groups continue to receive their shares of the profits. The difficulties in reducing the defense budget are similar to those of converting our current health budget into one in which prevention and the treatment of chronic disease get a greater share.

Currently, only 3.2 percent of all health expenditures are for prevention and education, both major means to reduce demand on current resources for treatment (Knowles, 1977: 65). Changing priorities in health care in the current organization is not easy. The conversion of the production of pharmaceuticals into mass screenings for hypertension or disseminating information about the importance of exercise and diet for health requires hard decisions that need mass support because earnings from investments and jobs are affected. Today, profits from investments in the drug industry are among the highest in the country.

The problem of defining adequate health care for the American public is not a difficult one. Low-cost health care services can be provided so that everyone, regardless of income, education, and occupation, has a fair chance of survival. Along with these services, it may be necessary to alter the physical and social environment so that the causes of disease are better controlled, particularly in the food we eat and the air we breathe. The problem is not one of technical expertise but of political sophistication. Probably, the majority of Americans would opt for a system of low-cost, federally financed and operated health services if they had a familiar model for comparison.

What seems to be more likely to occur is the establishment of a national health insurance program, using existing private and public third party payers. The establishment of any national health insurance program should be limited by a review process in which legislators can evaluate over a five-year period of operation whether or not the system is able to provide equal access to health care, limit the liability of patients, *and* control spending. Then the Congress can ascertain what social changes will make all three goals attainable.

The question will still remain a political one. To find out what social changes are necessary requires examining how various coalitions of providers and consumers support and maintain the status quo. In other words, an ideology that justifies their interests shapes the plans. Humanly constructed arrangements are sometimes given a permanence and universal character so that it appears that plans are made in the interests of all. Each solution involves dedication to the public well-being and a self-serving set of assumptions about the best way to run services.

Health care is not merely a social necessity; it is a business enterprise. Investors are attracted because of the possibility of realizing large profits, and providers are attracted on the basis of gaining remuneration for their services (Lee, 1974). Any plans that attempt to diminish the established patterns of spending will also diminish the flow of dollars to investors and providers. Most plans for national health insurance continue to guarantee that no existing interests will get less from the system than they are getting now. Thus a structural reform that changes the terms of the relationship between provider and consumer might be resisted vehemently by physicians.

Similar programs that limit the marketing of private health insurance or pharmaceuticals might receive a similar reaction from those interests. The creation of a unified system of health services under a national directorship might deeply affect the sales of drug companies, since each one markets a slightly different version of the same basic formulas (Fuchs, 1974: 109–12). Ordering for an entire region or even the entire country might be based on a centralized purchasing system, with costs reduced by buying in such large quantities of the same product for the entire area. As one might guess, the drug companies might be reluctant to see this kind of policy instituted since each has a share of the market the way the system is currently established.

Physicians might also raise serious objections to a national health service because they earn more as independent private practitioners paid on a fee-for-service basis than when they are salaried. Even salaried physicians are handsomely remunerated and have time to keep up with their field because there is an upper limit to their workload. The third-party payment system has made physicians more prosperous than in the past because patients are less reluctant to seek out services when they know that they will have some limit on their out-of-pocket expenses. Currently, few patients realize the dangers of undergoing unnecessary procedures and do not object to them when they do not directly pay for their services.

A national health service would not necessarily eliminate the right of physicians to practice privately, but it would cut down on the financial incentive to do so. A national health service would negotiate with the physicians' representatives to set the terms of their contract. A ceiling would be placed on the number of patients in a panel seen by a physician on an outpatient basis, or alternatively the specialist might be paid on the basis of the number of hours spent providing outpatient services, caring for a fixed number of patients in hospitals, or consulting with providers of primary care or with other specialists. There would probably be an end to solo practice, since sufficient evidence suggests that solo practitioners do not keep up with their fields as well as those in group practice (Rensberger, 1976). Therefore opportunities to increase one's income simply by seeing more patients would be less possible within the confines of the program, even when physicians have some private practice. Aside from a reduced workload, there are other advantages, such as more open communication with patients; a willingness to admit that they don't know everything; and less willingness to tolerate patients who generate income but who don't really need care. On the other hand, physicians would lose some of the tax advantages gained from being in private practice.

Hospitals might be forced to decrease the number of beds available since ambulatory care services would be increased. In addition, a national health service would discourage unnecessary hospitalization for elective surgery, extensive testing, and hospitalization of chronically ill patients who could be better served through a home care program. Administrators could be rewarded for encouraging the development of programs that limit hospitalization. They could also be evaluated on their ability to encourage other health care personnel to become involved in planning and implementation of innovations in service delivery and in cutting costs. The participation in planning might also encourage a similar sharing of responsibility toward the achievement of goals set by work units. Each particular region would encourage planning that would direct demands and goals back to national planning agencies, encouraging a recombination of decision making, job design, and the delivery of services. Such a decentralized system discourages the development of desensitized allocation that is sometimes found in national health services in other countries. But the United States is so diversified and enormous that regional inputs would be necessary.

PROFESSIONAL SUPPORT FOR A NATIONAL HEALTH SERVICE

There is already evidence of support in the field of health care for a national health service. In 1977, the national meetings of the American Public Health Association expressed approval for such a program. This is an organization made up of more than 50,000 professionals, including many physicians on fixed salaries. Some members are also involved in planning services and recognize the necessity for change in the social form of health care financing and delivery. The members have come to the realization that health is a social value equal to safety, a thought similar to that put forth by Abraham Flexner sixty years ago. Do we permit police and firefighters to be funded from private sources to protect only affluent areas?

Professionals who favor a national health service need to combine consumer groups seeking the same thing in order to sway public opinion in the direction needed to create a strong lobby.

This kind of program should be appealing to new practitioners because any national health service would almost certainly guarantee greater responsibility and opportunities to plan patient care as methods for reducing unnecessary hospitalization. Physician assistants and nurse practitioners would also be given greater opportunity to have their skills compared against physicians, and career ladders could be established. Some labor unions may support such a proposal in preference to the national health insurance proposals of Senator Kennedy and others because it will generate more jobs.

The one missing element is a mass-based national party to tie national health service to the goals of working people. The Democratic and Republican parties represent many of the interests of big business within their broad scopes. Such parties could hardly campaign for this social change because a national health service would exclude some of their largest supporters.

The consequences of establishing a national health service may be even more disruptive to economic and social arrangements than has already been suggested. A national health service ends the unrestricted use of public and nonprofit resources for private ends. The nationalization of health care facilities and the use of salaries for physicians calls into question the right of all private entrepreneurs to use public resources for profit-making ends, including radio and television networks, transportation, and others who make use of free facilities or pay low taxes for their use. An act of this kind is a symbolic transformation of public facilities for the public good rather than benefitting some private interests more than others.

A national health service also could involve some acquisition of private property, establishing a model and legal precedent for peaceful socialization of the means of production in other industries. Would socialization stop with health care? Why not nationalize the troubled steel industry or the coal and gas industries? If this happened in one sector, there would be less reluctance to do it in other parts of the economy, particularly if better services were provided.

A national health service can serve a capitalist society as well as a socialist society. Welfare-state measures such as social security pensions or free medical care for workers encourage contentment with government as providing something for their tax money; savings also become less of a needed bulwark against financial disaster produced by long-term illness or loss of earnings. Moreover, equal access to health care may mean a healthier labor force. Finally, keeping up the morale of the work force may be encouraged by the fairness of a system of care in which wealth and income matter little in decisions related to health. People can feel part of something larger than themselves when such measures end the privileges of social class.

Currently, the needs of people serve the institutions, rather than institutions serving the needs of people. The major purpose of a national health service would be to free these means of production to create general well-being.

Some Americans are beginning to redefine health care as a right rather than a privilege, given our dependence on providers for care. This idea is in sharp contrast to the conventional wisdom: that you only get what you pay for. This version of competitive individualism has some merit. Publicly-owned services are deliberately kept inferior so that they do not compete with private facilities. Even when private enterprise lives off the public treasury, as in the case of defense spending and Medicare and Medicaid, public facilities are treated as places where paupers get care. The desire for personal well-being increases the viability of the private sector of the economy, rather than the private sector fulfilling needs for personal well-being.

SOCIOLOGY AND HEALTH CARE

While sociology helps us to understand how we work and live, it can also reveal what is possible and make alternate solutions visible.

First, an examination of the markedly different ways in which different health care practitioners perform the same tasks reveals much about the range of behavior that is permissible in carrying them out. Second, sociology permits an examination of the interdependent relationship between provider and patient as a context for understanding nonbiologic or environmental factors in determining and maintaining health statuses. Finally, the discovery of how human beings create and re-create social institutions in their roles as patients and providers helps us understand the impact of health care institutions and also suggests new ways of controlling them.

Sociology can show that institutions are not unalterable, and such knowledge can be used in planning health care services or in predicting the behavior of providers and consumers. Further, it can help to establish guidelines and rules for the treatment of disease and the outcomes of different forms of intervention. Studies of procedures can demonstrate how failure to follow standardized treatment protocols results in poor health care. In so doing, sociological knowledge can help to make the allocation of resources based on effectiveness rather than on traditional practices and beliefs. And finally, it can shed some light on the potential and actual impact of various plans to make health services available to all Americans.

The question of national health insurance versus a national health service is as much an emotional as an intellectual problem because it sparks a wider debate on the questions related to who controls production and wealth and for what purposes.

Any extension of the welfare state in American society can be viewed as "creeping socialism" or a way of "buying the working class into consensus." There are evident benefits for maintaining class relationships by introducing extensive health and welfare measures. Broad-based support for further social change could emerge after a vigorous conflict between advocates of a national health service and the opposition, led by the AMA, the American Hospital Association, and drug manufacturers. The struggle would have some long-term consequences for relations between labor and management and owners.

Any organized effort to promote reform creates organization. A core of politically active organizers could provide a cutting edge for further social reforms. For example, the end of American involvement in Vietnam meant an end of the antiwar movement, but it did not mean an end to organizing around other political issues. The antinuclear-power movement is evidence of these continuities.

Basic sociological research can uncover differences in the relationship between provider and patient in different health care delivery systems. Thus it can be determined how these different arrangements encourage or discourage adequate prevention or utilization of treatment techniques. Results could be used to improve services and reward competency. Knowledge can be used in a reflexive way, increasing self-awareness of the provider and the patient as well.

Given a model of how to work with a patient in developing prevention and treatment plans could result from such research on the utility of involving patients as collectors of data about themselves. In fact, transmitting knowledge and technology to patients is also a way of saving money. Such a development means that knowledge and technique are used to gain greater control over one's life, and that they are in the hands of the user. Let the exchange between provider and patient enrich the provider through the knowledge that a genuine effort was made to help, and let the patient be enriched through the personal growth that resulted from this encounter.

REFERENCES

Alford, Robert R. 1975. *Health Care Politics: Ideological and Interest Group Barriers to Reform.* Chicago: University of Chicago Press.

Birenbaum, Arnold. 1968. "Noninstitutionalized Roles and Role Formation: A Study of the Adaptations of Mothers of Mentally Retarded Children." Ph.D. dissertation, Columbia University.

Breo, D. 1977. "In Socialist Cuba, primary care now reaches rural areas." *American Medical News,* July 25: 11–12.

Brooks, Thomas R. 1964. *Toil and Trouble: A History of American Labor.* New York: Delta.

Cambridge Research Institute. 1976. *Trends Affecting U.S. Health Care System.* Washington, D.C.: Department of Health, Education, and Welfare.

Chinoy, Eli. 1955. *The Automobile Worker and the American Dream.* New York: Doubleday.

Cutting, C. 1971. "Historical development and operating concepts." Pp. 17–22 in Anne R. Somers, ed., *The Kaiser-Permanente Medical Care Program.* New York: Commonwealth Fund.

Freidson, Eliot. 1970. *The Profession of Medicine: A Study of the Sociology of Applied Knowledge.* New York: Dodd, Mead.

Fuchs, Victor. 1972. *Who Shall Live: Health, Economics and Social Choice*. New York: Basic Books.

Geiger, H. J., and V. W. Sidel. 1976. "M.D.s for everyone." *New York Times*, August 9, p. 23.

Glaser, W. A. 1972. " 'Socialized medicine' in practice." Pp. 65–81 in Eliot Freidson and Judith Lorber, ed., *Medical Men and Their Work: A Sociological Reader*. Chicago: Aldine.

Guttmacher, S., and R. Danielson. 1976. "Changes in the delivery of health care: Sequel of a social revolution: Case study, Cuba." Presented at the 71st Annual Meeting of the American Sociological Association, September 3.

Horn, Joshua S. 1969. *Away with All Pests: An English Surgeon in People's China: 1954–1969*. New York: Monthly Review.

Keene, C. 1971. "Kaiser Industries and Kaiser-Permanente health care partnership." Pp. 13–16 in Anne R. Somers, ed., *The Kaiser-Permanente Medical Care Program*. New York: Commonwealth Fund.

Klaw, Spencer. 1975. *The Great American Medicine Show: The Unhealthy State of U.S. Medical Care, and What Can Be Done About It*. New York: Penguin Books.

Knowles, John H. 1977. "The responsibility of the individual." *Daedelus* 106 (Winter): 57–80.

Lee, Philip R. 1974. *Pills, Profits and Politics*. Berkeley: University of California Press.

Mechanic, David. 1968. *Medical Sociology: A Selective View*. New York: The Free Press.

Miller, Stephen J. 1970. *Prescription for Leadership: Training for the Medical Elite*. Chicago: Aldine.

Navarro, V. 1975. "Women as producers of service in the health sector of the United States." Proceedings of the International Conference on Women in Health. Washington, D.C.: DHEW Publication (HRA 76–51): 175–83.

Rensberger, B. 1976. "Unfit doctors create worry in profession." *New York Times*, January 26, pp. 1, 20.

Rogers, David E. 1977. "The challenge of primary care." *Daedalus* 106 (Winter): 81–104.

Sehnert, Keith W. 1975. *How to Be Your Own Doctor (Sometimes)*. New York: Grosset and Dunlap.

Sidel, Victor, and Ruth Sidel. 1978. *A Healthy State: An International Perspective on the Crisis of United States Medical Care*. New York: Pantheon Books.

Sidel, V. W. 1973. "Medical personnel and their training." Pp. 161 in Joseph R. Quinn, ed., *Medicine and Public Health in the People's Republic of China*. Washington, D.C.: Department of Health, Education, and Welfare.

Weissman, A., and R. Anderson. 1971. "Characteristics of health plan membership." Pp. 33–43 in Anne R. Somers, ed., *The Kaiser-Permanente Medical Care Program*. New York: Commonwealth Fund.

Wildavsky, Aaron. 1977. "Doing better and feeling worse: The political pathology of health policy." *Daedalus* 106 (Winter): 105–24.

15

Health Care with a Human Face

The sociological focus of this book has been on the changing patterns of health care and the new providers and programs that can create the working formula for a more equitable distribution of resources and greater belief in and reliance on health institutions for prevention and education. Any change will involve some disruption of services, and disappointments. A national health service or national health insurance could involve longer waits before patients are seen by a doctor, more paperwork on the part of the patient and physician, and limited availability of hospital beds for the less serious cases. More important, the doctor-patient relationship would be affected, becoming less personalized but perhaps more honest, since income and the size of a practice would not be dependent on performing procedures or scheduling unnecessary office visits.

When health care becomes more bureaucratized, as it is likely to become under either financial arrangement, providers will not only have to be technically proficient but will *still* have to come to terms with human concerns of patients. These concerns may take new, even sharpened forms of expression: the generalized dynamics of the careerlike sequence of roles available to the patient; new concerns over patient rights to information; the movements toward self-care and their ideological underpinnings; and finally, the recognition that while life crises involve suffering, they also bring opportunities for personal growth.

Every person in contemporary American society faces these changes. Those who work daily with the sick must recognize the social and psychological dynamics of the patient, despite their best efforts to save lives and reduce physical and mental suffering. The health care practitioner may be a limited partner in these various episodes, yet must increase patients' understanding and thereby give greater control over their lives.

Change is not always for the better unless greater sharing of decision making and respect for individual rights are considered. The title of this chapter, "Health Care with a Human Face," tries to reflect these values. It is borrowed from the brave socialists of Czechoslavakia who tried to reconstruct their society so that the coercive quality of the past regime could be eliminated. They called it socialism with a human face. The Russian occupation of 1968 ended their dreams but not their faith in humanity and socialism.

The idea of health care as a right and not a privilege is a similarly noble idea. If it comes into being in the United States as public policy, planners and practitioners will still have to deal with the indifference sometimes engendered in publicly funded programs. This chapter will show *why* this must be done. Sociological concepts can have great practical utility; they are often more important than specific findings because epochs and people change, rendering data meaningless.

By taking the role of the other, a well-recognized technique for learning about the effect of social relationships on behavior, it is possible to understand how health care providers can become better equipped for fulfilling their mission. Healing is strongly dependent on the belief in the efficacy of the healer, and patients acquire this belief when they feel that providers understand their concerns. The entry of a person into what medical sociologists have identified as the "sickness career" (Twaddle and Hessler, 1977: 122) demonstrates the validity of this proposition.

THE SICKNESS CAREER

Persons who become ill face a number of uncertainties: how they will be regarded by others, whether they will be permanently impaired, and whether they will be able to lead normal lives. While it might appear that these uncertainties are strictly psychological consequences of disease, they also imply that individuals manage to develop similar strategies of survival. Moreover, these strategies change over time. Group living encourages this patterning as a way of extracting standardized interpretations and strategies that can be used by others in their personal struggles.

Health and illness, then, have a larger meaning than simply the personal consequences of becoming ill. On the level of how culture interprets natural events, illness represents many undesired outcomes of relations with others, including malice or unrequited love. These interpretations are ways of coping with tensions in social life and things beyond our control. While culture eases the burden of having to reinvent anew all strategies of survival, cultural directives do not always work. The world of health and illness provides dramatic evidence of this. Moreover, iatrogenic disorders (sickness caused by medical intervention) are a major source of concern because they occur as a result of treatment.

The social consequences of disability provide further evidence that following cultural directives does not always prevent undesired circumstances. Disability is rarely acquired consciously, rather, it is acquired because the culture could not predict a fortuitous event or the onset of an illness so that it could be avoided. Acquiring a handicapping condition involves little intentional choice and can be conceived of as the crystallization of involuntary deviance into roles now performed by previously voluntary conformists. Since it is a competent person who becomes disabled, the rules defining competency are often called into question. Moreover, if this disabled person is still *psychologically* competent, he or she may start to question these rules, since they proved to be unreliable.

A second cultural dimension of illness and disability should be evident in the modern focus on certain diseases as sources of evil. Susan Sontag has demonstrated how TB has currently been replaced by cancer as the symbol of all evil in American culture (1978b: 31). Diseases for which there are no cures often become regarded as apt metaphors to refer to one's enemies or a sense of dissatisfaction with the state of society. William James, the noted modern philosopher, suggested that society needs a "moral equivalent of war" to create social solidarity, and diseases are excellent substitutes. Associating the victim and the disease occurs in other ways, making the individual accountable. Some lines of investigation into the causes of cancer, perhaps as a result of their failure to actually locate the specific triggering mechanisms in nature, have suggested that it can be willed (Sontag, 1978b: 29). Perhaps this is a new version of scapegoating, a practice with ancient roots in human society.

Whatever people believe about illness and disability will have real consequences, whether on an interpersonal or societal level. Much was made of the crusade against cancer initiated by President Nixon in 1971, with the fanfare preceding the establishment of a national institute for study of its causes and treatment. Despite the political maneuvering, this highly complicated effort at biomedical research has had demonstrably little impact on the nation's health (Rettig, 1978). Movements of this kind, moreover, often diffuse efforts at prevention through the promotion of environmental improvements, such as the elimination of asbestos from water supplies and curtailing the production of other carcinogens. Rather than encouraging people to refrain from smoking the possibility of an imminent cure may minimize their motivation to stop.

It is against this cultural background that an individual suffering from a disease must maintain a definition of self and project that self into future situations. Goffman's concept of a "moral career" goes beyond sickness, providing the practitioner, or anyone else coming into contact with a sick person, with a way to become sensitized to emergent problems or dilemmas in impression management. A moral career is defined by Goffman as

> . . . any social strand of any person's course through life. The perspective of natural history is taken: unique outcomes are neglected in favor of such changes over time as are basic and common to the members of a social category, although occurring independently to each of them. [1961: 127]

The concept of career focuses on the linkage between persons to institutions established to serve them, ongoing membership in such groups as family and community, and the strategies of adaptation of the sick and disabled to their new social identities. Biographical information is instructive in understanding the social consequences of sickness and handicap insofar as it helps to make visible the conditions that make for uniform patterns of conduct. The strategies patients adopt are real factors that affect their recovery from illness or management of disability, and they cannot be ignored because they are not physical phenomena. Most important, there are clear indications that the formulation of a strategy *is* rehabilitating: that is, it is a way of getting others to recognize the disabled or sick person's common humanity, and it may help the person maintain favorable definitions of self.

The first contact with health care providers is a pivotal testing ground for new concepts of self. Since personality remains intact, although shaken, every handicapped, disabled, or sick person seeks "social contacts which give him greatest subjective status, and avoids those in which he has lowest status," and playing the role of the patient is an ambivalently valued opportunity, at best, for anyone (Collins, 1975: 73). It follows that contacts with health care providers will produce some negotiation, or even struggle, over the definitions of illness used and the options offered by practitioners, particularly in the central areas of family life and vocational opportunity.

Those who work in organizations such as hospitals may possess a more matter-of-fact perspective on disease and disability than the general population, but they still seek to gain the cooperation of patients. Since hospitals and other health agencies control medical services, accepting the doctor's or rehabilitation worker's view of things often occurs without a demur.

These inequities of power are most evident in the case of physically handicapped people and the agencies where they receive services. Many of these agencies control scarce resources and are able to encourage the disabled person to accept a certain definition of himself, or at least say so in the presence of rehabilitation workers (Scott, 1969). The attitudes of the disabled assume a central importance in the perspectives held on handicaps by such workers: If they are to inculcate "acceptance" of the handicap and continued use of the agency they must be certain that the client will not question his or her fate. The segregated character of these agencies is enhanced by the failure of nonspecialized health services to treat the disabled for common problems; lack of contact with those who are not handicapped or who are not part of the organized world of rehabilitation reinforces this sense of differentness.

PATIENT RIGHTS

Increasingly, as medical and health care become organized into teams and systems, and as these mechanisms become responsible to outside funding sources, individuals feel they have less immediate control over their own fate. At the same time, most individuals who have access to third-party payer plans or prepaid care are less subject to the fate of poverty as a barrier to care. The extension of health care as a basic right of all citizens constitutes an event equal to other civil rights, such as voting. Rights can extend beyond eliminating financial barriers to care. What rights do patients have once in the presence of a health care team? How much information does a patient require to give informed consent for complicated and life-risking procedures? Can patients determine on the basis of the information they receive that they would rather have further medical intervention stopped?

Questions dealing with patient rights and medical ethics are now being discussed among medical and nursing students as well as full-fledged practitioners. Providers now recognize the social consequences of technological advances that prolong life but with great suffering or confinement. Several books present complicated cases dealing with medical intervention, for which there are no completely "right" answers (Veatch, 1977; Veatch and Branson, 1976).

Patients' views of their own care are becoming part of the problem-solving process. There is a growing willingness in medicine to allow patients to choose between alternative courses of action. One advocate of this position argues that patient compliance is possible only when there is active involvement in decision making.

> It seems to me that communication between patients and doctors should not be used to persuade patients to do what physicians want them to do; rather it should be used to outline the possible plans of action, so that patients can decide clinical matters for themselves. Some patients may not wish to assume this responsibility, and there is no reason for the physician to force them to do so. Such patients are likely to do what they are told and are probably not among the growing ranks of the "noncompliant." On the other hand, those who are not doing what they are told should be more likely to do what they tell themselves; I suggest that these patients will elect to make their own medical decisions and will be more faithful to them than the dictates of their physicians. [Slack, 1977: 240]

The evenhandedness of this statement is far distant from the usual take-charge attitude found among members of the medical profession. Recognizing that patients are competent human beings is a long way from the paternalistic attitude of doctors. Furthermore, acknowledging that patients have a *right* to choose imputes to them an active role in the process of receiving health care. The acceptance of patient rights involves physicians giving up the belief that they are omnipotent.

> If physicians were willing to let go of the notion that they are responsible for controlling their patients; if like electricians, accountants, and others with special knowledge, they were willing to present possible plans of action in a step-by-step manner, patients who wanted to could make informed decisions on the basis of their own values. Patients would not have to learn the pathophysiology of disease, although enlightenment on matters of health is generally beneficial; they would have to be told what could be expected from the available options. [Slack, 1977: 240]

The physician, however, still remains the expert. But patients treated in this manner might be more candid if useful information became part of the treatment plan.

SICKNESS AND INDIVIDUAL RESPONSIBILITY

The high cost of health care has led some planners and even advocates of patients' rights to suggest that more of the burden of prevention be placed on the shoulders of individuals. Now government economic experts see health care costs as putting a serious strain on the economy, wastefully using up capital that could be put to better use in different economic sectors (Schabecoff, 1978: 1).

Placing a greater responsibility on the individual makes sense, but it avoids looking at economic and social inequities found in the United States today. Blaming lifestyle for disease and such habits as smoking, drinking, and eating junk food is a safe target because few people will defend them. What do these behaviors mean to the person? Lifestyle preferences represent different forms of status and membership to a poor person or even to a relatively affluent person. Spending money for cigarettes may be viewed as a special form of security for people who previously had to do without or roll their own. To be able to offer a drink to a friend, or even drink in a bar, is a sign of caring for others and a basic standard for membership in many communities. Even eating junk food represents advancement for people previously on a tight food budget.

In peasant societies, life was often built around a combination of two or three foods. However, modern culture has often disparaged such fare, making us consumers of products sold by multinational corporations with little or no recognition of the consequences to those societies.

A shocking example of the lack of corporate responsibility is found directly in the area of health and nutrition. Corporations marketing formula for infants in Latin America and Africa have promoted their products in many ways, claiming that these premixed or packaged preparations are as healthy as mother's milk as well as more sanitary and convenient (Greiner, 1975). Since people in traditional societies nurse their infants, and since there is a strong desire among some in modernizing societies to dissociate themselves from traditional ways, the message is strong and persuasive (Wray, 1975). In South America, for example, an Indian woman might think if she used the formula, she would be able to pass as a Hispanic (*New York Times,* 1978). In addition to this appeal, the new mother who delivers in a hospital may be given free samples of formula for her newborn. Once the child is started on formula (a practice that was recently on the decline in advanced industrial societies), the mother's supply of milk diminishes, then disappears and there is no alternative but to buy formula, and often at high prices. Also, to reduce costs, parents may add water to the formula, which results in malnourished infants. Malnourishment also weakens the child's capacity to withstand infection. Under these social conditions of marketing, it is difficult to see how individual responsibility can reduce this health problem (Wray, 1975).

A second health problem emerges either when water is added from impure sources or formula requires mixing and the sterilization of bottles.

The use of formula that requires water is based on the assumption that water and facilities for sterilization are available. The poorer families of many newly developing nations, living in suburban slums, may have neither. Consequently, infectious diseases are transmitted to infants, a mechanism that would not exist if the traditional practices of breast feeding were continued. (*New York Times*, 1978).

Who is responsible for these health problems? The focus on lifestyle does not examine the relationship of individuals to their environment and their aspirations. The underlying social causes of disease are found within the way institutions are organized and controlled. These basic social factors affect health and safety. Since rates of accident, disease, injury, and death vary from periods of prosperity to periods of depression, and different industries have different rates of disease among their workers, it would follow that the social relationships and physical conditions found in different times and places can deeply affect the fate of individuals. Crawford, a socialist observer of the politics of health care, sees the movement toward individual responsibility as a counterattack on governmental regulation of health and safety standards.

> Industrial corporations are beginning to feel the pressure generated by a growing recognition of the social factors involved in disease. The deepening fear of cancer is now combined with a widely reported scientific and popular critique of environmental and occupational sources of carcinogens, a constant flow of environmental warnings and disasters, and a growing environmental consciousness and occupational safety and health movement. Even though there is a great difference between awareness and the sense of political efficacy required for a broad-based political movement, the issue of public health has become politicized. Government agencies are expanding their programs, the courts are being flooded with cases, and the Environmental Protection Agency, the Occupational Safety and Health Administration have become the most embattled agencies of the 1970s. [Crawford, 1978: 14]

The ideological component of the movement toward individual responsibility or even self-care movements notwithstanding, outright dismissal of these concerns for how individuals can better take care of themselves and free themselves from the high cost of being sick, would be a serious mistake. Equal access or entitlement may encourage altruistic individualism (Titmuss, 1970). Viewing health care as a societal responsibility means establishing new relationship between individuals and institutions.

Individual responsibility without social responsibility, however, cannot produce well-being. To provide people with the knowledge for self-care and fail collectively to clean up the environment and workplaces, or eliminate the social causes of stress found in job-related situations, is giving people a false sense of security. Many people have fatalistic arguments to justify smoking or drinking: The carcinogens in the atmosphere will do them in first. Perhaps this is more realistic than the pretense that one alone can save one's own life. Individuals not only have the right to make *personal* choices (i.e., how to treat a tumor), but to make *collective* choices (i.e., how to prevent U.S. Steel from polluting the air and water around Gary, Indiana, and endangering the lives of employees through failure to implement safety standards and decent management practices).

PATIENTHOOD AND SELFHOOD

The establishment of a patient-oriented health care system with fair access for all is not at odds with the idea of individual responsibility for health maintenance. The latter, however, should not be used as an excuse for the reluctance of our political leaders to establish a national health service. Even the most health-conscious person can be struck down by disease or accident.

Few governments can promise an end to death and disease by decree, permanent revolution, or an optimistic view of human nature. Even the socialists and communists in Nazi death camps could not deny their denial of imminent death with their slogan, "never say you are walking the last way." Staying alive under extreme conditions produces the strongest evidence of the failure of the Nazis to dehumanize their victims, since mutual aid and social solidarity were the sources of self. The men and women of the death camps healed each other while denying to their official murderers the right to select their next round of victims for the gas chambers (DesPres, 1977).

Under the conditions of everyday life, becoming sick can be a time for reflection. Hospitalization, in particular, creates a hiatus from the demands of family and work, making it possible for patients to see themselves under new circumstances. While it might be an exaggeration to suggest that a fateful career follows the onset of every illness, sometimes becoming sick is the only way people can find some space for themselves. Vittorio DeSica's last film, *A Brief Vacation,* beautifully demonstrates the time *gained* from hospitalization, rather than the loss.

While serious illness is a time of trial and suffering, ending in hope or despair, the return to normal life, a transition familiar to all of us at the end of a vacation period, can be a moment that marks a life's progress. The passage from being a patient to an ordinary citizen can be similar to any turning point in a person's life, indicating the loss of known and certain surroundings and routines.

Alexandr Solzhenitsyn's novel *The Cancer Ward* reveals how leaving a hospital bed can be as emotional an experience as entering a sickness career.

> Just as an old man who has outlived his generation feels a depressing emptiness—It's time I, too, took my leave"—so Kostoglotov no longer felt at home in the ward that evening, though all the beds were occupied and the patients were like any others and raised the same questions all over again as if they had never been asked: Is it cancer or not? Will they cure it or not? What other curatives might help? [1968: 547]

Not everything in this world can be controlled or accounted for by looking at social forces, and Solzhenitsyn reminds us that each individual goes through sickness with the same private questions. Moreover, social explanations, he deftly shows, cannot shock the common conscience into a single moral response as well as individualized attributions of gratuitous destruction. Even more magically, his protagonist enjoys his first day out of the hospital, born again to marvel at the simple enchantments of living in a world where the senses are enticed, a far remove from the antiseptic world of the hospital.

> The fragrance, a mingling of the aromas of smoke and meat was breath-taking. The meat on the skewers was not charred or even dark brown, but the soft rose-grey color that meat takes on as it begins to reach perfection. . . .
>
> He tested each bite with lips and tongue to see how the juice of the meat trickled, how the meat smelled, how perfectly it was done—not a bit burnt—how much of the original attraction each bite still retained. [1968: 568–69]

Recognition of the pivotal interaction between life career and sickness career is most evident in literature. Becoming sick represents a life crisis; at best, it represents an opportunity to find out more about oneself. In a small way, because of the cultural ambivalence to sickness and the player of the sick role, sickness may come to rival religious experiences as the acceptable basis for life changes in the middle of the road, often restoring a renewed zest for life.

A person who survived Hodgkin's disease candidly expresses his feelings about the experience of uncertainty and his struggle to go on living.

> Cancer has given me a sense of myself that I didn't have. A friend told me: "Having cancer was the best thing that ever happened to you," and my friend was right. I have been to a place where I couldn't control what happened to me, how much pain I felt, how much energy I would have. I didn't want to go there, and if I could avoid doing it again, I would. But all of us must deal with that same "emotional scar," that fear of death. I will, as we all will at some point, die. The cancer has made it easier for me to understand that life here on earth is limited and that I should make the best use of my time while I'm here. [Solkoff, 1978: 118]

The health care encounter, a clumsy phrase to describe a moment in the relationship between provider and patient, can be radically transformed by the opportunities within it for human and social development. One of the great novels of our time, Thomas Mann's *Magic Mountain* (1927), conveys this idea convincingly. The setting is the period before World War I, when Hans Castorp, a young man of the professional classes, visits a cousin at a tuberculosis sanitorium just before entering a life of responsibility as an employee of a ship-building firm. At the end of his visit, Castorp finds that he himself has tuberculosis, and he is forced to remain in a remote Swiss village, far from the busy world of Germany and its industrial development. Instead of mindlessly building the economic might of his country, Castorp is forced to encounter others and even to recognize in himself the opportunity to perfect his personality. Without the protection of societal positions and the concomitant power and prestige, the inhabitants of the sanitorium must face each other directly. Their sexuality and their intellect become refined forms of manifesting their selves. In addition, the sick person is given the opportunity to review the past, present, and future in great detail, a luxury that few human beings outside of monastic retreats can enjoy. This respite from the busy world results more from a socially assigned status than from the physical and mental suffering that accompanies disease.

Susan Sontag captures the potential of being trapped in this role of the sick person.

> Illness is the night-side of life, a more onerous citizenship. Everyone who is born holds dual citizenship, in the kingdom of the well and in the kingdom of the sick. Although we all prefer to use only the good passport, sooner or later each of us is obliged at least to identify ourselves as citizens of that other place. [1977: 10]

Recognizing the distinct character of the sick role may or may not make others disvalue or stigmatize the person suffering from disease, but for the individual, it is always an event. By virtue of the words associated with sickness, which make us feel less desirable or less competent, few people learn to use the time given when sick to be free of everyday responsibilities.

In addition, the passive nature of the self assigned to the sick role, perhaps the result of the extreme use of technology in diagnosis and treatment, limits the patient's involvement in his or her own cure. Health care providers should recognize the value of patient involvement for recovery in the process itself. But to do this, they would first have to recognize their own feelings of losing control over the situation when the patient gets involved. In addition, providers would have to avoid imputing to the sick person (as most healthy people do) an impaired personality to go along with the physical state of disease. The removal of this barrier to communication would promote a much greater sense of individual responsibility for maintaining health.

In so doing, the provider encourages the patient to share responsibility jointly for treatment, rather than be a passive recipient. Given the particular type of disease and the state of medical knowledge, *mutual participation* may or may not be possible. Some observers of doctor-patient relationships have suggested this type of involvement as one among several possibilities (Szasz and Hollender, 1956: 585).

The direct personal experiences of patients who shared involvement in their own diagnosis and treatment reveal the strength of the individual's capacities for survival and recovery. Literary critic Norman Cousins, after describing his recovery from a serious crippling disease, collagen illness, aptly pays tribute to this partnership.

> If I had to guess, I would say that the principal contribution made by my doctor to the taming and possible conquest of my illness was that he encouraged me to believe I was a respected partner with him in the total undertaking. He fully engaged my subjective energies. He may not have been able to define or diagnose the process through which self-confidence (wild hunches securely believed) was somehow picked up by the body's immunologic mechanisms and transmitted into anti-morbid effects. But he was acting, I believe, in the best tradition of medicine in recognizing that he had to reach out in my case beyond the usual verifiable modalities. In so doing, he was faithful to the first dictum in his medical education: *primum non nocere*. He knew that what I wanted to do might not help, but it probably would do little harm. Certainly, the threatened harm being risked was less, if anything, than the heroic medication so routinely administered in extreme cases of this kind. [1976: 14]

What the health care provider can discover through sociology is similar to what the self-aware patient can provide the practitioner—recognition of the importance of using one's self as a source of knowledge, not through introspective or mystical flights from social and physical reality, but by instituting ways of getting more involved with others. Medicine and all of health care can then be redefined, as the nineteenth-century physician Virchow advocated, as a social and not a natural science.

REFERENCES

Collins, Randall. 1975. *Conflict Sociology: Toward an Explanatory Science.* New York: Academic Press.

Cousins, Norman. 1976. "Anatomy of an illness." *New England Journal of Medicine* 295 (December 23): 1458–63.

Crawford, R. 1978. "Sickness as sin: A health ideology for the 1970s." *Health/PAC Bulletin* 80 (January/February): 10–16.

DesPres, Terrance. 1977. *The Survivor.* New York: Pocket Books.

Goffman, Erving. 1961. *Asylums: Essays on the Social Situation of Mental Patients and Other Inmates.* Garden City, N.Y.: Doubleday Anchor.

Greiner, Ted. 1975. *The Promotion of Bottle Feeding by Multinational Corporations: How Advertising and the Health Professions Have Contributed.* Cornell International Nutrition Monograph. Ithaca, N.Y.: Cornell University Press.

Mann, Thomas. (1927)(1952) *The Magic Mountain.* Trans. H. T. Lowe-Porter. New York: Vintage.

New York Times. May 28, 1978; p. 6E. "A formula for malnutrition."

Rettig, Richard A. 1978. *Cancer Crusade: The Story of the National Cancer Act of 1971.* Princeton, N.J.: Princeton University Press.

Schabecoff, P. 1978. "Soaring price of medical care puts a serious strain on economy." *New York Times,* May 7, pp. 1, 69.

Scott, Robert A. 1969. *The Making of Blind Men.* New York: Russell Sage.

Slack, W. V. 1977. "Points of view: The patient's right to decide." *Lancet* 2 (July 30): 240.

Solkoff, J. 1978. "Learning to live again." *New York Times Magazine* (June 4): 100–101, 112–13, 116–18.

Solzhenitsyn, Aleksandr I. 1968. *The Cancer Ward.* Trans. Rebecca Frank. New York: Dell Books.

Sontag, Susan. 1978. "Illness as metaphor." *New York Review of Books* (January 26): 10–16.

———. 1978. "Disease as political metaphor." *New York Review of Books* (February 23): 29–33.

Szasz, T. S., and M. H. Hollender. 1956. "A contribution to the philosophy of medicine: The basic models of the doctor-patient relationship." *Archives of Internal Medicine* 97 (May): 585–92.

Titmuss, Richard. 1970. *The Gift Relationship: From Human Blood to Social Policy.* London: Allen and Unwin.

Twaddle, Andrew C., and Richard M. Hessler. 1977. *A Sociology of Health.* Saint Louis: Mosby.

Veatch, Robert M., and Roy Branson, eds. 1976. *Ethics and Health Policy.* Cambridge: Ballinger.

Veatch, Robert M. 1977. *Case Studies in Medical Ethics.* Cambridge: Harvard University Press.

Wray, Joe. 1975. "Health maintaining behavior of mothers in traditional transitional and modern society." Paper presented at meeting of American Association for the Advancement of Science, New York.

INDEX OF NAMES

INDEX OF SUBJECTS